The Fountain of Youth

The Fountain of Youth

CULTURAL, SCIENTIFIC, AND ETHICAL PERSPECTIVES ON A BIOMEDICAL GOAL

....

Edited by

STEPHEN G. POST
ROBERT H. BINSTOCK

....

OXFORD
UNIVERSITY PRESS

OXFORD
UNIVERSITY PRESS

Oxford   New York
Auckland   Bangkok   Buenos Aires   Cape Town   Chennai
Dar es Salaam   Delhi   Hong Kong   Istanbul   Karachi   Kolkata
Kuala Lumpur   Madrid   Melbourne   Mexico City   Mumbai
Nairobi   Sao Paulo   Shanghai   Taipei   Tokyo   Toronto

Copyright © 2004 by Oxford University Press, Inc.

Published by Oxford University Press, Inc.
198 Madison Avenue, New York, New York 10016
www.oup.com

Oxford is a registered trademark of Oxford University Press

Library of Congress Cataloging-in-Publication Data
The fountain of youth:
cultural, scientific, and ethical perspectives on a biomedical goal/
edited by Stephen G. Post and Robert H. Binstock.
p. cm.   Includes bibliographical references and index.
ISBN 0-19-517008-3
1. Longevity.
I. Post, Stephen Garrard, 1951-II.
Binstock, Robert H.
RA776.75.F675 2004   612.6'8—dc22   2003014910

9 8 7 6 5 4 3 2 1
Printed in the United States of America
on acid-free paper

Preface

In March 2000, the John Templeton Foundation supported a select, focused conference on the subject of this volume hosted by the Center for Bioethics at the University of Pennsylvania. Stephen G. Post participated as a speaker and was sufficiently inspired by the thoughtful, probing discussions to conceive this book project and to secure funding for its development through a generous grant from the John Templeton Foundation. Charles L. Harper, Jr., Executive Director and Senior Vice President of the Foundation and a visionary thinker, encouraged this project from its inception. Pamela M. Bond, Special Projects Consultant to Dr. Harper, facilitated implementation of the grant and contributed her time and talent as the project moved forward.

Dr. Post's interest in this subject also led him to encourage his colleague Eric T. Juengst to submit a successful research grant on the topic to the National Institutes of Health. While the work on this book was unfolding, the grant (1RO1-AGHG20916-01) from the National Institute on Aging and the Human Genome Research Institute provided support for a team of researchers at the Department of Bioethics of the School of Medicine, Case Western Reserve University, of which the editors and several other chapter contributors are a part. Dr. Juengst, the Principal Investigator on this grant, was a source of insight and creativity throughout the 2 years spent shaping and editing this book. Roselle S. Ponsaran, research assistant for the grant, conducted helpful literature searches and contributed an annotated bibliography to this volume.

After work on the book was underway, Post enlisted his colleague Robert H. Binstock as coeditor. Binstock and Post had collaborated successfully as editors on two earlier volumes, *Too Old for Health Care? Controversies in Medicine, Law, Economics, and Ethics* (1991) and *Dementia and Aging: Ethics, Values, and Policy Choices* (1992). This project served as an exciting venue in which to renew their collaborative relationship.

Appreciation is due to the Institute for Research on Unlimited Love—Altruism, Compassion, Service, a research institute also funded through the generosity of the John Templeton Foundation and for which Post serves as President. Ours is an age that is seriously beginning to consider *transhuman* possibilities through biotechnological enhancements in human biological capacities. What will be the status of the altruistic generativity that Erik Erikson associated with old age as adventurous human beings begin to experiment with efforts to alter their life span? Will altruistic love be left behind in favor of the biotechnological pursuit of prolongevity and unfading beauty? Or is altruistic love the ultimate human enhancement? The Institute, which has funded a number of scientific studies on altruism and benevolence toward the young in older adults, sees this book project as integral to its ongoing efforts.

Catharine Carlin, our editor at Oxford University Press, was remarkably supportive as the book's prospectus was reviewed by no fewer than seven reviewers and approved by no fewer than five Oxford editors, a process mandated by the interdisciplinary nature of the topic. Throughout, Ms. Carlin was very patient and offered salutary guidance.

Finally, we thank the Department of Bioethics at Case Western Reserve University's School of Medicine, which provided a hospitable and creative environment for this project; and St. Paul's School in Concord, New Hampshire, where Post was a Dickey Visitor in Science and Religion in April of 2001 addressing anti-aging and the humanities.

Cleveland, Ohio   S.G.P.

                                                                R.H.B.

Contents

II   The Science of Prolongevity

III   Ethical and Social Perspectives
on Radical Life Extension

Contributors

....

Mark B. Adams, Ph.D., currently serves as Associate Professor and Graduate Chair in the Department of History and Sociology of Science at the University of Pennsylvania. Dr. Adams received his A.B. (1966), A.M. (1968), and Ph.D. (1973) in the History of Science from Harvard University. Since 1970 he has taught at the University of Pennsylvania, where he helped to found the Department of the History and Sociology of Science. He has won the Lindback Award for Distinguished Teaching, has held the Bers Chair in Social Science, and has been a Mellon Fellow at the Aspen Institute of Humanistic Studies. In 1982–1983, he organized the university's Darwin Centennial, which included a weekly lecture series and two international conferences. Dr. Adams' teaching and research have covered the general history of Western science, the history of biology, Russian science, science and politics, and the history of science fiction. He has published widely on genetics, population genetics, evolutionary theory, morphology, Darwinism, eugenics, medical genetics, and the nature–nurture controversy. His recent publications include *The Wellborn Science: Eugenics in Germany, France, Brazil, and Russia* (Oxford University Press, 1990) and *The Evolution of Theodosius Dobzhansky* (Princeton University Press, 1994). The winner of recent awards from the National Science Foundation and the National Endowment for the Humanities, he is currently engaged in two projects—an analysis of the science and politics of human heredity in Russia (1900–1990) and *Visionary Biology*, a history of twentieth-century biological futurism in science and literature.

DIOGENES ALLEN, PH.D., is the Stuart Professor of Philosophy at Princeton Theological Seminary. Dr. Allen, a former Rhodes Scholar and Princeton National Fellow, received his B.A. from the University of Oxford and his M.A. and Ph.D. from Yale University. He is also the past recipient of the Pew Evangelical Scholarship (1991–1992) and the Research Fellowship of the Center of Theological Inquiry (1994–1995). Dr. Allen has served as Visiting Professor at Drew University (1978) and the University of Notre Dame (1980, 1994). As a philosopher of religion, he has a long-standing interest in the grounds for religious belief, the problem of evil, and the nature of spirituality. Dr. Allen has published extensively and is author of *Christian Belief in a Postmodern World: The Full Wealth of Conviction* (Westminster John Knox Press, 1989); *Philosophy for Understanding Theology* (Westminster John Knox Press, 1985); *Spiritual Theology: The Theology of Yesterday for Spiritual Help Today* (Westminster John Knox Press, 1997); and *Primary Readings in Philosophy for Understanding Theology* (coedited with Eric O. Springsted; Westminster John Knox Press, 1992). Dr. Allen currently serves on the Board of the American Weil Society and the Advisory Committee of the Center of Theological Inquiry; he also is a member of the Executive Board of *Theology Today* and a former member of its Editorial Council.

ROBERT ARKING, PH.D., is Professor of Biological Sciences and a Faculty Associate of the Institute of Gerontology at Wayne State University. He received his B.S. in Biology from Dickinson College, obtained his Ph.D. in Biology from Temple University, and completed a post-doctoral fellowship at the University of Virginia. Dr. Arking has served on the editorial board of the *Journal of Anti-Aging Medicine* since 1998. In 1999, he served as Chair of the Biological Sciences Section and as Vice President of the Gerontology Society of America; he continues to serve on the GSA as a Council Executive Committee Member. In addition to his research papers and invited chapters and talks, Dr. Arking has written, *Biology of Aging: Observations and Principles,* now in its second edition (Sinauer Associates, 1998). His research has focused on understanding the biological mechanisms involved in delaying the onset of senescence and thus extending the longevity of fruit flies. This work has led to an appreciation of the importance of regulating the genes that defend our bodies against oxidative stress and of the important role that mitochondria play in the metabolic changes characteristic of extended longevity. Genetic homologies suggest that these findings may have a wider application.

ROBERT H. BINSTOCK, PH.D., received his A.B. and Ph.D. degrees in political science from Harvard University. He is Professor of Aging, Health, and Society at Case Western Reserve University. His primary appointment is in the Department of Epidemiology and Biostatistics in the School of Medicine. He holds secondary appointments as Professor in the Departments of Medicine, Political Science, and Sociology; the Center for Biomedical Ethics; and the School of Nursing. A former President of the Gerontological Society of America, Dr. Binstock has served as Director of a White House Task Force on Older Americans and as chairman and member of a number of advisory panels to the U.S. government, state and local governments, and foundations. He has testified before the U.S. Congress on about two dozen occasions. Dr. Binstock also is former Chair of the Gerontological Health Section of the American Public Health Association. He is the author of more than 200 articles and book chapters, most dealing with the politics and policies affecting aging. His 22 books include *Home Care Advances: Essential Research and Policy Issues,* Johns Hopkins University Press (2000); *The Lost Art of Caring: A Challenge to Health Professionals, Families, Communities, and Society,* Johns Hopkins University Press (2001); and five editions of the *Handbook of Aging and the Social Sciences* (the most recent one published in 2001 by Academic Press). Among the honors he has received for contributions to gerontology and the well-being of older persons are the Kent and the Brookdale Awards from the Gerontological Society of America; the Key Award from the American Public Health Association; the American Society on Aging Award; and the Arthur S. Flemming Award from the National Association of State Units on Aging.

ARTHUR L. CAPLAN, PH.D., has served since 1994 as Director of the Center for Bioethics at the University of Pennsylvania School of Medicine, where he is also the Emmanuel and Robert Hart Professor of Bioethics. In addition, he is Professor of Philosophy and Chair of the Department of Medical Ethics at the University of Pennsylvania

Medical Center. Dr. Caplan has published 23 books as author or editor, including *Assisted Suicide: Finding Common Ground* (coedited with Lois Snyder; Indiana University Press, 2001); *The Ethics of Organ Transplants: The Current Debate* (coedited with Daniel Coelho; Prometheus, 1999); *Am I My Brother's Keeper?* (Indiana University Press, 1998); *Due Consideration: Controversy in an Age of Medical Miracles* (Wiley Sons, 1997); *Moral Matters: Ethical Issues in Medicine and the Life Sciences* (Wiley, 1995); *Prescribing Our Future: Ethical Challenges in Genetic Counseling*, (Aldine Press, 1993); *If I Were a Rich Man Could I Buy a Pancreas and Other Essays on Medical Ethics* (Indiana University Press, 1992); and *When Medicine Went Mad: Bioethics and the Holocaust* (Humana, 1992). He has written more than 475 articles and reviews in professional journals in philosophy, medicine, health policy, and the biological sciences. Dr. Caplan served as Chairman, Advisory Committee to the Department of Health and Human Services, Centers for Disease Control and Food and Drug Administration on Blood Safety and Availability (1997–2001). He has been a Member of the Presidential Advisory Committee on Gulf War Veterans' Illnesses, the Scientific Advisory Board of the National Holocaust Museum, and the Clinton Health Care Task Force and chairman of various panels for the Office of Technology Assessment of the U.S. Congress. He was named the first President of the American Association of Bioethics and served as a Fellow of the American Association for the Advancement of Science (1993–1995), the New York Academy of Medicine (1997), and The College of Physicians in Philadelphia. He has won the Brandeis University Alumni Achievement Award (1995) and the McGovern Medal from the American Medical Writers Association (1998).

BRUCE A. CARNES, PH.D., received a B.S. in biology from the University of Utah in 1973, an M.S. in Population, Biology from the University of Houston in 1975, an M.A. in Statistics and a Ph.D. in Theoretical Ecology from the University of Kansas in 1980. Dr. Carnes spent 19 years as a research scientist in the Division of Biological and Medical Research at Argonne National Laboratory. After 4 years as a Senior Research Scientist in the Center on Aging at the National Opinion Research Center, located at the University of Chicago, he joined the Donald W. Reynolds Department of Geriatric Medicine, University of Oklahoma College of Medicine. Dr. Carnes is interested in why organisms die, why they die when they do, and whether age patterns of death are similar for different kinds of animals. These research interests have led Dr. Carnes to develop and pursue two separate but related research agendas. In research funded by the Department of Energy (DOE) and the National Aeronautics and Space Administration (NASA), Dr. Carnes has developed mathematical models to predict human mortality caused by radiation from historical data on comparably exposed laboratory animals. For example, he is using exposure data for mice to predict mortality among the A-bomb survivors in Hiroshima and Nagasaki, and his research will contribute to NASA's preparations to protect astronauts from radiation in space when they travel to Mars. Dr. Carnes is using his funding from the National Institute on Aging (NIA) to expand on the scientific contributions that he has already made to the emerging field of biodemography. By melding together biology and demography, Dr. Carnes has applied his interests in comparing mortality within and between species to such problems as forecasting human mortality, estimating biologically imposed upper limits to the longevity of individuals and the life expectancy of populations, and exploring how much influence the genetic constitution of organisms has on their longevity.

GEMMA CASADESUS, PH.D., graduated from Tufts University with a B.S. in Biopsychology in 1996 and received an M.S. in Physiological Psychology from the same university in 1999 for work exploring behavioral changes in animal models of aging and oxidatives stress. After 1999, Dr. Casadesus became actively involved with the neuroscience team at the U.S. Department of Agriculture–Human Nutrition Research Center on Aging at Tufts University, examining the effects of fruit and vegetable supplementation on cognition and brain plasticity. Dr. Casadesus received her Ph.D. in Physiological Psychology from Tufts University in 2003 for her research on the modulation of hippocampal neurogenesis, cognition, and cell signaling activation of fruits and vegetables in aged animals. Later in 2003, Dr. Casadesus accepted a position as a Research Associate at the Institute of Pathology at Case Western Reserve University, where she continues to explore molecular mechanisms involved in behavioral and neuronal changes associated with aging and neurodegenerative disorders.

AUDREY R. CHAPMAN, PH.D., serves as the Director of the Science and Human Rights Program of the American Association for the Advancement of Science (AAAS). Formerly the World Issues Secretary of the

United Church Board for World Ministries, Dr. Chapman coordinated justice, peace, and human rights programs for the international agency of the United Church of Christ. She was a Member and then Chair of the National Council of Churches Human Rights Committee. Dr. Chapman has been on the faculty of Barnard College, the University of Ghana, and the University of Nairobi. Dr. Chapman coauthored two recent AAAS reports: *Stem Cell Research and Applications: Monitoring the Frontiers of Biomedical Research* and *Human Inheritable Genetic Modifications: Assessing Scientific, Ethical, Religious and Policy Issues.* She works closely with the United Nations Office of the High Commissioner for Human Rights and the United Nations Committee on Economic, Social and Cultural Right and provided assistance in drafting the Committee's 2000 general comment on the right to health. She has also been the principal investigator for a multiyear research project evaluating the impact of the South African Truth and Reconciliation Commission. She is the author, coauthor, or editor of 14 books and numerous articles and monographs related to human rights and religious ethics. Recently published books include *Unprecedented Choices: Religious Ethics on the Frontiers of Genetic Science* (Fortress Press, 1999) and *Perspectives on Gene Patenting: Science, Religion, Industry, and Law in Dialogue* (AAAS, 1999).

AUBREY D.N.J. DE GREY, PH.D., is Research Associate in the Department of Genetics at the University of Cambridge, where he received his B.A., M.A., and Ph.D. His primary areas of research are the role and etiology of oxidative damage in mammalian aging, including both mitochondrial and extracellular free radical production and damage, and the design of interventions to retard and reverse the age-related accumulation of oxidative and other damage. Dr. de Grey holds editorial board memberships on the *Journal of Anti-Aging Medicine, Antioxidants and Redox Signaling,* and *Mitochondrion* (associate editor). Among his principal books and chapters are *The Mitochondrial Free Radical Theory of Aging* (Landes Bioscience, 1999) and "Time to talk SENS: Critiquing the Immutability of Human Aging" (coauthor), *Increasing Healthy Life Span: Conventional Measures and Slowing the Innate Aging Process* (Annals of the New York Academy of Sciences, 2002). Dr. de Grey's articles include "A proposed refinement of the mitochondrial free radical theory of aging" (*BioEssays,* 1997); "A mechanism proposed to explain the rise in oxidative stress during aging" (*Journal of Anti-Aging Medicine,* 1998); "The non-correlation between maximum longevity and enzymatic antioxidant levels among homeotherms; implications for retarding human aging," (*Journal of Anti-Aging Medicine,* 2000); "The reductive hot-spot hypothesis: An update," (*Archives of Biochemistry and Biophysics,* 2000); "Mitochondrial gene therapy: An arena for the biomedical use of inteins," (*Trends in Biotechnolooy* 2000); and "A proposed mechanism for the lowering of mitochondrial electron leak by caloric restriction" (*Mitochondrion,* 2001).

CAROL C. DONLEY, PH.D., is the Andrews Professor of Biomedical Humanities at Hiram College, Hiram, Ohio, where she codirects the Center for Literature, Medicine and the Health Care Professions. She has directed two National Endowment for the Humanities Institutes on Humanities and Medicine and has helped lead 11 summer seminars on literature, bioethics, and medicine offered annually at Hiram for health-care professionals, humanities scholars, and others interested in such interdisciplinary work. The summer seminar for 2003 focused on anti-aging and the search for immortality. Her publications include five books: *Einstein as Myth and Muse,* coauthored with Alan Friedman Cambridge University Press, 1985; *Literature and Aging: An Anthology,* coedited with Martin Kohn and Delese Wear (Kent State University Press, 1993); *The Tyranny of the Normal,* coedited with Sheryl Buckley (Kent State University Press, 1996); *What's Normal? Narratives of Mental and Emotional Disorders,* coedited with Sheryl Buckley (Kent State Univesity Press, 2000); and *Recognitions: Doctors and Their Stories,* coedited with Martin Kohn (Kent State University Press, 2002). She has published many articles, book chapters, and annotated bibliographies of literature and medicine, the latest of which will be in the third edition of the *Encyclopedia of Bioethics.* She team-teaches interdisciplinary courses with physicians in the Biomedical Humanities program at Hiram College.

NEIL GILLMAN, RABBI, PH.D., is the Aaron Rabinowitz and Simon H. Rifkind Professor of Jewish Philosophy at The Jewish Theological Seminary of America. A native of Quebec City, Canada, Dr. Gillman graduated from McGill University in 1954, was ordained at the Seminary in 1960, and received his Ph.D. in Philosophy at Columbia University in 1975. His dissertation, *Gabriel Marcel on Religious Knowledge,* was published by the University Press of America in 1980. Dr. Gillman has published extensively in the fields of modern Jewish thought, Jewish philosophy and theology, and liturgy. He has served as scholar-in-residence in Conservative and Reform congregations around the country. Dr. Gillman's second book, *Sacred Fragments: Recovering Theology for the Modern Jew* (The Jewish Publication Society of America 1992), won the National Jewish Book Award in Jewish Thought. His other books include *Conservative Judaism: A New Century* by (Behrman House, 1993); *The Death of Death: Resurrection and Immortality in Jewish Thought* (Jewish Lights Publishing, 1997); *The Way Into Encountering God in Judaism* (Jewish Lights Publishing, 2000). Dr. Gillman is one of three regular contributors to the "Sabbath Week" column in the *Jewish Week*, New York's Anglo-Jewish newspaper. He was a member of the Commission on the Philosophy of Conservative Judaism that wrote *Emet Ve'Emunah*, the first Statement of Principles of Conservative Judaism. Dr. Gillman serves as Chair of the Advisory Committee of the periodical *Sh'ma*. He also is a member of the editorial board of the quarterly *Conservative Judaism* and of the board of Cross Currents, an association of men and women who seek to integrate their religious commitments with issues of concern in the academy.

JAMES A. JOSEPH, PH.D., received his Ph.D. in Behavioral Neuroscience from the University of South Carolina in 1976. He was a Postdoctoral Fellow at the Gerontology Research Center at the National Institute of Health from 1976 to 1982 and a Senior Scientist at Lederle Research Laboratories from 1982 to 1985, when he joined the Armed Forces Radiobiology Institute. In 1988 he returned to the Gerontology Research Center as a Senior Scientist and in 1993 joined the U.S. Department of Agriculture Human Nutrition Research Center on Aging at Tufts University as the Chief of the Neuroscience Laboratory. He is the author or coauthor of more than 175 publications and has shared in the Sandoz Award in Gerontology, received the Stephanie Overstreet Award in Alzheimer Research from the Alzheimer Foundation, the Alex Wetherbee Award from the North American Blueberry Council, and the 2002 Glenn Foundation Award for Aging Research. He has also been nominated for the Linus Pauling Award. In addition to his scientific recognition, Dr. Joseph's work has been cited in every major health magazine in the United States, and in newspapers such as the *Wall Street Journal* and the *New York Times*.

ERIC T. JUENGST, PH.D., is an Associate Professor of Biomedical Ethics at the Case Western Reserve University School of Medicine in Cleveland, Ohio. He received his B.S. in Biology from the University of the South in 1978 and his Ph.D. in Philosophy from Georgetown University in 1985. He has taught medical ethics and the philosophy of science on the faculties of the medical schools of the University of California, San Francisco, and Penn State University. His research interests and publications have focused on the conceptual and ethical issues raised by new advances in human genetics and biotechnology, and from 1990 to 1994 he was the first Chief of the Ethical, Legal and Social Implications Branch of the National Center for Human Genome Research at the National Institutes of Health (NIH). Since 1995, Dr. Juengst has served on the Ethics Committee of the American Society for Gene Therapy, the National Ethics Committee of the March of Dimes, the U.S. Recombinant DNA Advisory Committee, the DNA Advisory Board of the Federal Bureau of Investigation, and the editorial boards of the *Journal of Medicine and Philosophy*, *Human Gene Therapy*, the *American Journal of Medical Genetics*, *Medical Humanities Reviews*, and *Community Genetics*. He was elected a Fellow of the Hastings Center in 2000 and serves as the Genetics Area Editor for the *Encyclopedia of Bioethics*. Research for his contribution to this volume was jointly supported by the NIH National Institute of Aging and the NIH National Human Genome Research Institute under Grant No. R01-AG/HG20916.

LEON R. KASS, M.D., PH.D., is Addie Clark Harding Professor of the Committee on Social Thought and the College at the University of Chicago, where he has taught since 1976, and, beginning in 2002, the Hertog Fellow in Social Thought at the American Enterprise Institute in Washington, DC. A native of Chicago, Dr. Kass was educated at the University of Chicago, where he earned his B.S. and M.D. degrees, and at Harvard University, where he earned a Ph.D. in Biochemistry. Following this, he did research in molecular biology at the National Institutes of Health while serving at the U.S. Public Health Service. Shifting from doing science to thinking about its human meaning, he has been engaged for more than 30 years with ethical and philosophical issues raised by biomedical advance and, more recently, with the ethics of everyday life. He is a Founding Fellow (and was for 26 years a Board member) of the Hastings Center and is a Senior Fellow of the MacLean Center for Clinical Medical

Ethics at the University of Chicago. His numerous books include *Toward a More Natural Science: Biology and Human Affairs* (Free Press, 1985); *The Hungry Soul: Eating and the Perfecting of Our Nature* (Free Press, 1985); *The Ethics of Human Cloning* (with James Q. Wilson) (AEI Press, 1998); and *Wing to Wing, Oar to Oar: Readings on Courting and Marrying* (with Amy A. Kass) (University of Notre Dame Press, 1998). In 2001, President George W. Bush appointed him to chair the President's Council on Bioethics.

RICHARD A. MILLER, PH.D., is Professor of Pathology at the University of Michigan Medical School and Associate Director of the Geriatrics Center. In addition, he is a research scientist at the Ann Arbor Department of Veterans Affairs Medical Center and Senior Research Scientist at the Institute of Gerontology at the University of Michigan. He and his laboratory colleagues study the genetics of aging in mice. The laboratory group maps genes that regulate longevity and immune function and develops new mouse lines with extended longevity in the hope that these will provide clues to the mechanisms that regulate aging rates in mammals.

S. JAY OLSHANSKY, PH.D., received his Ph.D. in Sociology at the University of Chicago in 1984. He is currently a Professor in the School of Public Health at the University of Illinois at Chicago and a Research Associate at the University of Chicago's Center on Aging and the London School of Hygiene and Tropical Medicine. Dr. Olshansky was a faculty member of the Department of Medicine at the University of Chicago from 1989 to 2000. The focus of his research to date has been on estimates of the upper limits to human longevity, exploring the health consequences of individual and population aging and the global implications of the reemergence of infectious and parasitic diseases. During the past 10 years, Dr. Olshansky has been working with colleagues in the biological sciences to develop the modern "*biodemographic paradigm*" of mortality—an effort to understand the biological nature of the dying-out process of living organisms. President of the Society for the Study of Social Biology, in 2003, Dr. Olshansky is Associate Editor of the *Journal of Gerontology: Biological Sciences and Biogerontology* and on the editorial board of several other scientific journals. He has spoken before the President's Council on Bioethics and has testified several times before the trustees of the Social Security Administration, where his research has influenced forecasts of the nation's entitlement programs. Dr. Ol-shansky has been invited to lecture on aging throughout the world, and has participated in a number of international debates on the future of human health and longevity. He is the lead author of *The Quest for Immortality: Science at the Frontiers of Aging* (W.W. Norton, 2001).

CHRISTINE OVERALL, PH.D., FRSC, is Professor of Philosophy and Associate Dean in the Faculty of Arts and Science at Queen's University, Kingston, Ontario, Canada. She was elected to the Royal Society of Canada in 1998. Dr. Overall is the coeditor of *Feminist Perspectives: Philosophical Essays on Method and Morals* (University of Toronto Press, 1988) and *Perspectives on AIDS: Ethical and Social Issues* (Oxford University Press, 1991). She is the editor of *The Future of Human Reproduction* (Toronto Women's Press, 1989). Dr. Overall is also the author of *Ethics and Human Reproduction: A Feminist Analysis* (Allen & Unwin, 1987); *Human Reproduction: Principles, Practices, Policies* (Oxford University Press, 1993); *A Feminist I: Reflections from Academia* (Broadview Press, 1998); and *Thinking Like a Woman: Personal Life and Political Ideas* (Sumach Press, 2001). Her book on longevity issues, *Aging, Death, and Human Longevity: A Philosophical Inquiry*, was published by the University of California Press in 2003. Dr. Overall is also the writer of a weekly feminist column, "In Other Words," which has been published for 9 years in the *Kingston Whig-Standard* and other Canadian newspapers.

GEORGE PERRY, PH.D., obtained his B.A. in Zoology from the University of California at Santa Barbara in 1974 and completed his Ph.D. in marine biology from the Scripps Institution of Oceanography, University of California, San Diego, in 1979. After postdoctoral studies in cell biology at Baylor College of Medicine, Dr. Perry joined the faculty of Case Western Reserve University in 1982 where he is a professor in the Departments of Pathology and Neurosciences and has served as Interim Chair of the Department of Pathology. Additionally, he was named a Fellow by the American Association for the Advancement of Science in 1998 and is an internationally known invited lecturer, with numerous papers, presentations, and publications to his credits. Dr. Perry's studies are focused on the mechanism of formation and physiological consequences of the cytopathology of Alzheimer's disease. Dr. Perry's group has shown that oxidative damage is the initial cytopathological abnormality in Alzheimer disease. They are working to determine the sequence of events leading to neuronal oxidative damage and the source of increased oxygen radicals. Current studies focus on three issues: (*1*) the metabolic basis for the mitochondrial damage restricted to vulnerable neurons; (*2*) the effects of RNA oxidation on protein synthesis rate and fidelity; and (*3*) the role of phosphorylation in controlling oxidative adduction.

ROSELLE PONSARAN, M.A., is a Research Assistant in the Department of Bioethics at Case Western Reserve University's School of Medicine. In 1997 she received a B.A. in English from the University of San Francisco, and in 2001 she received an M.A. in medical anthropology from Case Western Reserve University, where she is currently working on a Ph.D.

STEPHEN G. POST, PH.D., is Professor and Associate Director for Educational Programs, Department of Bioethics, School of Medicine, Case Western Reserve University. Dr. Post has served as Senior Research Scholar in the Becket Institute at St. Hugh's College, University of Oxford. He received his Ph.D. in Philosophical and Religious Ethics from the University of Chicago, where he was an elected university Fellow.

With regard to his work in cognitive disabilities and dementia, Dr. Post is a member of the Medical and Scientific Advisory Panel of Alzheimer's Disease International. He serves on the National Ethics Advisory Board for the Alzheimer's Association and was presented with the special recognition award by the American Geriatrics Society for service on its Ethics Committee (2001). He was recognized for distinguished service by the Association's National Board for educational efforts in bringing ethical issues to Association chapters and families throughout the United States (1998). His book, *The Moral Challenge of Alzheimer Disease: Ethical Issues from Diagnosis to Dying*, 2nd (Johns Hopkins University Press, 2000), is considered a benchmark in the field. Dr. Post's research on issues surrounding dementia and aging has been funded by R01 grants from the National Institute on Aging and the National Human Genome Research Institute of the National Institutes of Health. Currently, he is focusing on issues surrounding persons with the dual diagnoses of Down's syndrome and Alzheimer's disease, as well as on the implications of anti-aging research. He is

Associate Editor for Ethics of the *Encyclopedia of Aging* (Macmillan Reference, 2002) and Editor-in-Chief of the definitive *Encyclopedia of Bioethics*, 3rd ed. (Macmillan Reference, 2003). Dr. Post has published more than 120 articles in the leading medical, scientific, philosophical, and religious studies journals.

MICHAEL R. ROSE, PH.D., is Professor of Ecology and Evolutionary Biology at the University of California, Irvine. A Canadian born in Germany, Michael Rose finished his education at the University of Sussex, England. The subject of his doctoral research was the evolution of aging. A NATO Science Fellowship took Dr. Rose to the University of Wisconsin—Madison. In 1981 he became Assistant Professor at Dalhousie University, Halifax, Nova Scotia, where he and his students showed that resistance to stress was a key factor in postponed aging. Dr. Rose also worked on the evolution of sex and the evolution of the human brain. In 1987 he returned to the United States as Associate Professor in the School of Biological Sciences at the University of California, Irvine, and was promoted to Professor in 1990. In 1991 he published *Evolutionary Biology of Aging*, a book that ranged from mathematical genetics to cell biology. This work offered a view of aging that was a complete departure from the views that had dominated the field of aging since 1960. The journal *Evolution* described the field of aging research as "after Rose." In 1997, Dr. Rose received the Busse Prize of the World Congress of Gerontology. His book *Darwin's Spectre*, a popular introduction to the history and significance of evolutionary biology, was published in 1998. Dr. Rose has been on the editorial boards of a variety of scientific journals and is currently working on a general textbook for his field, *Evolution and Ecology of the Organism*.

MARK A. SMITH, PH.D., is a Professor of Pathology in the School of Medicine at Case Western Reserve University. His research involves investigating the pathological mechanism(s) underlying selective neuronal death in neurodegenerative disease such as Alzheimer's disease. This research includes a variety of techniques ranging from histological to molecular biology to cellular models. The major hypothesis ranging from histological to molecular biology to cellular models. The major hypothesis being pursued by his group is that oxidative stress plays a pivotal role in disease pathogenesis. Therefore, current work is directed to elucidating triggers of oxidative stress including

(*1*) fundamental metabolic alterations; (*2*) homeostatic dysregulation of transition metals; (*3*) signal transduction alterations; and (*4*) inappropriate reentry into the cell cycle. Dr. Smith has authored over 250 peer-reviewed articles and chapters. He is the recipient of several awards including the Ruth Salta Junior Investigator Achievement Award from the American Health Assistance Foundation, the Young Scientist Lectureship Award from the International Society for Neurochemistry, the Nathan Shock New Investigator Award from The Gerontological Society of America, the Zenith Award from the Alzheimer's Association, and the Jordi Folch-Pi Award from the American Society of Neurochemistry.

CAROL G. ZALESKI, PH.D., is Professor of Religion in the Department of Religion and Biblical Literature at Smith College. She received her B.A. from Wesleyan University and her M.A. and Ph.D. in the Study of Religion from Harvard University. Dr. Zaleski is the author of *Otherworld Journeys: Accounts of Near-Death Experience in Medieval and Modern Times* (New York: Oxford University Press, 1987; revised ed., 1989); *The Life of the World to Come: Near-Death Experience and Christian Hope* (New York: Oxford University Press, 1996); and, with Philip Zaleski, *The Book of Heaven: An Anthology of Writings from Ancient to Modern Times* (New York: Oxford University Press, 2000). Her current work in progress includes *The Language of Paradise: Prayer in Human Life and Culture*, with Philip Zaleski, for Houghton-Mifflin; *On Seeing Angels: A Theory of Religious Experience*, for Oxford University Press; *The Book of Hell*, with Philip Zaleski, for Oxford University Press, as well as articles on heaven, hell, and purgatory for *The Encyclopaedia Britannica*. Dr. Zaleski's articles and reviews have appeared in *First Things, The New York Times Book Review, Parabola*, and various scholarly journals. She writes a monthly column for *The Christian Century* and is one of the coeditors of *Second Spring: A Journal of Faith and Culture*, published by the Centre for Faith and Culture, Oxford. At Smith, Dr. Zaleski teaches courses in philosophy of religion and comparative study of world religions. In March 2000 she delivered the annual Ingersoll Lecture on Human Immortality at Harvard Divinity School.

The Fountain of Youth

Introduction

....

Stephen G. Post and Robert H. Binstock

Anti-aging interventions—a wide variety of ambitions and measures to slow, arrest, and reverse phenomena associated with aging—have been part of human culture and societies since early civilizations. An obsession with immortality is a central theme in a Babylonian legend about King Gilgamesh, who ruled southern Mesopotamia in about 3000 B.C. In the third century B.C., adherents of the Taoist religion in China developed a systematic program for prolonging life (Olshansky and Carnes, 2001). Perhaps the oldest written record of attempts to reverse aging is in an Egyptian papyrus, circa 1600 B.C., which provides instructions for preparing an ointment that transforms an old man into a youth of 20 and claims that it has been "found effective myriad times" (quoted in Hayflick, 1994, p. 267). Through the centuries, a variety of anti-aging approaches have recurred. Among them have been alchemy, the use of precious metals (e.g., as eating utensils) that have been transmuted from baser minerals; *shunamatism* or *gerocomy* (cavorting with young girls); grafts (or injected extracts) from the testicles, ovaries, or glands of various animal species; cell injections from the tissues of newborn or fetal animals; consumption of elixirs, drugs, hormones, dietary supplements, and specific foods; cryonics; and rejuvenation from devices and exposure to various substances such as mineral and thermal springs and the classic Fountain of Youth that the governor of Puerto Rico,

1

Juan Ponce de León, searched for in Florida in the early sixteenth century (Hayflick, 1994; Cohen, 2000; Gruman, 2003).

Many of these practices continue in modern times, and some new ones have been added. As one critic of contemporary anti-aging interventions has observed, "Yesterday's prolongevists who searched for the fountain of youth, advocated sleeping with young virgins, encouraged grafting of monkey testicles, and ate yogurt simply have been replaced with modern equivalents" (Hayflick, 2001–2002, p. 25). The marketing and use of anti-aging products and services claiming to prevent, retard, or reverse aging have skyrocketed in recent years (e.g., Shelton, 2000; U.S. General Accounting Office, 2001), accelerated by the advent of the Internet (e.g., Youngevity, 2003). Increased consumer interest in them appears to be fueled by their appeal to baby boomers trying to preserve their youthfulness as they approach old age as well as older persons attempting to rejuvenate themselves. In response, various governmental entities and members of the gerontological professional community have issued public health warnings about the risks and ineffectiveness of various anti-aging products and services (Binstock, 2003).

Yet, contemporary developments in anti-aging interventions are not confined to the efforts of charlatans and quacks. As this volume will demonstrate, many biogerontologists (biologists in the field of aging) are substantially funded by government and the private sector to conduct research that they believe will lead to effective anti-aging interventions. In a broad metaphoric sense, they are searching for modern equivalents to the Fountain of Youth. Some of their anti-aging goals are relatively modest; others are extraordinarily ambitious in terms of achieving *prolongevity*—significant extension of the length of human life, free from the diseases and disabilities now associated with old age (Gruman, 2003). (None of these scientists is seeking to create a prolonged senescence characterized by dependence and chronic illness.) Today's biogerontological quests to achieve prolongevity can be summarized by three models.

Contemporary Models of Prolongevity

One model is commonly described as *compressed morbidity*, a term first promoted by a Stanford physician, James Fries, a quarter of a century ago (Fries, 1980). In this scenario humans live long and vigorous lives, terminated by a sharp decline in functioning mandated by senescence, followed relatively swiftly by death. "The basic syllogism of the compression of morbidity is that since the age of first infirmity can be postponed but the lifespan itself is genetically fixed, the period of infirmity can be shortened" (Fries, 1987, p. 6). The ideal envisioned by Fries is for all of us to lead long lives free of chronic disease and disability, and then die rather quickly as we reach the limits of the human life span because we are "worn out" from the fundamental processes of aging. Compressed morbidity includes the possibility of increases in average life expectancy, but not in maximum life span for the human species.

Another model is *decelerated aging*, in which the processes of aging are slowed and average life expectancy and/or maximum life span are increased. In contrast to the compression of morbidity ideal, late-life functional disabilities are not eliminated but occur at a more advanced age than has been the case historically. The University of Cambridge geneticist Aubrey de Grey and colleagues argue that this phenomenon is already taking place in the context of greater average life expectancy; they do so by drawing on data showing that the onset of late-life frailty is occurring at later ages than previously, but the period of time for which it is experienced is not becoming shorter (de Grey et al., 2002b). Richard Miller (2002), a University of Michigan pathologist, suggests that it may be possible through decelerated aging to "produce 90-year-old adults who are as healthy and active as today's 50-year-olds" (p. 155), as well as "increase the mean and maximal human life span by about 40 percent, which is a mean age at death of about 112 years for Caucasian American or Japanese women, with an occasional winner topping out at about 140 years" (p. 164). Roy Walford (1983), a UCLA biologist, has also suggested that a maximum life span of 140 years can be achieved through decelerated aging.

A third model of prolongevity is *arrested aging*, in which the processes of aging are reversed in adults. In contrast to slowing the rate of aging, the goal of reversing aging is to *restore* vitality and function— akin to the rejuvenation theme that has been present in prolongevity myths and quests for millennia. Some scientists believe that reversal could be accomplished through strategies that remove the damage inevitably caused by basic metabolic processes and thereby attain "indefinite postponement of aging" (de Grey et al., 2002a, p. 670) or negligible senescence (de Grey et al., 2002a). Success in achieving arrested aging would be tantamount to bringing about "virtual immortality"—that is, an increase in the healthy adult life span of such great magnitude that the consequence would be societies in which no one dies except from accidents, homicides, and suicides, or from choosing to forego or being excluded from the interventions that bestow continuing vigorous life. A leading proponent of the likelihood that interventions to arrest aging will be achieved asserts that it is "inevitable, barring the end of civilization, that we will eventually achieve a 150-year mean longevity" (de Grey, 2000, p. 369). Moreover, he hypothesizes that in a world with universally available engineered negligible senescence, "life expectancies of around 1000 years" would be attained (personal communication to R.H. Binstock, October 15, 2002).

The Need for Debate and Dialogue

When one first encounters these models of anti-aging intervention, the goals they embody may seem incredible and unlikely to be realized—even those of the most conservative model, compression of morbidity. Yet many biomedical developments that long seemed improbable have caught society unawares, such as the cloning of mammals (Bonnicksen, 2002).

Research on measures to significantly extend human life expectancy and the maximum life span is now a mainstream activity sponsored and supported, for instance, by the U.S. National Institutes of Health (NIH) (Masoro, 2001; National Institute on Aging, 2001). Biogerontologists and society at large would benefit from anticipatory deliberations concerning the potential consequences of this research (Watson and Juengst, 1992; de Grey et al., 2002).

If such anti-aging interventions are achieved, they could bring about profound alterations in the experiences of individual and collective life. Moreover, serious ethical issues would arise if anti-aging interventions were not universally available, but were distributed in response to status (economic, social, or political), merit, nationality, or other criteria. If access to anti-aging interventions were unlimited, radical changes would take place in virtually every social institution.

Until recently, the potential consequences of anti-aging interventions were discussed only rarely and in venues that do not reach a wide audience (e.g., Moody, 1995, 2001–2002; Seltzer, 1995; Hackler,

2001–2002). However, the important need for debate and dialogue on this topic is now becoming more widely recognized. In late 2002 and early 2003, the U.S. President's Council on Bioethics, aided by testimony from biogerontologists, began debating the promise and moral challenges of research on aging and on what a Council staff paper termed *age retardation* (President's Council on Bioethics, 2002, 2003; Mooney, 2003).

Meanwhile, NIH has begun to fund research on the ethical and policy implications of anti-aging interventions (Juengst, 2002; Binstock, 2003; Binstock et al., 2003). And our colleagues and we published an article in *Science* (Juengst et al., 2003) calling upon NIH to establish a program that engenders sustained and widespread public dialogue on the implications of the anti-aging research for which it is providing its cachet and public funds. Our scientific institutions should take the lead in ensuring that public discussions of this topic are as deliberate and farsighted as the research itself, perhaps addressing how our societal institutions and policies might be shaped to cope with the profound implications of achieving prolongevity. Success in achieving prolongevity would make the ramifications of most other current biomedical policy issues—such as the ethics of research on embryonic stem cells—seem relatively minor. Whether NIH does take on the challenge of promoting broad debate and dialogue regarding the implications of anti-aging interventions remains to be seen.

The Purposes of This Book

This book is intended to extend knowledge, promote discussion, and engender open debate concerning the biomedical goal of prolongevity to a much wider circle of laypersons, professionals, and students than has been reached until now. It is designed to present differing views and to foster communication among scientists, philosophers, religious thinkers, bioethicists, historians, social scientists, and students and citizens who have a sense of responsibility concerning the nature of life in the future. The volume comprises three parts.

Part I, The Perennial Quests for Extended and Eternal Life, introduces a range of historical and contemporary ideas about prolongevity and immortality. The opening chapter by Robert H. Binstock provides an overview of the contentiousness that has characterized the modern arena of research on the biology of aging. Succeeding chapters probe ideas about the quest for immortality as expressed in literature (Mark B. Adams), the desirability of "drinking from" the Fountain of Youth (Stephen G. Post), and additional religious perspectives on extended life and immortality (Neil Gillman and Carol Zaleski).

The six chapters in Part II focus on The Science of Prolongevity. The first of these (by S. Jay Olshansky and Bruce C. Carnes) deals with the historical and contemporary science of understanding senescence. Then two chapters (by Michael R. Rose and Robert Arking, respectively) explore the biological possibilities and probabilities of human life extension. Gemma Casadesus and associates explore the role of diet in aging and how it can affect longevity. The two final chapters deal with more radical approaches to prolongevity. Richard A. Miller discusses achieving decelerated aging through caloric restriction—particularly through the development of a pill that mimics the biochemical effects of caloric restriction (rather than through limited dietary intake). Aubrey D.N.J. de Grey explains how arrested aging might be achieved through a strategy for "engineering negligible senescence."

The final part of the volume, Ethical and Social Perspectives on Radical Life Extension, treats a series of issues raised by the prospect of achieving prolongevity—whether through compressed morbidity, decelerated aging, or arrested aging. It opens with a chapter by Arthur L. Caplan, arguing that it is not inherently wrong to pursue extended, healthy life. Then Christine Overall employs a feminist construct to make a case that increases in life expectancy and maximum life span are worth seeking. Next, Leon R. Kass presents a series of arguments against prolongevity. Eric T. Juengst considers a number of ethical issues that effective anti-aging interventions would pose for the profession of medicine. Audrey R. Chapman examines the social and justice implications of extending the human life span. And Binstock explores the possible political ramifications of a "long-lived society" that includes the "prolonged old."

The book concludes with an epilogue and two annotated bibliographies on prolongevity. In the epilogue, Diogenes Allen presents an existential theological discourse on the merits of aging and death as venues to virtue. The first bibliography, by Roselle S. Ponsaran, has four sections: (A) science, (B) ethics, (C) secondary analyses of literature and mythology, and (D) history. The second, by Carol A. Donley, presents selected primary literary sources.

References

Binstock, R.H. (2003). The war on "anti-aging medicine." *The Gerontologist*, 43, 4–14.

Binstock, R.H., Juengst, E.T., Mehlman, M.J., and Post, S.G. (2003). Anti-aging medicine and science: An arena of conflict and profound societal implications. *Geriatrics and Aging*, 6(5), 61–63.

Bonnicksen, A.L. (2002). *Crafting a Cloning Policy. From Dolly to Stem Cells*. Washington, DC: Georgetown University Press.

Cohen, G.D. (2000). *The Creative Age: Awakening Human Potential in the Second Half of Life*. New York: Avon Books.

de Grey, A.D.N.J. (2000). Gerontologists and the media: The dangers of over-pessimism. *Biogerontology*, 1, 369.

de Grey, A.D.N.J., Ames, B.N., Andersen, J.K., Bartke, A., Campisi, J., Heward, C.B., McCarter, R.J., and Stock, G. (2002a). Time to talk SENS: Critiquing the immutability of human aging. *Annals of the New York Academy of Science*, 959, 452–462.

de Grey, A.D.N.J., Baynes, J.W., Berd, D., Heward, C.B., Pawelec, G., and Stock, G. (2002b). Is human aging still mysterious enough to be left only to scientists? *BioEssays*, 24(7), 667–676.

Fries, J.F. (1980). Aging, natural death and the compression of morbidity. *New England Journal of Medicine*, 303, 130–136.

Fries, J.F. (1987). An introduction to the compression of morbidity. *Gerontologica Perspecta*, 1, 5–8.

Gruman, G.J. (2003). *A History of Ideas about the Prolongation of Life*. New York: Springer.

Hackler C. (2001–2002). Troubling implications of doubling the human lifespan. *Generations*, XXV(4), 15–19.

Hayflick, L. (1994). *How and Why We Age*. New York: Ballantine Books.

Hayflick, L. (2001–2002). Anti-aging medicine: Hype, hope, and reality. *Generations*, XXV(4), 20–26.

Juengst, E.T. (2002). Growing pains: Bioethical perspectives on growth hormone replacement research. *Journal of Anti-Aging Medicine*, 5, 73–79.

Juengst, E.T., Binstock, R.H., Mehlman, M.J., and Post, S.G. (2003). Antiaging research and the need for public dialogue. *Science*, 299, 1323.

Masoro, E.J. (Ed.). (2001). Caloric restriction's effects on aging: Opportunities for research on human implications. *Journals of Gerontology: Biological Sciences and Medical Sciences*, 56A (Special Issue 1).

Miller, R.A. (2002). Extending life: Scientific prospects and political obstacles. *The Milbank Quarterly*, 80, 155–174.

Moody, H.R. (1995). The meaning of old age: Scenarios for the future. In: Callahan, D., ter Meulen, R.H.J., and Topinková, E., eds. *A World Growing Old: The Coming Health Care Challenges*. Washington, DC: Georgetown University Press, pp. 9–19.

Moody, H.R. (2001–2002). Who's afraid of life extension? *Generations*, XXV(4), 33–37.

Mooney, C. (2003). Panel politics. Retrieved May 23, 2003, from http://www.sagecrossroads.net/news_042103.cfm

National Institute on Aging. (2001). *Action Plan for Aging Research: Strategic Plan for Fiscal Years 2001–2005*. Washington, DC: U.S. Department of Health and Human Services.

Olshansky, S.J. and Carnes, B.A. (2001). *The Quest for Immortality: Science at the Frontiers of Aging*. New York: W.W. Norton.

President's Council on Bioethics. (2002). The promise and the challenge of aging research. Staff background paper. Retrieved May 23, 2003, from http://www.bioethics.gov/background/agingresearch.html

President's Council on Bioethics. (2003). Age-retardation: Scientific possibilities and moral challenges. Staff background paper. Retrieved May 23, 2003, from http://www.bioethics.gov/background/age_retardation.html

Seltzer, M. (Ed). (1995). *The Impact of Increased Life Expectancy: Beyond the Gray Horizon*. New York: Springer.

Shelton, D. (2000). Dipping in the fountain of youth. *AMA News*, Dec. 4, 25.

U.S. General Accounting Office. (2001). *Health Products for Seniors: "Anti-Aging" Products Pose Potential for Physical and Economic Harm*. (GAO-01-1129). Washington, DC: U.S. Government Printing Office.

Walford, R.L. (1983). *Maximum Life Span*. New York: W.W. Norton.

Watson, J.D. and Juengst, E.T. (1992). Doing science in the real world: The role of ethics, laws, and the social sciences in the human genome project. In: Annas, G. and Elias, S. eds. *Gene Mapping: Using Law and Ethics as Guides*. New York: Oxford University Press, pp. xv–xix.

Youngevity. (2003). The youngevity story. Retrieved May 24, 2003, from http://www.youngevity.com/the_ygy_story_fs.htm

I

THE PERENNIAL QUESTS FOR EXTENDED AND ETERNAL LIFE

1

The Search for Prolongevity: A Contentious Pursuit

Robert H. Binstock

N early 40 years ago, historian Gerald Gruman (1966) created the term *prolongevity* to encompass the multiple goals of anti-aging interventions over the years, defining it as significant extension of the human life span and/or average life expectancy without suffering and infirmity. In doing so, however, he observed that the idea of prolongevity and those who pursue it have tended to be

> relegated to a limbo reserved for impractical projects or eccentric whims not quite worthy of serious scientific or philosophic consideration. One reason for this neglect is that there is, in philosophy, science, and religion, a long tradition of apologism, the belief that the prolongation of life is neither possible nor desirable. . . . Another reason is the fact that there are few subjects which have been more misleading to the uncritical and more profitable to the unscrupulous; the exploitation of this topic by the sensational press and by medical quacks and charlatans is well known.
>
> (p. 6)

Today, however, the search for prolongevity is a far more respectable activity. It is undertaken by a community of biologists in the field of aging (gerontology)—biogerontologists—based on their scientific studies of the fundamental biological processes of aging. In the United States, for instance, their work is pursuant to an official strategic plan of the National Institutes of Health (National Institute on Aging, 2001), and they receive research funds from both private and public organizations. Yet, their efforts to attempts to achieve effective anti-aging interventions remain contentious, in large measure for the reasons suggested by Gruman.

The purpose of this chapter is to elucidate the social forces, ideas, and concerns that confront the contemporary scientific search for prolongevity. It traces the twentieth-century struggle of biogerontologists to attain scientific legitimacy and obtain adequate funding for their research efforts, a struggle that is ongoing. Then it examines the controversy on whether achieving prolongevity is a desirable goal.

The Ongoing Struggle for Legitimacy and Funding

Although a modern U.S. community of biogerontological scientists (as well as geriatricians and gerontologists more generally) began to develop in the late 1930s, some 40 years later it was still stigmatized by the historical legacy of mythology and charlantanism that has characterized prolongevity aspirations and practices. In her history of the development of federal support for research on aging, published over 20 years ago, political scientist Betty Lockett observed: "Those who would study aging in order to retard or halt the process have been considered on the fringe of biomedical research, looking for the fountain of youth . . . a marginal area . . . with so little backing from the scientific community" (Lockett, 1983, p. 5).

Following the establishment of the National Institute on Aging (NIA) in the mid-1970s, biogerontology gradually began to distance itself from this legacy and attain a substantial measure of scientific legitimation and funding. Yet, the legitimacy of the field is still not secure, as evidenced by current contentious efforts of biogerontologists to distinguish themselves from contemporary promoters of anti-aging products and therapies. This contemporary war against *anti-aging medicine* parallels disputes in many other areas of science in which rhetorical demarcations are employed to maintain legitimacy and power. As Taylor (1996) observes, "Practicing scientists, consciously or otherwise, discursively construct working definitions of science that function, for example, to exclude various non- or pseudo-sciences so as to sustain their (perhaps well-earned) position of epistemic authority and to maintain a variety of professional resources" (p. 5; also see Gieryn, 1983). Such is the case with biogerontology.

Achieving Status and Funding at the National Institutes of Health

As Lockett (1983) and historian W. Andrew Achenbaum (1995) detail, the early development of the modern research enterprise in the biology of aging in the United States, and in geriatrics as well, was to a significant degree stimulated by the Josiah Macy Foundation. During the late 1930s it supported surveys on aging and commissioned a seminal volume on *Problems of Aging: Biological and Medical Aspects* (Cowdry, 1939) that reviewed research knowledge and issues regarding how to prolong human life and how to reduce disabilities and chronic diseases in old age. The Foundation also funded a series of professional conferences that brought together researchers from a variety of disciplines and professions who formed a Club for Research on Ageing. In 1940, the Surgeon General of the United States, who had attended a meeting of the Club, took the lead in establishing a small intramural research program in gerontology at the National Institutes of Health (NIH).

Over the next three decades the broad field of gerontology grew, but the biomedical research enterprise in gerontology stagnated. In 1945, the two dozen members of the Club for Research on Ageing incorporated themselves as a professional association, the Gerontological Society (known since 1980 as the Gerontological Society of America), began publishing a *Journal of Gerontology*, and grew 100-fold over the next 25 years to comprise nearly 2400 members from a wide variety of academic disciplines and professions (C.A. Schutz, executive director of the Gerontological Society of America, personal communication based on organization records, June 19, 2002). In addition, the NIH intramural program was given a line item budget in 1948 and eventually blossomed into a longitudinal study of aging men that became the prime element of NIH intramural research on aging (Achenbaum, 1995). But NIH administrative support and funding for the growth of extramural biomedical research explicitly focused on aging from the 1940s through the early 1970s was quite limited.

Although an NIH Gerontological Study Section for reviewing extramural research applications was created in 1946, it was abolished in 1949. Lockett's documentary research and interviews reveal that this review panel was perceived by some NIA officials as too favorably biased toward applications because there were so few researchers in the field of aging that many of them were members of the Study Section and were evaluating their own research proposals. Ironically, according to one member of the Study Section, the community of gerontological researchers had fought for their own study section because they thought that there was a bias *against* them—"they felt that other study sections automatically turned down proposals that had the word 'aging' in them" (quoted in Lockett, 1983, p. 36). In any event, gerontological applications were subsequently reviewed by other study sections that, according to one NIH staff member, "downgraded gerontology research," and the percentage of approvals "went from one extreme to another" (Lockett, 1983, p. 37).

During the 1950s and 1960s, extramural research on aging gained little ground at NIH. During this period, in order to mollify several members of Congress who were interested in the development of gerontological research, five regional multidisciplinary centers for aging research and training were funded through NIH's program project mechanism. Only one of these centers ultimately survived, and an internal NIH evaluation of the work of these centers was pointedly uncomplimentary concerning the "mediocre scientific competence" of gerontological research (quoted in Lockett, 1983, p. 41). Meanwhile, a Senate subcommittee issued a report "disparaging the quality of gerontologic research" (Achenbaum, 1995, p. 200).

When the National Institute of Child Health and Human Development (NICHD) was established in 1963, aging was designated as one of its five program areas and existing NIH programs on aging became part of NICHD's Adult Development and Aging Branch. Over the next 10 years, gerontologists consistently expressed their disappointment with the NICHD arrangement, especially the low proportion of that institute's funds earmarked for research on aging (e.g., Eisdorfer, 1968; U.S. Senate Subcommittee on Aging of the Committee on Labor and Public Welfare, 1973).

By the late 1960s, frustrated by NIH's lack of funding for research on the basic mechanisms of aging, biogerontologists set in motion the forces that ultimately led to the creation of a separate National Institute on Aging in order to ensure that earmarked funds for gerontological research would be adequate. They drafted a bill in 1968 that called for a new NIH institute with a 5-year research plan "to promote intensive coordinated research on the biological origins of aging" (Lockett, 1983, p. 85). In order to gain the support of the Gerontological Society, however, the bill was subsequently broadened to include the medical, behavioral, and social sciences.

During the subsequent political processes that finally led to the establishment of NIA in 1974, themes suggesting the marginal status of biogerontology persistently emerged. For one thing, the key political actor in the successful lobbying effort, Florence Mahoney, was an ardent pursuer of anti-aging interventions. Mahoney was a powerful Washington insider with politically elite connections, a long-time behind-the-scenes effective advocate for expanded government support for biomedical research. She was very interested in rejuvenation therapies offered by an institute in Bucharest, Romania, and was accustomed to taking serum treatments that were purported to slow or prevent aging. As noted in her biography, Mahoney's "accuracy in separating real science from charletan [sic] science was not precise; she occasionally backed a rejuvenation expert who had mastered promotion and mystique" (Robinson, 2001, p. 237). At the point when biogerontologists attempted to persuade her to make legislation for a separate institute her prime objective, she was more than happy to do so. Her receptiveness to their cause was nourished not only by her personal interest in anti-aging interventions, but also by her experience from 1963 to 1967 as a citizen member of the NICHD Advisory Council, where she felt that gerontological research was shortchanged. Regarding her NICHD experience, Mahoney observed:

> Every time a grant came up about aging, it was turned down. . . . Everyone said aging came naturally. I never believed the effects of old age were irreversible. . . .
> I kept telling them not to discourage those grants, or they would have to have another institute.
>
> (Robinson, 2001, pp. 237–238)

Throughout the protracted legislative history of NIA's establishment, from 1969 through 1974, various opponents of such an institute were quite candid regarding their negative views of the quality and promise of gerontological research. At a Senate hearing in 1971, for instance, an assistant secretary in the Department of Health,

Education, and Welfare argued that the field of aging was not ripe for the injection of major new resources because it lacked "a substantial body of interested and competent research investigators, plus enough research leads, or promising ideas within the field to challenge the researchers to productive endeavors" (quoted in Lockett, 1983, p. 98). Similarly, in a House of Representatives hearing in 1972, the president of the Association of American Medical Colleges asserted that "there is a paucity of trained researchers and valid ideas in the field of aging research" (quoted in Lockett, 1983, p. 122). And when one version of the bill passed in 1972, a memo from the Office of Management and Budget to President Richard Nixon urged him to veto it—which he ultimately did—because an NIA "could raise false expectations that the aging process can somehow be controlled and managed through biomedical research" (quoted in Lockett, 1983, p. 139).

Despite Nixon's veto—and consistent opposition from high-level NIH officials who apparently did not want to have a new institute carving out its own share of NIH appropriations (e.g., U.S. Senate Subcommittee on Aging of the Committee on Labor and Public Welfare, 1973; Lockett, 1983)—Mahoney, the gerontologists, and several key members of Congress persisted in their efforts. In 1974, in the midst of calls for his impeachment, Nixon signed the legislation creating NIA (P.L. 93-296).

The creation of a separate institute on aging began a process that legitimated research on aging both as more of a mainstream subject for biomedical research than it had been regarded by the broader scientific community in the past and as an appropriate area in which to invest sizable amounts of public funds. Since then, a number of important scientific frontiers have been opened up in research on the fundamental biological processes of aging (see, e.g., Martin et al., 1996; Melov et al., 2000; Masoro, 2001a; Masoro and Austad, 2001; Partridge, 2001; Cristofalo and Adelman, 2002; Johnson, 2002; Lin et al., 2002; Wright and Shay, 2002). Moreover, the NIA budget, which was only about $20 million in 1976, its first year of operation (Lockett, 1983, p. 169), has grown rapidly over the years to reach just under $1 billion by fiscal year 2003 (National Institute on Aging, 2002a). To be sure, biogerontologists argue that they require a larger share of this budget in order to purse their promising and exciting lines of research. They contend that NIA invests a disproportionately large share of its resources in disease-oriented research, especially on

Alzheimer's disease (Adelman, 1995), while marginalizing basic biological research on aging in terms of both strategic planning and
actual research funding. The consequence, they argue, is that the sector of research that has the greatest promise for improving health in
old age is being shortchanged, because the fundamental mechanisms
of aging are the underlying and leading risk factors for virtually all
age-associated diseases (Hayflick, 2002; Miller, 2002; Martin, 2003).
Nonetheless, the establishment and growth of NIA has provided for
biogerontology the kind of institutionalization that confers scientific
stature and power (Cozzens, 1990).

The Anti-Aging Medicine Movement versus the "Gerontological Establishment"

Even as biogerontological research achieved scientific and political
legitimacy in the late twentieth century, however, a new challenge to
its reputation was developing in the form of an *anti-aging medicine*
movement in the 1990s. Perhaps historian Carole Haber (2001–2002)
is correct in suggesting that the contemporary emergence of this
movement lies in the appeal of its promises to aging baby boomers
who grew up in a youth-oriented cultural period; recent scientific discoveries that seemingly (though not necessarily) have potential relevance to slowing the rate of aging in humans; and concerns about
negative economic consequences for society associated with the baby
boomers reaching old age. In any event, the use of anti-aging products, particularly dietary supplements, soared following the enactment of the Dietary Supplement Health and Education Act of 1994,
which relaxed regulation of such products (U.S. General Accounting
Office, 2001). During the same period, several dozen books on anti-
aging were published (e.g., Pierpaoli et al., 1995; Fossel, 1996; Carper,
1996; Chopra, 2001; Shostak, 2002). A refereed scientific journal, the
Journal of Anti-Aging Medicine, began publishing in 1998 and now has
a circulation of about 1000 comprising biomedical researchers and
clinicians from a variety of disciplines and specialties (V. Cohn, Mary
Ann Liebert, Inc., which publishes the *Journal of Anti-Aging Medicine,*
personal communication, July 17, 2002). Two nonrefereed publications with similar-sounding names— *The Journal of Longevity* and *The
International Journal of Anti-Aging Medicine*—have also appeared (de
Grey et al., 2002c). And a website for Youngevity: The Anti-Aging Company markets products such as "The Vilcabamba Mineral Essence" to

enable people to "live their lives in a state of youthfulness" (Youngevity, 2002).

The element of the anti-aging movement that has most directly challenged the established gerontological community, however, is the American Academy of Anti-Aging Medicine (A4M), which proclaims that "anti-aging medicine is ushering in the Ageless Society" (American Academy of Anti-Aging Medicine, 2002a, p. 8). Founded in 1993 by "pioneering anti-aging physicians and researchers" (Klatz, 1999, p. 4), A4M claims that it now has "11,000 member physicians, health practitioners, and scientists representing 65 countries, [and] is the undisputed leader in advancing anti-aging medicine around the world" (American Academy of Anti-Aging Medicine, 2002b). Although the organization is not recognized by the American Medical Association, A4M has established three board certification programs under its auspices—for physicians, chiropractors, dentists, naturopaths, podiatrists, pharmacists, registered nurses, nurse practitioners, nutritionists, dietitians, sports trainers and fitness consultants, and Ph.Ds. (American Academy of Anti-Aging Medicine, 2002c). According to A4M, it has organized more than two dozen international conferences on anti-aging medicine and has "conducted educational meetings on Capitol Hill for the purpose of informing key legislators about the necessity of funding anti-aging research into clinical anti-aging therapies" (American Academy of Anti-Aging Medicine, 2002d).

The president and the chairman of this organization, Ronald Klatz and Robert Goldman, respectively, are Chicago-based osteopaths. In the 1980s they published books on the subject of drugs and training regimens intended to enhance performance in sports (Goldman et al., 1984; Goldman and Klatz, 1988). But since the inception of A4M, they have turned to a different subject matter, publishing nearly a dozen books with such titles as *7 Anti-Aging Secrets* (Goldman and Klatz, 1996); *Stopping the Clock: Why Many of Us Will Live Past 100— and Enjoy Every Minute* (Klatz and Goldman, 1996); and *Grow Young with HGH: The Amazing Medically Proven Plan to Reverse Aging* (Klatz and Kahn, 1988). The cover of one of Klatz's books, *Ten Weeks to a Younger You*, promises "age reversing benefits of the youth hormones" such as "enhance IQ," "eliminate wrinkles," "increase memory," and "enhance sexual performance" (Klatz, 1999).

The American Academy of Anti-Aging Medicine states that it does not sell or endorse any commercial product or promote or endorse any specific treatment. But, "prompted by the numerous inquires received each day" (American Academy of Anti-Aging Medicine, 2002e), it actively solicits and displays numerous advertisements on its website for products and services (such as cosmetics and alternative medicines and therapies), anti-aging clinics, and anti-aging physicians and practitioners, some of them listing board certification by A4M. The website also has an "A4M Longevity Store" where anti-aging medicine publications and individual and organizational memberships in A4M can be purchased.

Although what A4M terms "the traditional, antiquated gerontological establishment" (Arumainathan, 2001) may disagree with many of the organization's messages and the measures it promotes, most elements of A4M's broadly stated goals seem, on the surface, to be the same as those of many biomedical researchers and practitioners in gerontology and geriatrics (Klatz, 2001–2002). The stated mission of A4M is

> the advancement of technology to detect, prevent, and treat aging related disease and to promote research into methods to retard and optimize the human aging process. A4M is also dedicated to educating physicians, scientists, and members of the public on anti-aging issues. A4M believes that the disabilities associated with normal aging are caused by physiological dysfunction which in many cases are ameliorable [sic] to medical treatment, such that the human life span can be increased, and the quality of one's life improved as one grows chronologically older.
>
> (American Academy of Anti-Aging Medicine, 2002f)

(Use of the term *life span* by A4M in this and other statements in which it describes historical improvements in longevity seems to refer to what is customarily termed *life expectancy* rather than life span, defined as "the maximum amount of time that a member of a species is known to have lived" [Hayflick, 2002, p. 417]).

To be sure, most, if not all, biogerontologists would probably quarrel with A4M's notion that *at present* human life expectancy for adults can be significantly "increased" or "prolonged" (Olshansky et al., 2002a). But many of them believe that *in the future*, on the basis of further research, both average life expectancy and maximum life span can be extended through biomedical interventions (see, e.g., de Grey et al., 2002a; Holden, 2002; Lane et al., 2002; Miller, 2002).

Although there is a superficial resemblance between the broad goals of A4M and those of the established community of gerontologists and geriatricians, the organization presents anti-aging medicine as a "new health care paradigm" (American Academy of Anti-Aging Medicine, 2002g), actively promoting itself as a challenger to the established gerontological community. For instance, A4M has produced a document entitled "Intellectual Dishonesty in Geriatric Medicine— Truth versus Fallacy" in which it berates NIA for its public information campaign regarding anti-aging therapies, characterizing it as anti-competitive censorship:

> As the worldwide popularity of anti-aging medicine grows, the NIA has scrambled to brand their own flavor of anti-aging medicine as "successful aging," healthy aging," and "aging gracefully." The only perceptible difference between these terms seems to be that the latter phrases are somehow politically correct, mirror-image clones of anti-aging as put forth by A4M's trailblazing work in this field. . . . *NIA wishes to absorb what it cannot contain: by discrediting "anti-aging-medicine" in lieu of its notion of "healthy aging" they silence the most visible outside source of innovations in aging research and education. The status quo of research funding, academic interests, and—most importantly to NIA— the consolidation of power—is thereby maintained.*
>
> (Arumainathan, 2001)

The National Institute on Aging has not responded to this diatribe. Indeed, publicly, NIA has appeared to ignore A4M altogether. Although the institute lists and describes over 250 organizations that may be helpful resources for older people, A4M is not among them (National Institute on Aging, 2002b). Individuals in the field of gerontology, however, have certainly responded to the marketing of anti-aging products and therapies by A4M and others.

Maintaining Legitimacy: Responses from Gerontologists

The active promotion of anti-aging medicine has elicited a flurry of responses from established biological and medical researchers in the field of aging. The most widely publicized of these to date has been an article published in *Scientific American* entitled "No Truth to the

Fountain of Youth," written by S. Jay Olshansky, Leonard Hayflick, and Bruce A. Carnes (2002a), three scientists who have undertaken research on aging for many years. They declared that:

> The hawking of anti-aging "therapies" has taken a particularly troubling turn of late. Disturbingly large numbers of entrepreneurs are luring gullible and frequently desperate customers of all ages to "longevity" clinics, claiming a scientific basis for the anti-aging products they recommend and, often, sell. At the same time, the Internet has enabled those who seek lucre from supposed anti-aging products to reach new consumers with ease.
>
> (p. 92)

They went on to assert that "no currently marketed intervention—none—has yet been proved to slow, stop, or reverse human aging, and some can be downright dangerous" (pp. 92–93). They also presented their interpretations of various lines of biological research relevant to the underlying nature of aging and their promise, or lack of promise, for slowing the progression of aging.

This *Scientific American* article was a summary of a lengthier position statement that had been posted a month earlier on the website of the magazine (Olshansky et al., 2000b) and explicitly endorsed there by an international roster of 51 scientists and physicians that Olshansky, Hayflick, and Carnes had organized and worked with for about a year in order to achieve a text that was mutually acceptable to a group comprising a wide range of views (S.J. Olshansky, personal communication, July 18, 2002; also see Smith and Olshansky, 2002). Shortly after the article appeared, the full position statement, under a slightly different title (Olshansky et al., 2000c), was also posted online at the Science of Aging Knowledge Environment (SAGE KE), a subdivision of the website of the American Association for the Advancement of Science and the journal *Science*. Arrangements were also made to have the statement reprinted in the biological sciences journal of the Gerontological Society of America (Olshansky et al., 2002d) and published (in translation) in Chinese, French, German, Korean, and Spanish journals (S.J. Olshansky, personal communication, July 18, 2002). The scientists' message also reached a very large audience when the *AARP Bulletin* (published by AARP, formerly The American Association of Retired Persons), which has a circulation of more than 35 million, made the *Scientific American* article the lead story in its next issue (Pope, 2002).

At one level, the statement signed by the 51 scientists can be seen as a public health effort, an attempt to educate health professionals and the public regarding the harmful and misleading aspects of anti-aging interventions and claims. In this respect, it joins other efforts of this kind that have been made in recent years. For instance, Robert N. Butler, the first director of the NIA, convened a workshop that produced a consensus report entitled "Is There an 'Anti-aging' Medicine?" (International Longevity Center-USA, 2001) and is responsible for two subsequent journal articles with the same title (Butler, 2001–2002; Butler et al., 2002). The U.S. Senate Special Committee on Aging (2001) held a hearing focused on fraudulent marketing tactics for anti-aging medicines, entitled "Swindlers, Hucksters and Snake Oil Salesmen: The Hype and Hope of Marketing Anti-aging Products to Seniors." The U.S. General Accounting Office (2001) issued a report on the physical and economic harms wrought by anti-aging products. The editor-in-chief of *Experimental Gerontology* has written a similar denunciation of both anti-aging products and treatments (Wick, 2002), and two geriatricians have published an editorial entitled "Antiaging Medicine: The Good, the Bad, and the Ugly" (Fisher and Morley, 2002). The National Institute on Aging has produced an "Age Page" entitled "Life Extension: Science or Science Fiction?" in which it discredits "very much exaggerated" anti-aging claims for pills containing anti-oxidants, DNA, and RNA, as well as for dehydroepiandrosterone (DHEA) and growth hormone (National Institute on Aging, 2002c). And the website of NIA promotes a free fact sheet on "'anti-aging' miracle drugs" (National Institute on Aging, 2002d) as part of "an education effort urging consumers to use caution when it comes to 'anti-aging' hormone supplements" (National Institute on Aging, 1997).

At another level, the statement can be viewed as an attempt to provide its audience with an informed understanding of the potential and limitations of biological research for leading to future interventions in the processes of aging. A number of articles in professional and scientific journals have also done this in the past several years, some of them very optimistic about such interventions (e.g., de Grey et al., 2002a; Miller, 2002) and others who regard them as most unlikely and question their desirability (e.g., Hayflick, 2000). A more popularized examination of the possibilities for anti-aging interventions was presented by reporters in a special issue of *Scientific American* entitled "The Quest to Beat Aging" (Fischetti and Stix, 2000), in which some of the 51 signers of the 2000 position statement were quoted as authorities.

At a third level, the position statement can be interpreted as an attempt by established gerontological researchers to preserve their scientific and political legitimacy, which took many years to achieve, as well as to maintain and enhance funding for research on the basic biological mechanisms of aging. As such, it is *boundary work* that parallels disputes in many other areas of science in which rhetorical demarcations are employed to maintain legitimacy and power (Gieryn, 1983). The superficial resemblance between the broad goals of those who promote anti-aging products and therapies and those of established biological and medical researchers in the field of aging have clearly led members of the latter group to become worried about being confused with the former. As a consequence, they have striven to distance the field of gerontological science from the anti-aging medicine movement. Although different strategies have been employed in these efforts, one common goal has been to ensure that the hard-won respectability attained by the community of gerontological researchers is not tainted by the anti-aging movement. As the position statement acknowledges, *"Our concern is that when proponents of anti-aging medicine claim that the fountain of youth has already been discovered, it negatively affects the credibility of serious scientific research efforts on aging"* (Olshansky et al., 2002d, p. B295; emphasis added).

One approach to maintaining the legitimacy of research on aging has been to invent new terminology to describe its possible benefits. As some gerontological researchers put it in a letter to *Science*, "Misuse of the term 'anti-aging medicine' has led many scientists . . . to shy away from using the term at all, for fear of guilt by association" (de Grey et al., 2000c). Butler argues that in order to ensure that research on aging does not lose credibility and funding, "we should rename the field of aging medicine 'longevity medicine,' to differentiate it from anti-aging practitioners and their nostrums" (Butler, 2001–2002, p. 64). Similarly, in a workshop convened by Butler, participants selected "Longevity Science and Medicine" as an alternative term to "anti-aging [which] has acquired a tarnished image" (International Longevity Center-USA, 2001, p. 12). It is not evident, however, why it is desirable or necessary to invent a new term. *Anti-aging* therapies and products have been around for a long time without any indication that they are confused with *research on aging* (or *aging research* or *geriatric medicine*). Moreover, many who conduct biomedical research on aging are not undertaking *longevity* research.

A second approach has been to discredit the anti-aging medicine movement by disparaging it for making a "quick profit" by fraudulently "exploiting the ignorance and gullibility of the public" (Hayflick, 2001–2002, p. 25). To this end, Olshansky, Hayflick, and Carnes have constituted themselves as a committee to designate annual "Silver Fleece Awards" (emulating the practice of former U.S. Senator William Proxmire, who periodically announced "Golden Fleece Awards" to designate government funding for research projects that he regarded as devoid of any redeeming value to society). In early 2002, Olshansky arranged for his university's office of public affairs to publicize that he was announcing the first annual Silver Fleece Awards in "a light-hearted attempt to make the public aware of the anti-aging quackery that has become so widespread here and abroad" and presenting to the winners (in absentia) bottles of salad oil labeled "Snake Oil" (University of Illinois at Chicago, 2002). The Silver Fleece Award for "Anti-Aging-Quackery" went to Clustered Water for being the product "with the most ridiculous, outrageous, scientifically unsupported or exaggerated assertions about aging or age-related diseases." The Silver Fleece Award for an Anti-Aging Organization went to A4M, which Olshansky characterized "as responsible for leading the lay public and some in the medical and scientific community to the mistaken belief that technologies already exist that stop or reverse human aging" (University of Illinois at Chicago, 2002). This strategy was continued in 2003, when two more Silver Fleece Awards were announced (University of Illinois at Chicago, 2003).

A third and more subtle approach has been to mobilize the adjective *legitimate* to modify research on aging and thereby distinguish it from anti-aging medicine. Thus, in an article reporting an increase in funding for NIA, the newsletter of Butler's organization exhorts, "It is essential in the years ahead, however, that our nation continue to maintain a strong financial commitment to *legitimate* research in the field of aging and longevity . . . *Legitimate* aging research is particularly important due to the prevalence of 'anti-aging therapies' being peddled in the marketplace that are not based on any scientific evidence and could possibly be dangerous" (Nyberg, 2002, p. 1; emphasis added). The position statement signed by the 51 scientists also presents this contrast: "The misleading marketing and the public acceptance of antiaging medicine is not only a waste of health dollars; it has also made it far more difficult to inform the public about *legitimate* scientific research on aging and disease" (Olshansky et al., 2002d, p. B293; emphasis added).

Understandably, the various attacks on anti-aging medicine have engendered very strong ripostes from A4M. Although some of the responses have been personal, they have been primarily aimed at discrediting gerontology for the purpose of legitimizing anti-aging medicine. In rejoinder to the press release announcing its receipt of the Silver Fleece Award, A4M characterized Olshansky as "part of a 'multibillion gerontological machine' that, without any basis in truth or fact, seeks to discredit tens of thousands of innovative, honest, world-class scientists, physicians, and health practitioners" (American Academy of Anti-Aging Medicine, 2002g, p. 1). In response to the *Scientific American* position statement signed by the 51 scientists, A4M set forth 10 alleged "gerontological biases" and purported to refute each of them by describing various articles and data (often in a misleading pseudoscientific fashion). In conclusion, it asserted:

> Simply put, the death cult of gerontology desperately labors to sustain an arcane, outmoded stance that aging is natural and inevitable. . . . Ultimately, the truth on aging intervention will prevail, but this truth will be scarred from the well-funded propaganda campaign of the power elite who depend on an uninterrupted status quo in the concept of aging in order to maintain its unilateral control over the funding of today's research in aging.
> (American Academy of Anti-Aging Medicine, 2002b)

(It is interesting to note that this attack on the establishment of gerontologists is directed at the very people who could further A4M's purported mission, anti-aging, through their research discoveries.)

Assessing the Present Controversy

Few, if any, in the gerontological community would quarrel with the goals of those gerontologists who have recently focused their attention on the anti-aging movement. One goal has been to disseminate a public health message to "scientists and health care workers because they should be on the front warning the public about the possible dangers associated with the use of anti-aging substances"

(S.J. Olshansky, personal communication, July 18, 2002). This effort complements the public health messages disseminated by NIA, the U.S. Senate Special Committee on Aging, and the U.S. General Accounting Office (described above).

Another goal, clearly—and more important in its ramifications for the biogerontological community (and ultimately, perhaps, for society)—is to prevent the anti-aging movement from stigmatizing research on aging, once again, with the charlatanic baggage it had carried until the establishment of NIA ushered it into the mainstream of science in the last quarter of the twentieth century. As Butler observes, "Unfortunately, anti-aging medicine is often confused with serious research. Consequently, public and private philanthropic organizations are less interested in funding serious aging research" (Butler, 2001–2002, p. 64). It is certainly ironic that the field for which the major stride toward legitimacy and funding was largely achieved through the political influence of Florence Mahoney—a woman responsive to the marketing of anti-aging charlatans—is now understandably trying to distinguish itself from pseudoscientific entrepreneurs and practitioners.

But will the war on anti-aging medicine succeed in preventing erosion of the scientific and political legitimacy of research on aging and reduction of funds for conducting it? Or will it boomerang as gerontologists become engaged with the anti-aging movement, much as Brer Rabbit became inextricably embroiled with Tar Baby in the Uncle Remus tale (Johnson, 1997)?

From evidence available in the short run, it is possible to argue that efforts to criticize the anti-aging movement have provided it with greater visibility. When the *AARP Bulletin* published its lead story on the *Scientific American* position statement, the president of A4M, Ronald Klatz, was enabled to reach a readership of more than 30 million persons, gaining attention for his organization and issuing a strong indictment of gerontologists. The American Academy of Anti-Aging Medicine was described at some length in the article, and Klatz was quoted as saying: "The A4M is the first serious affront to the gerontological establishment in 30 years and they want to kill anyone with a competing philosophy . . . The old-line philosophy was aging is inevitable, nothing can be done, get used to it, grow old and die" (Pope, 2002, p. 3).

To be sure, the publication of this and other Klatz quotations and the description of A4M in the *AARP Bulletin* was not the first recognition that A4M and Klatz had received from long-established organizations in the field of aging. In 1997, A4M received a grant from the Retirement Research Foundation to expand its "educational program and to establish the American Board of Anti-Aging Medicine" (Donors Forum of Chicago—Philanthropic Database, 2002). In early 2002, *Generations*, the journal of the American Society on Aging, published an issue on the topic of anti-aging (Cole and Thompson, 2001–2002); in it, Klatz (2001–2002) was provided the same platform to spread his message as was provided to Butler (2001–2002) and Hayflick (2001–2002), two of the most distinguished and senior figures in the field of gerontology. Moreover, the very fact that the author of the *AARP Bulletin* story felt that it was appropriate to get several quotes from Klatz and display his photo in a sidebar–even though neither he nor A4M was mentioned in the *Scientific American* article or position statement—was an indication that his organization had already attained some measure of legitimacy in the larger society. But the new exposure that Klatz received through the publication of his quotes was surely a major escalation in recognition for A4M because of the bulletin's huge circulation. One wonders how many AARP members who learned about A4M by reading this story subsequently attempted to access the website of Klatz's organization to pursue an interest in anti-aging products and therapies. Indeed, the *AARP Bulletin* story featuring the "No Truth to the Fountain of Youth" message provoked a substantial backlash on AARP member online message boards, condemning the biogerontologists' warning as a scare tactic to keep consumers away from anti-aging medicine (AARP Community Message Boards, 2002).

In addition to providing some limelight for A4M, the war on anti-aging medicine might also have had the unintended consequence of blurring public understanding of the difference between the anti-aging movement and the anti-aging aspirations of some biogerontological researchers that could eventually lead to significant improvements of health conditions in old age. Consider that among highly respected biogerontologists—including three who signed the position statement attached to the "No Truth to the Fountain of Youth" article in *Scientific American*—there are those who maintain that substantive progress toward "engineered negligible senescence," or aging *reversal*, will be feasible "within about a decade" and urge investment in its development (de Grey et al., 2002a). One wonders if public (and thereby) financial support for researchers in this camp, as well as those who have somewhat less ambitious goals for modifying aging (e.g., Masoro, 2001b; Lane et al., 2002; Miller, 2002), will be inadvertently weakened by confusion with the objects of attacks on anti-aging medicine. After all, a highly visible sidebar in the *AARP Bulletin* quotes Olshansky (somewhat out of context) as saying, "Anyone who claims that they can stop or reverse the aging process is lying" (Pope, 2002, p. 4).

Yet, regardless of any unintended consequences, it was inevitable that gerontologists would launch a war on the pseudoscientific elements of the contemporary anti-aging movement sooner or later. For one thing, the gerontological community has an ethical responsibility to do so. As Olshansky says:

> The anti-aging entrepreneurs are taking advantage of the legitimate scientists by taking our research, extending and exaggerating our findings well beyond our own views, and then selling their false anti-aging potions to the public with the claims that there is science behind them. By ignoring them, we're indirectly supporting them, and that had to stop.
>
> (S. J. Olshansky, personal communication, July 18, 2002)

More importantly, as indicated by the early history of U.S. biogerontology, it is probably essential for biogerontologists to debunk anti-aging products and therapies so that the image of research on aging will not become blemished once more. Hayflick expresses the situation in an extremely cogent fashion: "After some 25 years of legitimizing the field of biogerontology, it is our responsibility to maintain that legitimacy so that public support for research that advances understanding of the fundamental biology of aging and longevity determination will be sustained and enhanced" (L. Hayflick, personal communication, July 22, 2002).

Are the Goals of Prolongevity Desirable?

The contemporary challenge of maintaining legitimacy and funding extends, however, to more than the goal of simply understanding the basic mechanisms of aging and longevity determination. As indicated above, many biological researchers in the field of longevity are focused on prolongevity, or applied biogerontology—pursuing the goals of compressing morbidity, decelerating aging, or arresting aging.

For example, a great deal of research has established that caloric restriction in various species of experimental animals increases the life span and slows aging-associated changes (Masoro, 2001a). One experiment in caloric restriction in humans that went on for nearly 2 years, undergone by the eight crew members of Biosphere 2, showed physiological, hematological, hormonal, and biochemical changes resembling those of rodents and monkeys on such a diet, accompanied by excellent health and high levels of physical and mental activity (Walford et al., 2002). By 1999, NIA and the National Institute of Diabetes, Digestive, and Kidney Diseases regarded work in this area to be sufficiently important to jointly convene a Caloric Restriction Clinical Implications Advisory Group to explore the implications "for the development of interventions to affect human age-related changes and diseases" (Hadley et al., 2001, p. 5). The 52 scientists that composed this group, working in six panels, produced a substantial agenda of opportunities for research on the human implications, including aspirations to slow fundamental processes of aging and extend the maximum life span (Masoro, 2001b).

Although such efforts are legitimated by the NIH, however, the modern quest for prolongevity is not without its critics. The concerns expressed by the critics depend somewhat on which of the models of prolongevity—described in the Introduction to this volume—they seem to have in mind.

Not surprisingly, hardly any of the contemporary scientists, physicians, social scientists, or humanists who have commented on the desirability of prolongevity has expressed favorable views of attempts to achieve arrested aging or virtual immortality. One exception is Michael Fossel, a clinical professor of medicine at Michigan State University and editor of the *Journal of Anti-Aging Medicine*. He has written a book (Fossel, 1996) about the "promise of a time when we will live longer and much healthier lives—of one hundred, two hundred, possibly five hundred years" (p. 1), in which he tells the reader that "your life span can be extended by several hundred years" (p. 171). Perhaps another exception is John Harris, a bioethicist in the United Kingdom. After reviewing a number of possible arguments against immortality, he argues that "it is doubtful that we can produce coherent ethical objections" to achieving it, and urges that we "start thinking now about how we can live decently and creatively with the prospect" (Harris, 2000, p. 59; also see Harris and Holm, 2002).

In sharp contrast to Fossel and Harris, U.S. bioethicist Leon Kass, chairman of the President's Council on Bioethics, appointed by President George W. Bush in 2001, rejects the goal of arrested aging and virtual immortality—as well as the goal of decelerated aging—on philosophical grounds. He believes that "the finitude of human life is a blessing for every human individual, whether he knows it or not" (Kass, 2001, p. 20), and that "to covet a prolonged life span [he seems to mean *increased average life expectancy*] for ourselves is both a sign and a cause of our failure to open ourselves to . . . any higher . . . purpose" (Kass, 1985, p. 316). Kass argues that even if the human life span (read *life expectancy*) were increased by only 20 years, we would lose the benefits that finitude confers: (*1*) interest and engagement in life, (*2*) seriousness and aspiration, (*3*) beauty and love, and (*4*) virtue and moral excellence (Kass, 2001).

The philosophy of another prominent American bioethicist, Daniel Callahan, also rejects arrested aging and virtual immortality, as well as decelerated aging. Like Kass, he thinks that a sense of finitude to life is important for the individual and that "death is an inherent part of all life and is necessary for the continuation and vitality of species" (Callahan, 2000, p. 654). Indeed, he argues that the only "premature" deaths are those that occur before age 65. He also believes that prolonging life beyond "the natural life span" would have deleterious social consequences. In Callahan's view, even the sizable and growing contemporary population of older Americans is a "social threat" and "a demographic, economic, and medical avalanche . . . that could ultimately (and perhaps already do) [sic] great harm" (Callahan, 1987, p. 23).

Even biogerontologist Leonard Hayflick, regarded by many in the field as having laid the groundwork for contemporary research advances in molecular mechanisms of aging (Shay and Wright, 2000), sees "no value to society or to the individual in seeking to slow or stop the aging process or to achieve immortality" (Hayflick, 1994, p. 341). Among his concerns are that issues of distributional justice will arise if access to life-extending technologies were limited. To whom would they be available and on what terms? Even worse, if they were universally available, he fears an exacerbation of the consequences of worldwide overpopulation, ranging "from the indiscriminate destruction of the planet to mass starvation, wars, economic inequities, and health failures" (Hayflick, 1994, p. 339; also see Hayflick, 2000). Other biogerontologists—particularly, of course, those who are engaged in efforts to decelerate or to arrest aging—acknowledge such concerns but do not feel that they warrant a halt to the quest for prolongevity (e.g., de Grey et al., 2002a,b; Miller, 2002).

On the other hand, Hayflick joins with most other biogerontologists and gerontologists (e.g., Rowe and Kahn, 1998) in regarding as highly desirable the compression of morbidity—or, as he puts it, "active longevity free from disability and functional dependence" (Hayflick, 2002, p. 269). Indeed, he and others in the field believe that the possibilities for achieving compressed morbidity are the best argument for obtaining greater public funding for biogerontology, although Hayflick is "apprehensive about extending average life expectation beyond one hundred" (Hayflick, 1994, p. 335).

Callahan also strongly endorses the compression of morbidity, explicitly urging that research to achieve this goal be given a "status equivalent to that now given to the prolongation of life" (Callahan, 2000, p. 655). In his view, it is not death that is the enemy, but rather a painful, impaired, and unhealthy life before death.

Yet, as desirable as the compression of morbidity may seem, there are those who oppose it. Among bioethicists, Kass condemns compression of morbidity because it will deny individuals the blessings of anticipated mortality:

> it is highly likely that even a modest prolongation of life with vigor or even only a preservation of youthfulness with no increase in longevity would make death less acceptable and exacerbate the desire to keep pushing it away.
>
> (Kass, 2001, p. 20)

Among biogerontologists, de Grey et al. (2002b) argue against the goal of compression of morbidity for a different reason. They believe that it cannot be accomplished and, therefore, that to argue that it is achievable misleadingly diverts needed public attention, credibility, and funding from their own efforts to arrest aging.

Thus, even on a goal that one might expect to find universal agreement—achieving a virtually disease- and disability-free old age without increasing the maximum life span—there is no consensus. In short, each of the various goals of the search for prolongevity remains contentious in the twenty-first century, along with the boundary dispute between biogerontologists and the anti-aging medicine movement. And there is little to indicate that this contentiousness will fade in the decades ahead as biogerontologists pursue their research, anti-aging promoters attempt to draw on that research, and philosophers and other social commentators contemplate the implications of prolongevity.

Acknowledgments

Support for the preparation of this chapter was provided by the National Institute on Aging (NIA), the National Human Genome Research Institute (NHGRI), Grant No. 1R01AGHG20916-01 (Eric T. Juengst, Ph.D., Principal Investigator), and the John Templeton Foundation (JTF). The opinions expressed are solely those of the author and do not reflect those of NIA, NHGRI, or JTF. Portions of this chapter are adapted from R. H. Binstock, The war on "anti-aging medicine," *The Gerontologist*, 43 (2003), 4–14.

References

AARP Community Message Boards. (2002). Retrieved May 16, 2003, from http://community.aarp.org/n/mb/message.asp?webtage=rp-health&msg=45.1&maxT=7

Achenbaum, W.A. (1995). *Crossing Frontiers: Gerontology Emerges as a Science.* New York: Cambridge University Press.

Adelman, R.C. (1995). The Alzheimerization of aging. *The Gerontologist*, 35, 526–723.

American Academy of Anti-Aging Medicine. (2002a). Validating the facts and science of anti-aging medicine: A report on the state of the clinical specialty. AM4 white paper: The report of the Medical Committee on Aging Research and Care. Retrieved June 13, 2002, from http://www.worldhealth.net/whitepaper/index.htm

American Academy of Anti-Aging Medicine. (2002b). Official position statement on the truth about aging intervention. Retrieved June 13, 2002, from http://www.worldhealth.net/html/truth/html

American Academy of Anti-Aging Medicine. (2002c). Board certification programs. Retrieved June 13, 2002, from http://www.worldhealth.net/whitepaper/id24.htm

American Academy of Anti-Aging Medicine. (2002d). Achievements of the A4M. Retrieved June 13, 2002, from http://www.worldhealth.net/whitepaper/id23.htm

American Academy of Anti-Aging Medicine. (2002e). Find an anti-aging product or service. Retrieved June 13, 2002 from http://www.worldhealth.net

American Academy of Anti-Aging Medicine. (2002f). *About A4M—History and overview.* Retrieved June 13, 2002, from http://worldhealth.net/html/about_a4m_-_history_and-over.htm

American Academy of Anti-Aging Medicine. (2002g, February 22). The fleecing of academic integrity by the gerontological establishment: American Academy of Anti-Aging Medicine official response statement to February

12, 2002 "Silver Fleece Awards Target Anti-Aging Hype" (University of Illinois news release, February 12, 2002). Retrieved June 13, 2002, from http://www.worldhealth.net/html/fleecing_of_academic_ integrity.htm

Arumainathan, S. (2001). Intellectual dishonesty in geriatric Medicine—truth versus fallacy: A4M sets the record straight on a campaign of disinformation challenging the facts of the science of anti-aging medicine. Retrieved June 13, 2002, from http://www.worldhealth.net

Butler, R.N. (2001–2002). Is there an "anti-aging" medicine? *Generations*, XXV(4), 63–65.

Butler, R.N., Fossel, M., Harman, S.M., Heward, C.B., Olshansky, S.J., Perls, T.T., Rothman, D.J., Rothman, S.M., Warner, H.R., West, M.D., and Wright, W.E. (2002). Is there an antiaging medicine? *Journal of Gerontology: Biological Sciences*, 57A, B333–B338.

Callahan, D. (1987). *Setting Limits: Medical Goals in an Aging Society*. New York: Simon & Schuster.

Callahan, D. (2000). Death and the research imperative. *New England Journal of Medicine*, 342, 654–656.

Carper, J. (1996). *Stop Aging Now!: The Ultimate Plan for Staying Young and Reversing the Aging Process*. New York: HarperCollins.

Chopra, D. (2001). *Grow Younger, Live Longer: 10 Steps to Reverse Aging*. New York: Harmony Books.

Cohen, G.D. (2000). *The Creative Age: Awakening Human Potential in the Second Half of Life*. New York: Avon Books.

Cole, T.R. and Thompson, B. (Eds.). (2001–2002). Anti-aging: Are you for it or against it? *Generations*, XXV(4).

Cowdry, V.E. (Ed.). (1939). *Problems of Ageing: Biological and Medical Aspects*. Baltimore: Williams & Wilkins.

Cozzens, S.E. (1990). Autonomy and power in science. In: Cozzens, S.E. and Gieryn, T.F., Eds., *Theories of Science in Society*. Bloomington: Indiana University Press, pp. 164–184.

Cristofalo, V.J. and Adelman, R. (Eds.). (2002). *Focus on Modern Topics in the Biology of Aging: Annual Review of Gerontology and Geriatrics*, vol. 21. New York: Springer.

de Grey, A.D.N.J. (2000). Gerontologists and the media: The dangers of overpessimism. *Biogerontology*, 1, 369.

de Grey, A.D.N.J., Ames, B.N., Andersen, J.K., Bartke, A., Campisi, J., Heward, C.B., McCarter, R.J., and Stock, G. (2002a). Time to talk SENS: Critiquing the immutability of human aging. *Annals of the New York Academy of Science*, 959, 452–462.

de Grey, A.D.N.J., Baynes, J.W., Berd, D., Heward, C.B., Pawelec, G., and Stock, G. (2002b). Is human aging still mysterious enough to be left only to scientists? *BioEssays*, 24(7), 667–676.

de Grey, A.D.N.J., Gavrilov, L., Olshansky, S.J., Coles, L.S., Cutler, R.G., Fossel, M., and Harman, S.M. (2002c). Antiaging technology and pseudoscience. *Science*, 296, 656.

Donors Forum of Chicago—Philanthropic Database. (2002). Recipient: American Academy of Anti-Aging Medicine. Retrieved June 21, 2002, from http://homeless.cued.uic.edu/donors/forum

Eisdorfer, C. (1968). Patterns of federal funding for research in aging. *The Gerontologist*, 8(1, Part I), 3–6.

Fischer, A. and Morley, J.E. (2002). Antiaging medicine: The good, the bad, and the ugly. *Journal of Gerontology: Medical Sciences*, 57A, M636–M639.

Fischetti, M. and Stix, G. (Eds.). (2000). The quest to beat aging. *Scientific American*, 11(2).

Fossel, M. (1996). *Reversing Human Aging*. New York: William Morrow.

Gieryn, T.F. (1983). Boundary-work and the demarcation of science from non-science: Strains and interests in professional ideologies of scientists. *American Sociological Review*, 48, 781–795.

Goldman, B., Bush, P., and Klatz, R. (1984). *Death in the Locker Room: Steroids and Sports*. South Bend, IN: Hardwood Press.

Goldman, B. and Klatz, R. (1988). *The "E" Factor: Ergogenic Aids, the Secrets of New-Tech Training and Fitness for the Winning Edge*. Chicago: Elite Sports Medicine Publications.

Goldman, B. and Klatz, R. (1996). *7 Anti-Aging Secrets*. Chicago: Elite Sports Medicine Publications.

Gruman, G.J. (1966). A history of ideas about the prolongation of life: The evolution of prolongevity hypotheses to 1800. *Transactions of the American Philosophical Society*, 56(Part 9), 1–97.

Haber, C. (2001–2002). Anti-aging: Why now?—A historical framework for understanding the contemporary enthusiasm. *Generations*, XXV(4), 9–14.

Hadley, E.C., Dutta, C., Finkelstein, J., Harris, T.B., Lane, M.A., Roth, G.S., Sherman, S.S., and Starke-Reed, P.E. (2001). Human implications of caloric restriction's effects on aging in laboratory animals: An overview of opportunities for research. *Journals of Gerontology: Biological and Medical Sciences*, 56a(Special Issue 1), 5–6.

Harris, J. (2000). Intimations of immortality. *Science*, 288, 59.

Harris, J. and Holm, S. (2002). Extending human lifespan and the precautionary paradox. *Journal of Medicine and Philosophy*, 27, 355–368.

Hayflick, L. (1994). *How and Why We Age*. New York: Ballantine Books.

Hayflick, L. (2000). The future of aging. *Nature*, 408, 267–269.

Hayflick, L. (2001–2002). Anti-aging medicine: Hype, hope, and reality. *Generations*, XXV(4), 20–26.

Hayflick, L. (2002). Anarchy in gerontological terminology. *The Gerontologist*, 42, 416–421.

Holden, C. (2002). The quest to reverse time's toll. *Science*, 295, 1032–1033.

International Longevity Center-USA. (2001). *Is there an "Anti-Aging" Medicine?* New York: International Longevity Center-USA.

Johnson, J.P. (1997). *Brer Rabbit and the Tar Baby*. Memphis, TN: Troll Associates.

Johnson, T.E. (2002). A personal retrospective on the genetics of aging. *Biogerontology*, 3, 7–12.

Kass, L.R. (1985). *Toward a More Natural Science: Biology and Human Affairs.* New York: Free Press.

Kass, L.R. (2001). L'chaim and its limits: Why not immortality? *First Things*, No. 13, 17–24.

Klatz, R. (ed.). (1999). *Ten Weeks to a Younger You.* Chicago: Sport Tech Labs.

Klatz, R. (2001–2002). Anti-aging medicine: Resounding, independent support for expansion of an innovative medical specialty. *Generations*, XXV(4), 59–62.

Klatz, R. and Goldman, R. (1996). *Stopping the clock: Why Many of Us Will Live Past 100—and Enjoy Every Minute.* New Canaan, CT: Keats Publishers.

Klatz, R. and Kahn, C. (1998). *Grow Young with HGH: The Amazing Medically Proven Plan to Reverse Aging.* New York: Harper Perennial.

Lane, M.A., Ingram, D.K., and Roth, G.S. (2002). The serious search for an anti-aging pill. *Scientific American*, 287(2), 36–41.

Lin, S.-J., Kaeberlein, M., Andalis, A.A., Sturtz, L.A., Defossez, P.-A., Culotta, V.C., Fink, G.R., and Guarente, L. (2002). Caloric restriction extends *Saccharomyces cerevisiae* lifespan by increasing respiration. *Nature*, 418, 344–348.

Lockett, B.A. (1983). *Aging, Politics, and Research: Setting the Federal Agenda for Research on Aging.* New York: Springer.

Martin, G.M. (2003). Biology of aging: The state of the art. *The Gerontologist*, 43, 272–274.

Martin, G.M., Austad, S.N., and Johnson, T.E. (1996). Genetic analysis of ageing: Role of oxidative damage and environmental stresses. *Nature Genetics*, 13(1), 25–34.

Masoro, E.J. (2001a) Dietary restriction: An experimental approach to the study of the biology of aging. In: Masoro, E.J. and Austad, S.N., eds., *Handbook of the Biology of Aging* (5th ed.). San Diego, CA: Academic Press, pp. 396–420.

Masoro, E.J. (Ed.). (2001b). Caloric restriction's effects on aging: Opportunities for research on human implications. Journals of Gerontology: Biological Sciences and Medical Sciences, 56A(Special Issue 1).

Masoro, E.J. and Austad, S.N. (Eds.). (2001). *Handbook of the biology of aging* (5th ed.). San Diego, CA: Academic Press.

Melov, S., Ravenscroft, J., Malik, S., Gill, M.S., Walker, D.W., Clayton, P.E., Wallace, D.C., Malfroy, B., Doctrow, S.R., and Lithgow, G.J. (2000). Extension of life-span with superoxide dismutase/catalase mimetics. *Science*, 289, 1567–1569.

Miller, R.A. (2002). Extending life: Scientific prospects and political obstacles. *The Milbank Quarterly*, 80, 155–174.

National Institute on Aging. (1997, April 1). Media campaign cautions consumers about "anti-aging" hormone supplements [NIH news release].

Retrieved July 3, 2002, from http://www.nia.nih.gov/news/pr/1997/04%2D01.htm

National Institute on Aging. (2001). *Action Plan for Aging Research: Strategic Plan for Fiscal Years 2001–2005*. Washington, DC: U.S. Department of Health and Human Services.

National Institute on Aging. (2002a). National Institute on Aging: FY2003 budget. Retrieved July 17, 2002, from http://www.nia.nih.gov/fy2003_congress/justification.html

National Institute on Aging. (2002b). Resource directory for older people. Retrieved July 8, 2002, from http://www.nia.nih.gov/resource

National Institute on Aging. (2002c). Life-extension. Science or science fiction? Retrieved July 8, 2002, from http://www.nia.nih.gov/health/agepages/lifeext.htm

National Institute on Aging. (2002d). Looking for the fountain of youth? Retrieved July 3, 2002, from http://www.nia.nih.gov/health/ads/fount1.git

Nyberg, J.P. (2002). *The Importance of Aging Research. ILC Policy Report*, May, p. 1.

Olshansky, S.J. and Carnes, B.A. (2001). *The Quest for Immortality: Science at the Frontiers of Aging*. New York: W.W. Norton.

Olshansky, S.J., Hayflick, L., and Carnes, B.A. (2002a). No truth to the fountain of youth. *Scientific American*, 286(6), 92–95.

Olshansky, J.S., Hayflick, L, and Carnes, B.A. (2002b, May 12). The truth about human aging. Retrieved June 12, 2002, from http://sciam.com

Olshansky, J.S., Hayflick, L., and Carnes, B.A. (2002c, June 19). Position statement on human aging. Retrieved June 25, 2002, from http://scienceonline.org

Olshansky, S.J., Hayflick, L., and Carnes, B.A. (2002d). Position statement on human aging. *Journals of Gerontology: Biological Sciences and Medical Sciences*, 57A, B292–B297.

Partridge, L. (2001). Evolutionary theories of ageing applied to long-lived organisms. *Experimental Gerontology*, 36, 641–650.

Pierpaoli, W., Regelson, W., and Colman, C. (1995). *The Melatonin Miracle*. New York: Simon & Schuster.

Pope, E. (2002). 51 top scientists blast anti-aging idea. *AARP Bulletin*, 23(43), 3–5.

Robinson, J. (2001). *Noble Conspirator: Florence S. Mahoney and the Rise of the National Institutes of Health*. Washington, DC: Francis Press.

Rowe, J.W. and Kahn, R.L. (1998). *Successful Aging*. New York: Pantheon Books.

Shay, J.W. and Wright, W.E. (2000). Hayflick, his limit, and cellular ageing. *Perspectives*, 1, 72–76.

Shostak, S. (2002). *Becoming Immortal: Combining Cloning and Stem-Cell Therapy*. Albany: State University of New York Press.

Smith, J.R. and Olshansky, S.J. (2002). Editorial: Position statement on human aging. *Journal of Gerontology: Biological Sciences*, 57A, B291.

Taylor, C.A. (1996). *Defining Science: A Rhetoric of Demarcation*. Madison: University of Wisconsin Press.

University of Illinois at Chicago (2002, February 12). Silver Fleece Awards target anti-aging hype [Office of Public Affairs news release]. Retrieved June 21, 2002, from http://tigger.uic.edu/htbin/cgiwrap/bin/newsbureau

University of Illinois at Chicago Office of Public Affairs. (2003, March 13). Second annual "Silver Fleece" Awards aim to expose anti-aging propaganda. Retrieved March 19, 2003, from http://tigger.uic.edu/htbin/cgiwrap/bin/newsbureau/cgi-bin/indes.cgu

U.S. General Accounting Office. (2001). *Health Products for Seniors: "Anti-Aging" Products Pose Potential for Physical and Economic Harm* (GAO-01-1129). Washington, DC: U.S. Government Printing Office.

U.S. Senate Special Committee on Aging. (2001). Swindlers, hucksters and snake oil salesmen: The hype and hope of marketing anti-aging products to seniors. Hearing held in Washington, DC, September 10.

U.S. Senate Subcommittee on Aging of the Committee on Labor and Public Welfare. (1973). Research on Aging Act, *1973.* Washington, DC: U.S. Government Printing Office.

Walford, R.L. (1983). *Maximum Life Span.* New York: W.W. Norton.

Walford, R.L., Mock, D.M., Verdery, R., and MacCallum, T. (2002). Caloric restriction in Biosphere 2: Alterations in physiologic, hematologic, hormonal, and biochemical parameters in humans restricted for a 2-year period. *Journal of Gerontology: Biological Sciences,* 57A, B211–B224.

Wick, G. (2002). Anti-aging" medicine: Does it exist? A critical discussion of "anti-aging health products. *Experimental Gerontology* [online prepublication]. Retrieved September 16, 2002, from http://sciencedirect.com

Wright, W.E. and Shay, J.W. (2002). Historical claims and current interpretations of replicative aging. *Nature Biotechnology,* 20, 682–688.

Youngevity, (2002). The youngevity story. Retrieved July 29, 2002, from http://www.youngevity.com/the_ygy_story.htm

2

The Quest for Immortality: Visions and Presentiments in Science and Literature

Mark B. Adams

> Because biological immortality and the preservation of
> youth are such potent lures, men will never cease to search
> for them . . . undeterred by the unfortunate experience of
> Dr. Faust. It would be foolish to imagine that this search will
> never be successful, down all the ages that lie ahead.
> Whether success would be desirable is quite another matter.
> (Clarke, 1963, p. 208)

*T*he spectacular developments in current biotechnology have sprung from recent theoretical and experimental breakthroughs, and they have raised a range of issues relating to ethics, human destiny, and the relationship between science and religion. Yet, although many may be unaware of it, these developments have been historically shaped by a tradition of thought that arose roughly a century ago, at the birth of what was then called the *new biology*.

The turn of the twentieth century witnessed the birth of various new and exciting forms of experimental biology. Inspiring and underlying these new fields was a new vision of the human future—one in which the triumphs of the new science were seen as making possible the control of life, long-held dreams of human longevity, and new empowerment in determining our ultimate collective fate. That time also saw a nascent science of human destiny, one in which eugenics and rejuvenation research seemed to offer great hope for humans to escape from the constraints of Darwinian selection and seize control of their future.

This underlying vision infused and informed a whole generation of thinkers. They included H.G. Wells, philosophers Bertrand Russell and Olaf Stapledon, humanists Aldous Huxley, C.S. Lewis, and J.R.R. Tolkien, and many biologists, notably J.B.S. Haldane and Julian Huxley. Over the course of four decades, they conducted an active public debate exploring the scientific possibilities, social implications, and ethical quandaries of the new science. With the emergence of modern science fiction in the early 1940s, these same issues were taken up by a new generation of scientific visionaries, notably Robert A. Heinlein and Arthur C. Clarke, who brought to them a fresh and somewhat different perspective.

This chapter will sample the rich diversity of thought and experience of those earlier generations that surveyed and mapped the horizons we are now beginning to explore.

From Dismal Darwinism to the New Biology

The quest for human immortality is as old as civilization itself, with each successive culture giving it new, often culture-specific meanings and textures. But something happened in Western thinking around the turn of the twentieth century that would reconfigure that quest and give it new significance and urgency. The nature of that reconfiguration would shape the debate in the ensuing decades and still colors current discussions.

Problems with Progress:
The Dismal Darwinism of H.G. Wells

As the end of the nineteenth century approached, many works appeared celebrating its unparalleled achievements. The triumphs of the "century of progress"—the Industrial Revolution, the rise of scientific medicine, the heroic age of invention, and the creation and efflorescence of a host of new sciences—were everywhere evident. No wonder, then, that the major philosophers and social scientists of the century had been centrally preoccupied with explaining progress itself: such disparate thinkers as Auguste Comte, Herbert Spencer, and Karl Marx shared in common the effort to understand its causes and nature. For Spencer, for example, the "law of progress" was everywhere evident in the universe, and always, inevitably, led from the homogeneous to the heterogeneous, producing universal progress— of the solar system, from a nebular cloud to the planets; of the Earth, from a molten body to its current, marvelously accommodating state; of the organism, from the fertilized egg through the undifferentiated embryo into the complex and differentiated adult; of life itself, from the simple through increasingly advanced and complex forms of life, culminating in humankind; and of human society, from primitive tribal forms into nations and advanced scientific civilization.

Yet, many such works, even those of a celebratory tone, contained troubling worries based on the discoveries of nineteenth-century science. By the end of the century of progress, there was a widespread sense that progress was over. At the *fin de siècle*, in the words of one prominent witness, "the prevalent feeling is one of perdition and extinction" (Bergonzi, 1961, p. 5). Most troubling was not what science was saying about the past, but rather what science seemed to be saying about the future.

It was the work of Charles Darwin, probably more than any other, that both provided the progress theorists with their best scientific evidence and at the same time threw cold water on the idea of progress itself. Darwin's *theory of descent with modification*—that all current species are the modified descendants of other, earlier forms closely associated with them in time and space—caused no problems; it was his explanation—natural selection—that proved troubling. If the marvelous adaptations everywhere evident in animate nature were not the product of God's design but simply the result of over-population, variation, and natural selection—the *survival of the fittest*— then humanity's progress from the apes had occurred because less advantaged types had been outcompeted and outbred by fitter types. Darwin made it clear that there was nothing inevitable about progress in Spencer's sense: cave fish whose ancestors had eyes could lose them and become blind if doing so helped them survive in their lightless environment. Others drew stronger lessons: if humanity was "higher" than the apes, it was because the fitter had triumphed over the weaker through fierce competition—the fiercer the competition, the faster the "progress."

In one sense, then, Darwin's theory had made progress inevitable (almost by definition, those fittest to survive would do so), but, in a more profound sense, his theory seemed to destroy the very idea of progress altogether. Future human progress of the sort everyone was celebrating was not inevitable but contingent: there was no guarantee whatever that we would progress any further without the survival of the fittest. So, as thinkers gradually began to realize, humanity seemed to be in a kind of Darwinian cul-de-sac. Most major contemporaries agreed that altruism, civility, freedom, immunization, and charity toward the less fortunate were characteristics demonstrating a higher, more socially evolved form of civilization. Yet, drawing on Darwin, many had come to believe that, by sparing humans the struggles that weeded out the unfit, such advanced, civilized behavior would almost certainly lead to human degeneration and the undoing of civilization itself. Like that of any other species, our future—even our continued existence—was subject to natural laws beyond our control.

No one expressed these concerns more vividly, or to a wider audience, than that *fin de siècle* phenomenon Herbert George Wells (1866–1946). The scientific romances he published in the decade between 1895 and 1905 were translated into many languages and brought him international fame as a futurological guru. A onetime student of "Darwin's bulldog," T.H. Huxley, Wells used biological themes often in his scientific romances, but only as he used other sciences, to make a particular pessimistic point: humans were subject to inexorable natural laws beyond their control and were powerless to shape their individual and collective destiny.

The earliest and most widely read of these romances was *The Time Machine* (1895), which launched his career. Its unnamed narrator is a product of the scientific progress of the Victorian age. He builds a time machine and travels forward to the year 802,701 in order to observe the scientific marvels and social advancement he expects to find. Instead, he discovers that the human race has evolved into two degenerate species: the childlike Eloi, who graze innocently aboveground, and the Morlocks, who live underground, tend their machines without understanding them, and harvest the Eloi for food. Lest any reader miss the point, the time traveler voyages to a still more distant future, only to discover a dying planet with no trace of humanity or intelligence, a cold earth sitting motionless beneath a pale, red, dying sun.

Where did such a bleak picture of the human future come from? We can trace the elements of Wells's story in the history of nineteenth-century science. The split of humanity into the Eloi (derived from the ruling class) and the Morlocks (derived from the workers) followed the view that social evolution and class structure flowed from economics, a common theme in the bevy of new social sciences that had emerged in the late nineteenth century. That these two groups became biologically distinct followed from Darwinian evolution. The dying sun and the dying planet came out of nineteenth-century physics and astronomy: entropy, as embodied in the Second Law of Thermodynamics, implied that every energy source runs down; indeed, one of its formulators, Lord Kelvin, had used his knowledge of combustion to predict when the sun would go out (Burchfield, 1975). For Wells, then, the most glorious fruits of the century of progress—the astronomical, physical, biological, and social laws discovered by nineteenth-century science—suggested that progress itself is constrained, and that the likely ultimate destiny of humanity would be degeneration and extinction.

In this and other Wells stories, then, biological laws took their place beside cosmic, astronomical, physical, chemical, and social laws as the forces that control human destiny. Laws of history, evolution, geology, or astronomy were inexorable. Indeed, the pathetic characters for whom he reserves special ridicule are those, like Dr. Moreau, who believe in their pride and folly that they can use science and technology to change the human condition for the better.

For many who took the triumphs of nineteenth-century science seriously, then, the human future seemed bleak. Human destiny, both individual and collective, had been—and would be—beyond our control and subject to inexorable natural law. The apparent *design* in the world—which had seemed to many the proof of a benevolent Creator—was now seen as an artifact of natural struggle, one in which death played the central role. As a consequence, future human progress, which had once seemed inevitable, had come to seem unlikely, if not impossible.

The Quickening: Human Implications of the New Biology

A way out of the apparent Darwinian cul-de-sac was provided by the rise of a new kind of biology. The generation of H.G. Wells had known traditional zoology, botany, embryology, paleontology, and morphology as descriptive enterprises aimed at generalizing natural order and discovering natural laws. But the generation after Wells had witnessed the birth of "experimental biology." This new biology embraced an experimentalist concept of scientific law: it was laboratory law—directly observable, demonstrable, repeatable, predictable, and controllable. For many, the prospects for the new biology were summed up in the phrase *the control of life* (Pauly, 1987).

One of the fields that seemed to offer the most immediate promise for the human future in these years was *eugenics*—literally, "being well born"—directed at improving the biological quality of future human generations. Originally conceived by Darwin's cousin Francis Galton (1822–1911) as a civic religion whereby couples would voluntarily control their reproduction to fulfill their moral obligation to the biological future of the human race, eugenics gained new vigor with the emergence of the new science of genetics. In the period 1900–1925, eugenics movements developed in at least two dozen countries (Adams, 1990). Galton's ideas concerning negative eugenics—decreasing the reproduction of the physically, mentally, or morally "defective"—gained wide acceptance, leading to a series of laws in the United States and elsewhere restricting undesirable immigration and mandating the sterilization of the "unfit." These negative measures, however, were generally seen as a holding action at best: while they might halt the degeneration of the human race, they could hardly lead to its regeneration. Much more attractive—and more illusive—were the hopes for *positive* eugenics—increasing the reproduction of the hereditarily "gifted." To many, it appeared that, by controlling human breeding, the degeneration of the human race—which had seemed so inevitable a few years earlier—might well be halted and even reversed. Further improvement in the species could occur not through the suffering and death entailed in natural selection, but by the much more humane and morally satisfying procedures of voluntary control of human reproduction.

Galton's eugenic ideas appealed to the Irish dramatist George Bernard Shaw (1856–1950). In two well-known plays he dwelt on the theme of human evolutionary improvement, and both were published with lengthy prefaces detailing Shaw's view of the implications of the old and new biology for humanity. In *Man and Superman* (1901), Shaw scoffed at negative eugenics but held forth great hope for positive eugenics, lamenting the fact that, although humanity had wiped out millions of people, "we have never deliberately called a human being into existence for the sake of civilization." In *Back to*

Methuselah: A Metabiological Pentateuch (1921), Shaw portrayed humanity in five stages of its evolution, concluding with incredibly long-lived humans of the far future who are about to transcend the material world to become pure mentality.

Much of the new biology was ultimately directed at the problems relating to human longevity or, put another way, the scientific quest for human immortality. A list of the laboratories that grew up under the aegis of the new experimental biology in the period 1900–1920 would include a number of fields with which we are familiar (genetics and experimental embryology, for example), but also a number of others that may come as a surprise: experimental morphology, animal psychology, tissue culture, organ transplantation, sexology, eugenics, and rejuvenation. Meanwhile, comparable enthusiasms in the new scientific medicine were taking hold with the development of such fields as bacteriology, immunology, and hygiene. Many leading scientific figures in these various fields, including immunologist Ilya Mechnikov (1908) and experimental surgeon Alexis Carrel (both Nobel laureates), as well as "monkey gland" therapist Serge Voronoff (1926; Réal, 2001) and a host of others, explored in their research and popular writings the visionary implications of their work for lengthening the healthy human life span. Taken together, these new fields developing under the banner of the new biology held forth the promise that, through science, humankind would be able to intervene in natural processes to create a revolution in the health, quality, and length of human life.

The creation of this new biology had largely been the work of a generation born in the mid-1800s. Following World War I, however, the torch passed to a younger generation born around 1890. All had grown up entranced by the futurology of the early novels of H.G. Wells, which had achieved universal popularity during their youth. But this generation was also tantalized by the prospects of the new biology that was rapidly developing around them. And, in that new biology, this generation saw a way out of the dismal future Wells had so palpably portrayed. They shared Wells's futurology, then, but not his early pessimism about the inexorable human future. For them, the new biology was redefining the possible and empowering humankind with a new lease on its future.

The product of this blend was a consuming interest in a future-oriented biology aimed not only at preventing human degeneration and extinction, but also at shaping the human future to suit visionary ends. Others of the same generation saw vast implications of these developments for human freedom and society, not all of them good.

Immediately following World War I, members of this new 1890 generation began to actively discuss the potentials of the new biology for the human future, engaging in a structured public exploration during the interwar years of the possibilities for controlling human evolution, engineering human longevity, and deploying the new biology to seize control of human destiny. It was a remarkable group indeed, involving some of the leading scientists, philosophers, and writers of their generation. They included, among others, Julian Huxley (1887–1975), his younger brother Aldous Huxley (1894–1973), Olaf Stapledon (1886–1950), J.B.S. Haldane (1892–1964), C.S. Lewis (1898–1963), and J.R.R. Tolkien (1892–1973).

The Great Debate

The interwar period witnessed an intensification of the discourse on human biological futurism, pitting its most visionary advocates against their most severe critics. This intensification occurred in response to contemporary revolutions taking place in biology, physics, and astronomy, but also as a post–World War I response to the collapse of the old world order and a growing sense in many European societies that human social destiny had to be brought under social control. These trends were reinforced in the 1930s with the emergence of the ideological struggle between Soviet communism and German national socialism—two radical secular regimes with very different visions for the human future—and the challenge they posed to liberal democracies in economic crisis.

The postwar debate opened in 1920 with the appearance of a major popular work by H.G. Wells, *The Outline of History*. Now the pessimistic Wells of the early novels was gone, replaced by Wells the socialist utopian technocrat, a transformation prefigured by the appearance in 1905 of his nonfiction book *A Modern Utopia*, which had depicted a worldwide, monolingual, cooperative society run by a technocratic elite called the Samurai. The *Outline* was a human history unlike any that had appeared before, setting the human past in the context of the evolution of the solar system, the evolution of life, and the gradual emergence of humankind. The core of the book chronicles the advancement of human civilization as the result of the progress of science and technology, periodically obstructed by religion. It concludes with a contemplation of the human future and ends on a triumphal note: "Gathered together at last under the leadership of man, the student-teacher of the universe, unified, disciplined, armed with the secret powers of the atom and with knowledge as yet beyond dreaming, Life, for ever dying to be born afresh, for ever young and eager, will presently stand upon this earth as upon a footstool and stretch out its realm amidst the stars" (Wells, 1920, vol. 2, p. 595). Wells's work was immensely popular the world over, and its view of secular progress based on setting aside the old religions became a kind of rallying cry for a new generation—and occasioned major opposition from traditionalists and religious believers.

But Wells was of an older generation, and his solution was a social, not a biological, one. There soon emerged a spokesman for the new generation in the person of the biologist J.B.S. Haldane.

The Visionaries

The most daring voice of the new generation of visionaries, and its most controversial and confrontational advocate, was J.B.S. Haldane (Adams, 2000). The son of a renowned physiologist, Haldane in the 1920s began the work on evolutionary theory, human genetics, and biochemistry that would establish his fame as one of the century's greatest biologists. But to the public, he became best known for his many entertaining and provocative essays, and through them he became the chief lightning rod and spokesman for his visionary generation. In two enormously influential essays written in the mid-1920s, Haldane offered his view of the short- and long-term future of humanity—and a complete answer to the *fin de siècle* Darwinian dilemma Wells had so effectively expressed in his novels.

The first of these essays, published in 1924, was *Daedalus, or Science and the Future* (reprinted in Dronamraju, 1995). The work sold some 15,000 copies in its first year. Arguing that "the biologist is the most romantic figure on earth at the present day," Haldane noted: "They do not see themselves as sinister and revolutionary figures. They have no time to dream. But I suspect that more of them dream than would care to confess it" (pp. 77, 80). One of Haldane's own dreams was what he called *ectogenesis*—the in vitro fertilization and embryonic development of human eggs—and the eugenic transformation of human society that the technique would produce. To illustrate his vision, Haldane broke into a fictional format. He concocted a plausible college essay written by an undergraduate many years hence about how these biological developments during the period 1950–1990 had transformed civilization: "Had it not been for ectogenesis there can be little doubt that civilization would have collapsed within a measurable time owing to the greater fertility of the less desirable members of the population in almost all countries" (Haldane, 1924, pp. 66–67). As this excerpt makes clear, Haldane saw the new biology as a way of controlling the human future and, indeed, of saving humankind. We may note that Haldane's essay casts the outdated morality of organized religion as the main stumbling block to salvation.

Even more provocative was an essay Haldane published in 1927 called "The Last Judgment." The core of the essay is a fictional message from the future that embodies his visionary ideas—a 17-page "broadcast to infants on the planet Venus some forty million years hence." The intervening history is recounted briefly: Science has been harnessed to gratify all human desires. The development of synthetic food allows the population to grow. The continents and climate are remodeled to suit human tastes. Of special moment is the triumph over natural selection: with the development of the biological sciences, humans achieve almost complete control of life. Although they apply this knowledge to the sculpting of other life forms, the alteration of the human form is only minor, and largely directed at achieving "happiness." Teeth are eliminated, along with all disease; the healthy human life span is extended to 3000 years; and, since it is no longer needed, the human pain sense is almost completely abolished— "the most striking piece of artificial evolution accomplished," according to the message. As a consequence, by the year 5,000,000, "natural selection had been abolished" and "human evolution had ceased"— leading to millions of years of utopian stasis.

Soon, however, it becomes clear that the moon is falling and the Earth's days are numbered. The impending doom leads some to consider "the colonization of other planets." A small group of humans decide to forgo earthly pleasures in order to preserve humankind: they willingly undergo controlled human evolution in order to create a race capable of inhabiting Venus. After 10,000 years, a suitable human race is bioengineered; in the meantime, that planet is flooded with specially engineered bacteria designed to wipe out all native Venusian life forms and render the planet more habitable. Once on Venus, the settlers continue their modifications apace: "So rapid was our evolution," notes the message, "that the crew of the last projectile to reach Venus were incapable of fertile unions with our inhabitants, and they were therefore used for experimental purposes." Well before the Earth's destruction, then, there are in effect *two* human species: the "old" one on Earth—which, having "successfully cultivated human happiness," will be "destroyed by fire from heaven"—and a new, bioengineered humanity on Venus.

Thereafter, the new Venusian humanity "settled down as members of a super-organism with no limits to its possible progress." Before long, "the evolution of the individual has been brought under complete social control," and humans have undergone rapid controlled evolution, reacquiring the pain sense and also a sensitivity to wavelengths that "places every individual at all moments of life, both asleep and awake, under the influence of the voice of the community." Safe on Venus, these "evolved humans" escape the catastrophe on Earth. But they do not stop there. Plans are underway to colonize Jupiter: "A dwarf form of the human race about a tenth of our height, and with short stumpy legs but very thick bones, is therefore being bred. . . . They are selected by spinning them round in centrifuges which supply an artificial gravitational field, and destroy the less suitable members of each generation." If Jupiter is successfully occupied, attempts will be made to colonize Saturn, Uranus, Neptune, and Pluto, where "it is possible that under the conditions of life in the outer planets the human brain may alter in such a way as to open up possibilities inconceivable to our own minds." And further plans are underway to seed other stars and galaxies: "Our galaxy has a probable life of at least eighty million million years. Before that time has elapsed it is our ideal that all the matter in it available for life should be within the power of the heirs of the species whose original home has just been destroyed. . . . And there are other galaxies."

In *Daedalus*, Haldane had criticized H.G. Wells for being "behind the times": he had not realized the tremendous potential of the new biology. Wells apparently took Haldane's criticisms to heart. Alerted to the critical importance of the new biology and aware of his own weak grasp of it, Wells in 1926 drafted his son "Gip," a zoologist, and the young biologist Julian Huxley to prepare a popular and monumental work that would be a sequel to *The Outline of History*, a kind of "outline of biology."

Wells's selection of Julian Huxley as a collaborator was apt indeed. A member of the 1890s generation, grandson of T.H. Huxley, and a leading experimental biologist and bird ethologist, Julian had already made something of a name for himself as a science popularizer who focused on the implications of the new biology for religion and society. Indeed, he had tried his own hand at fiction, publishing a science fiction story about the implications of the work of Alexis Carrel in experimental surgery called "The Tissue Culture King" (1927). The Wells project was a memorable one for Huxley: impressed by *The Outline of History*, he accepted the challenge—resigning his London professorship in order to do so. Many years later, he devoted an entire chapter of his memoirs to the undertaking. As Sir Julian recalls: "[Wells] had forgotten much of his biology and what he remembered was by now old-fashioned—pre-Mendelian. . . . Thus the bulk of the scientific work would fall on my shoulders" (J. Huxley 1970, pp. 155–156). When the research and writing were well underway, Haldane's "The Last Judgment" appeared, and its effects can be clearly seen in the final product: the concluding section of *The Science of Life*, "The Biology of the Human Race," includes sections on "The Breeding of Mankind," "The Possibility of One Collective Human Mind and Will," and a final five-page section, "Life Under Control," which reprises ideas from "The Last Judgment." The 1500-page text enjoyed remarkable popularity and went through many reprintings.

Throughout his life, Julian Huxley remained true to his vision. In series of popular books and collected essays, including *Religion Without Revelation*, he continued to urge his version of *Evolutionary Humanism*, a faith based on the spiritual dimensions of Darwinian science. In various popular works, he argued for Darwinism, population control, and enlightened eugenics. After World War II, he became active in the United Nations, serving as a founder—and the first Director General—of UNESCO, where he became active in organizing efforts aimed at population control. With the "hardening" of the evolutionary synthesis in the postwar period, Huxley emerged as one of the founders of modern evolutionary theory, and in popular and public settings, he frequently used his standing to advocate the themes of his persistent credo. In his speech at the Darwin Centennial convocation in Chicago, on November 26, 1959, entitled "The Evolutionary Vision," he urged that we "jettison the democratic myth of equality" and undertake population control, advocated a new religion based on knowledge and Darwinian evolution, highlighted "the hidden treasure of fresh possibilities that could be realized in [humanity's] long future," and summoned man to fulfill "his evolutionary role in the universe," declaring the present "stage of evolving man" comparable in importance to that 300,000,000 years ago when "our amphibian ancestors were just establishing themselves out of the world's water" (J. Huxley, 1960).

But the power of Haldane's vision in "The Last Judgment" found even greater resonance in the works of another member of his generation: Olaf Stapledon (1886–1950). In 1930—the same year that the final volume of *The Science of Life* appeared—the ultimate implications for human destiny of Haldane's perspective were spelled out in panoramic detail in Stapledon's classic and influential book *Last and First Men: A Story of the Near and Far Future*—a philosophical pseudohistory of humanity from the world of 1930 through to the end of a habitable solar system (Stapledon, 1930; Fiedler, 1983; Crossley, 1994). In the course of this future history, human civilizations rise and fall, humankind almost becomes extinct several times, and some 18 distinct human species succeed one another—among them a musical species, a flying species, and giant brains. Throughout much of the book, the human future is depicted in a Wellsian fashion, with human evolution governed by natural forces largely outside of human control. However, beginning in the 10th chapter, Stapledon elaborates on Haldane's ideas and explores their consequences for society, religion, culture, survival, and for the question of what it means to be human.

The Third Men master the "plastic art" of controlling and shaping life. Worshipping mentality, they design a successor race of superbrains, who become the Fourth Men; realizing their limitations, these in turn experiment on the surviving specimens of the Third Men to produce a new race: their goal was a "normal human" but "perfected through and through," with a life span measured in thousands of years. These become the Fifth Men, who subsequently undergo the events described in Haldane's "Last Judgment" with remarkable precision. With the Earth's immanent end, a new race of experimentally engineered humans moves to Venus. There humanity degenerates into various populations, one of which eventually evolves into the Sixth Men, who design the Seventh, who in turn design the Eighth Men—a race that shares a communal mind. When it becomes clear that astronomical events on the sun will make life impossible except on the outer planets, that species turns its skills "to the production of a human being capable of carrying the torch of mentality into a new world." Eventually, various designed and naturally produced species lead to the Eighteenth Men, the final human species, with large, dexterous hands, an additional pair of occipital eyes—and a life span of a quarter million terrestrial years. These, in turn, contemplate seeding the galaxy before the solar system itself becomes uninhabitable.

In his preface to the 1930 English edition of *Last and First Men*, Stapledon wrote of his intention to present a "potent" possible future by creating "neither mere history, nor mere fiction, but myth":

> A true myth is one which, within the universe of a certain culture (living or dead), expresses richly, and often perhaps tragically, the highest admirations possible within that culture. A false myth is one which either violently transgresses the limits of credibility set by its own cultural matrix, or expresses admirations less developed than those of its culture's best vision. This book can no more claim to be true myth than true prophecy. But it is an essay in myth creation. The kind of future which is here imagined, should not, I think, seem wholly fantastic . . . to modern western individuals who are familiar with the outlines of contemporary thought.
>
> (pp. 11–12)

Stapledon expanded his vision in later works, first in *Last Men in London* (1932) and then in *Starmaker* (1937), which depicts a cosmos filled with civilized and utterly alien intelligences who, together with humans, form a kind of universal community in which the stars and the universe itself participate.

The new myth, or credo, largely shared by Wells, Huxley, Haldane, and Stapledon, was essentially this: Traditional religion is untenable. We live in a material, Darwinian world governed by the laws of science, and we must understand our existence and our future in an evolutionary, cosmic time scale. Humanity is at a crucial moment in its history as a species, with only a few centuries remaining for us to seize control of our destiny: left to natural law, humanity will degenerate and, like all other biological species, eventually become extinct; our planet (and later our sun) will die. But the new biology affords us a way out: In the short term, we can halt our degeneration through some form of negative eugenics, social experimentation, world government, and technocratic socialism. In the long term, using positive eugenics and bioengineering, we can create new kinds of humans for moving into space and colonizing other planets within—and, if possible, beyond—our solar system. In this way, human progress can proceed indefinitely, producing future descendants with even higher (perhaps telepathic or communal) forms of mentality. This is the science-based faith that will provide what Christianity and other religions cannot: scientific answers to the profound questions of ethics, human destiny, our place in the universe, and the meaning of life. To realize our true destiny, we must be guided not by a myth from our past but by a vision of our future (Adams, 2000, p. 476).

We should note that, for these visionaries, it was the immortality of the human race itself, not that of individual humans, that was at stake, and it was a goal worthy of individual sacrifice. True, once humans had mastered the "plastic art" of controlling life, they could ameliorate the human form and extend the human life span virtually without limit. Recall: Haldane's future humans, even before they migrate to Venus, have been engineered to have a healthy life span of 3000 years; Stapledon's Fifth Men have a life span of thousands of years; the Eighteenth Men have a life span of a quarter million years. But personal immortality itself is neither the goal nor even a realistic prospect. In *The Science of Life*, Wells and Huxley devote a section to the issue of human immortality where they make this clear:

> Individual death is one of the methods of life. . . . Every individual is a biological experiment, and a species progresses and advances by the selection, the rejection or multiplication of these individuals. Biologically, life ceases to go forward unless individuals come to an end and are replaced by others. The idea of any sort of individual immortality runs flatly counter to the idea of continuing evolution. Mr. Everyman makes his experiments, learns and teaches his lesson, and hands on the torch of life and experience. The bad habits he has acquired, the ineradicable memories, the mutilations and distortions that have been his lot, the poison and prejudice and decay in him—all surely are better erased at last and forgotten. A time will come when he will be weary and ready to sleep. It is the young who want personal immortality, not the old.
>
> Yet these considerations do not abolish the idea of immortality; they only shift it from the personality. In the visible biological world, in the world of fact, life never dies; only the

individuals it throws up die. . . . And our lives do not end with
death; they stream on, not merely in direct offspring, but more
importantly perhaps in the influence they have had on the rest
of life.

(Wells et al., 1934, pp. 1434–1435)

The meaning of our lives is the contribution we make to the survival of our species. It is also in the *communal mind* contemplated by
Haldane and Stapledon that prospects for relating and joining with
the universe in some spiritual way are contemplated.

This nexus of ideas among the visionaries was quite naturally
associated with certain philosophical and political orientations. As a
group, the visionaries tended to be on the political Left: some, such as
Haldane, became Marxists and members of the Communist Party;
others were simply socialists who foresaw our best hope in the emergence of a world government; all were fascinated by the "Soviet experiment," although some took longer than others to understand that
Stalinism was not what they had in mind. They also shared a faith in
rationalism and science, seeing it as the basis for true spirituality, and
were uniformly dismissive of established religions, preferring (if you
will) their own. Understandably, their vision provoked a reaction.

The Critics

"All happy families are alike," writes Leo Tolstoy at the beginning of
Anna Karenina, "but each unhappy family is unhappy in its own way."
So too with the visionaries and their critics: despite their differences,
Wells, Haldane, J. Huxley, and Stapledon shared, in the main, a com-
mon vision—but each of the major critics of that vision had his own
problems with it.

The appearance of *Daedalus* in 1924 brought forth critical responses almost immediately. One of the first, published the same year,
was a sobering essay by Bertrand Russell (1872–1970). At the time,
Russell was already one of the world's most distinguished mathemati-
cians, the author of *Russell's paradox*, and, together with Alfred North
Whitehead, the author of *Principia Mathematica* (1910–1913), which
helped to found modern symbolic logic. In *Icarus, or the Future of
Science* (1924), Russell spelled out some of the dystopian social possibilities in eugenics. Alluding to Haldane's essay, he remarked that
"much as I should like to agree with his forecast . . . I am compelled

to fear that science will be used to promote the power of dominant groups, rather than to make men happy" (p. 5). His critique of negative eugenics was portentous: "We may perhaps assume that . . . governments will acquire the right to sterilize those who are not considered desirable as parents. This power will be used, at first, to diminish imbecility, a most desirable object. But probably, in time, opposition to the government will be taken to prove imbecility, so that rebels of all kinds will be sterilized. Epileptics, consumptives, dipsomaniacs and so on will gradually be included; in the end, there will be a tendency to include all who fail to pass the usual school examinations" (pp. 48–49). He then turned his attention from negative to positive eugenics, dismissing its utopian prospects with a strong dose of realism: "If we knew enough about heredity to determine, within limits, what sort of population we would have, the matter would of course be in the hands of State officials, presumably elderly medical men. . . . I suspect that they would breed a subservient population, convenient to rulers but incapable of initiative" (pp. 51–52). Thus, in essay form, Russell spelled out some of the dystopian social possibilities of Haldane's ectogenetic eugenic vision.

Eight years later, Russell's reservations were given palpable fictional form by Julian Huxley's younger brother, Aldous Huxley (1894–1963). From Julian and family friends, he was fully up-to-date on the latest scientific possibilities and explored their human implications in many of his novels, ranging from the potential effects of consciousness-expanding drugs to the possible alteration of the human mating period. One of his better-known novels—*After Many a Summer Dies the Swan* (1939)—took up the problem of human rejuvenation and immortality. The story concerns a reclusive California millionaire who finances private research to produce a rejuvenating serum to extend his life indefinitely; unfortunately, the product causes him to regress into something like his evolutionary ancestors.

The work for which Aldous is chiefly remembered, however, is *Brave New World* (1932)—a novel aimed squarely at *Daedalus* that expanded on the reservations expressed by Russell. It portrays a future technocratic utopia based on the eugenic ectogenetic production of bottled babies, designed for their class and role in life to produce social stability, one in which social harmony is assured through the scientific control of human behavior. By genetic, embryological, psychological, hormonal, and chemical manipulations—bioengineering, conditioning, and drugs—each of its five social classes (Alphas, Betas,

Gammas, Deltas, and Epsilons) is shaped to perform, and to enjoy performing, its particular social role. The society is entirely ectogenetic. The novel opens with three chapters set in the Central London Hatchery and Conditioning Center, where the techniques of human production are detailed for a visiting group. "Take ectogenesis," remarks the Controller. "Pfitzner and Kawaguchi had got the whole technique worked out. But would the Governments look at it? No. There was something called Christianity. Women were forced to go on being viviparous" (A. Huxley 1932, pp. 30–31). The novel is often misread as dealing entirely with the dystopian implications of the new biology; actually, it is no less a critique of the ideas of technocracy, scientific management, industrial mass production, modern psychology, drugs, and the British class system. Only when taken together did such developments constitute the challenge to human individuality and freedom Huxley was warning us about.

If the ideas in Haldane's *Daedalus* evoked powerful critiques from Russell and Aldous Huxley, the vision in Haldane's second essay—"Last Judgment"—provoked even more reaction, although it took longer to play itself out. We have already noted that Haldane's credo constituted a new, future-oriented myth of human destiny intended to replace the old religions. That Haldane was advancing a new religion was a fact not lost on the orthodox, and it provoked memorable responses from two of his more devout contemporaries: C.S. Lewis, and J.R.R. Tolkien.

Clive Staples Lewis (1898–1963) was one of Britain's most prominent authors of the twentieth century, a religious philosopher, fantasy writer, and Oxford professor of medieval and Renaissance English literature. Today, he is chiefly remembered for his "Narnia" series for children and his book *The Screwtape Letters*, although a 1993 film (*Shadowlands*, with Lewis played by Anthony Hopkins) has immortalized his postwar romance with an American woman. Long an admirer of moral tales and "planetary fantasies" such as those of H.G. Wells, Lewis did not take at all kindly to the visions of Haldane and Stapledon. "What immediately spurred me to write," he noted to a student, "was Olaf Stapledon's *Last and First Men* and an essay in J.B.S. Haldane's *Possible Worlds*" (Green and Hooper, 1974, p. 163)— which he later identified as "the brilliant, though to my mind depraved, paper called 'The Last Judgment'" (Lewis, 1966, p. 65–66). Haldane had written an essay, Stapledon a book: Lewis responded with a trilogy of novels.

The first novel was *Out of the Silent Planet* (1938), a planetary romance built around Lewis's version of medieval Christian cosmogony. Its hero is Ransom, a British philologist; its villain, Weston, a physicist who embodies Haldane's philosophy. Weston has no problem experimenting on people in the name of science and kidnaps Ransom, taking him as a prisoner to Mars to offer him as a human sacrifice to its indigenous natives. Frightened at first of traveling through cold empty space, Ransom experiences instead an "empyrean warmth" that suffuses the heavens. As it turns out, Weston was mistaken: the universe is ruled by benevolent angels in a kind of harmony of the spheres, and it is the Earth—the "silent planet"—that had lost its rightful place in the cosmos as a result of the Bent One, the angel who ruled here but became mad. When Ransom is brought to the spirit ruling Mars, who seeks to understand Weston's behavior, the philologist is called upon to translate. Out of Weston's mouth comes Haldane's vision in "The Last Judgment," whose absurdity is revealed by Ransom's translation. A year after the book appeared, Lewis explained how he had come to write it:

> The danger of "Westonism" I meant to be real. What set me about writing the book was the discovery that a pupil of mine took all that dream of interplanetary colonization quite seriously, and the realization that thousands of people in one way and another depend on some hope of perpetuating and improving the human race for the whole meaning of the universe—that a "scientific" hope of defeating death is a real rival to Christianity.
>
> (Green and Hooper, 1974, p. 164)

Lewis was quite deliberate in his parallel: Weston was *meant* to be Haldane; it was "The Last Judgment" and *Last and First Men* that "embodied the desperately immoral outlook which I try to pillory in Weston" (Green and Hooper, 1974, p. 163).

Soon Lewis had produced a sequel to his novel, called *Perelandra* (1943). This time, Weston and Ransom contest on Venus, where Weston—now possessed by Satan—seeks to despoil the Venusian Garden of Eden that is unfolding. Weston's defeat there permits the establishment of Lewis's alternative to utopia, an idyllic pastoral that was the moral history of Man without the Fall. Here Lewis spells out once again his objections to Haldane's view.

Professor Weston had meant plenty of harm. He was a man obsessed with the idea which is at this moment circulating all over our planet in obscure works of "scientifiction," in little Interplanetary Societies and Rocketry Clubs, and between the covers of monstrous magazines, ignored or mocked by the intellectuals, but ready, if ever the power is put into its hands, to open a new chapter of misery for the universe. It is the idea that humanity, having now sufficiently corrupted the planet where it arose, must at all costs contrive to seed itself over a larger area: that the vast astronomical distances which are God's quarantine regulations, must somehow be overcome. This for a start. But beyond this lies *the sweet poison of the false infinite*—the wild dream that planet after planet, system after system, in the end, galaxy after galaxy, can be forced to sustain, everywhere and for ever, the sort of life which is contained in the loins of our own species—*a dream begotten by the hatred of death upon the fear of true immortality*, fondled in secret by thousands of ignorant men and hundreds who are not ignorant. The destruction or enslavement of other species in the universe, if such there are, is to these minds a welcome corollary. In Professor Weston the power had at last met the dream.

(pp. 81–82; emphasis added)

Meanwhile, Weston's philosophical justification has evolved into a notion of "emergent" or "creative" evolution, whereby his interplanetary efforts are actually serving religious purposes, preparing for the emergence of the Life Spirit. As we learn in the novel when Weston actually becomes possessed by the Bent One, however, this is simply Satanic sophistry.

Two years later, the trilogy was completed with *That Hideous Strength* (1945), where the battle was carried to Earth (actually, rural England, which, for Lewis, is much the same thing). Now Weston is the director of a scientific research institute—N.I.C.E.—ostensibly to better humanity but secretly (as we discover) to complete a diabolical plot to seize cosmic powers from the grave of Merlin. When Lewis completed his trilogy, Haldane reviewed all three novels in a stinging essay entitled "Auld Hornie, F.R.S." (1946; the title, meaning the devil, referring to himself as depicted by Lewis). The review attacked Lewis for scientific inaccuracies, the complete mischaracterization of science, and his disparagement of the human race. Lewis wrote a detailed rebuttal but put it away in a folder marked "Anti-Haldane"; it was published posthumously under a more suitable title (Lewis, 1966, pp. 74–85). It made clear, as did the Perelandra trilogy itself, that Lewis objected not only to specific proposals of the biological visionaries but to their central premise: he opposed all scientific attempts to manipulate or control life or nature for human purposes as contrary to the divine harmonious order and a source of great evil.

By the late 1930s, Lewis had gathered around him a small Oxford circle of like-minded literary friends, dubbed the Inklings, that met periodically to read each other their works. One notable Inkling was J.R.R. Tolkien (1892–1973), a fellow Oxford professor, first of Anglo-Saxon (1925–1945) and subsequently of English language and literature (1945–1959). Tolkien is principally remembered today as the author of *The Lord of the Rings* (1954–1955), a mythical fantasy of elves, wizards, and hobbits that became something of a cult classic for many young readers in the 1960s. Today's generation is becoming reacquainted with the work in the series of three films created by Peter Jackson, each based on one of the three works in his trilogy.

Tolkien had met Lewis in 1926 and shared much of his worldview (Carpenter, 1977). Although Lewis was an Anglican convert, whereas Tolkien was a lifelong devout Catholic, they shared a love of myth and the medieval Christian world. For both, the universe was an essentially moral place, and the secular religion of visionary science of the sort advocated by Haldane, Stapledon, and their ilk was profoundly immoral and corrupting. Lewis's trilogy makes much more explicit references to Haldane's vision of secular immortality than does Tolkien's. Nonetheless, one finds in Tolkien's work (and the films based on it) a powerful mythic embodiment of the same themes.

At the core of Tolkien's trilogy is the "One Ring," the "Ring of Power," forged by the dark lord, "Sauron the Deceiver," so that he may rule and bring darkness to the world forever—and the quest by an unlikely band of hobbits, aided by elves, a wizard, and assorted human allies, to destroy it. In forging the ring, we are told, Sauron has infused it with his "will to dominate all life." One of the ring's attributes, we learn, is that it gives its bearer "unnatural long life." It did so first for the unfortunate creature Gollum (Golem?), whom it consumed, and "poisoned his mind" for 500 years. By chance it then fell into the hands of Bilbo Baggins, a hobbit, and "for sixty years the Ring lay quiet, in Bilbo's keeping, prolonging his life, delaying old age"—although he is beginning to feel old in his heart, "thin, sort of stretched, like butter scraped over too much bread." The trilogy begins at the celebration of Bilbo's 111th birthday. With the help of Gandalf, a wizard, he overcomes considerable temptation and leaves the ring behind, to his nephew, the unsuspecting Frodo. Meanwhile, Sauron's evil forces are stirring and, learning of the ring's rediscovery, the race is on: for Frodo and his companions, to destroy the ring by casting it into the fires where it was forged; for Sauron's evil forces, to seize the ring and thereby achieve domination over the world.

As Peter Jackson (Jackson et al., 2001) has commented, there is little doubt that the One Ring represents science and technology. The ring seems to have "a will of it's own," tempting men—"who, above all else, desire power" and whose hearts "are easily corrupted"—away from what is "natural" with its promise of long life and the power over nature. Punctuating the trilogy are a series of tests, which most pass (but some fail), in which the ring is offered to various powerful characters, including the wizard, Gandalf, and Galadriel, queen of the elves. As Gandalf explains: "I dare not take it, even to keep it safe. Understand, Frodo, I would use this ring in a desire to do good. But through me, it would wield a power too great and terrible to imagine." Those who fall under its sway, like the Ringwraiths (former human kings), become "neither living nor dead." Meanwhile, the forces of evil use "foul craft" to create their armies. As Saruman (a powerful wizard who has succumbed to Sauron's temptation) notes, the evil orcs "were elves once—taken by the dark powers, tortured and mutilated, a ruined and terrible form of life . . . and now perfected." In turn, Saruman himself, using "foul craft," "has crossed orcs with goblin men" to breed an army in the caverns surrounding his castle, formed by ripping out all the trees with their deep roots. As the film splendidly portrays, wherever the ring holds sway, evil corrupts and destroys nature and replaces it with flames and the clanking of "dark Satanic mills" and workshops.

No wonder the film opens with Galadriel's lament: "The world is changed. I feel it in the water, I feel it in the earth, I smell it in the air. Much that once was is lost" (Jackson et al., 2001). In a way, it is the essential lament of both Lewis and Tolkien, two medievalists mythologically lamenting what science and technology have done to the world and the far greater harm they threaten to do if Haldane and his ilk have their way.

What are we to make of the responses of Lewis and Tolkien to the visionary biology of their generational contemporaries? The power of their writing, and of the views they espouse, might seem to suggest that their critiques embody many of the quite natural religious and moral qualms of humanists and the faithful alike concerning the devastations of the natural world and the human condition wrought by misguided scientism. Considering the time and place in which they wrote—when other scientistic civic religions such as Nazism and Stalinism were creating vast human miseries in the name of a brighter future—their qualms are understandable.

At the same time, theirs was a hardly a mainstream religious reaction. Each in his own way was proudly reactionary, fascinated by the medieval Christian worldview and devoutly devoted to his faith. Lewis and Tolkien understood full well what the visionaries were about—and that the prospect of their scientistic religion, stated as myth and holding forth the prospect of collective human immortality, posed a real challenge to traditional religion, with its emphasis on individual spiritual immortality. But, in opposing this view, what they proposed in its place was their version of a medieval worldview whose long-standing abandonment they elsewhere lamented.

A New Visionary Generation

It is sobering to reflect on the great debate in the interwar period between the British biological visionaries and their critics. In retrospect, it may come as a surprise in this age of the biotech revolution to realize that, beginning a century ago and culminating in the 1930s, some of the most fundamental issues concerning both the breathtaking implications of such developments, and also their troubling implications, had been hotly and thoroughly debated by some of the greatest minds of the time, including some of its leading biologists and philosophers, as well as some of its greatest writers.

Yet, stepping back and setting the debate in context, we may well wonder: was this simply a tempest in a British teapot? Its leading protagonists were members of the same British generation, and the character of the debate reflects the peculiarities both of the politics of "the Thirties," and of the peculiar tensions during that period within British intellectual elites—between Oxbridge and the redbrick universities, between the "visible college" of antireligious Marxist scientists

(Werskey, 1978) and the defenders of traditional British values and society. That the linkages and issues were framed as they were in those years may seem in retrospect overdetermined. At the same time, we may well wonder what intrinsic connection human longevity research has with worldwide socialist government, or whether moral concerns about the misuse of science or the destruction of nature necessarily entail a return to medieval Christianity as imagined to have been practiced on the British Isles.

A useful corrective may be provided by noting how these arguments and linkages, forged in a quite particular time and place, spread and became transformed as they moved into other places and times. A particularly revealing comparison involves the deployment of these ideas, so hotly debated by the generation of 1890, by subsequent generations. We can see this by looking at a new field that had not even been given its modern name when Haldane wrote his 1920s essays: science fiction. The pioneers of so-called classic science fiction were a new, younger generation, born some 20 years later, around 1910—for example, John W. Campbell (1910), Robert A. Heinlein (1907), Jack Williamson (1908), and A.E. Van Vogt (1912). Many of the giants of the Campbell style of science fiction were younger still, by roughly a decade—for example, Arthur C. Clarke (1917), Isaac Asimov (1920), Frank Herbert (1920), James Blish (1921), and Hal Clement (1922).

Classical American science fiction emerged in *Astounding Science-Fiction* in what has become known as its golden age (1939–1942). Largely abandoning the bug-eyed monster and space opera traditions of the earlier pulps, editor John W. Campbell, Jr. (1910–1971) catalyzed the emergence of a popular genre true to the tenets of science and widely read by current and would-be scientists and engineers. The spirit of golden age science fiction was nicely captured in a letter from a reader, a certain Seymour Kapetansky, that appeared in the October 1939 issue of *Astounding Science-Fiction* (pp. 155–156):

> We have a group of publications that profess to speak in the name of science, and science alone. . . . The reader of such magazines as Astounding Science-Fiction is ready, willing, and able to foresee vast improvements in the future of the human race. He is an incurable and narrow-minded optimist, because he believes that whatever will come, will be right; progress go forward. He is close to being a technocratic socialist, believing

with the forward march of civilization will come less work and more educated play for the average man, whether he has anything to do with it or not. The science-fictionist disregards submergence of the individual in the world of today and assumes that the world of tomorrow will have an entirely democratic foundation. . . . The wealth of the Universe shall be transformed into a storehouse of blessings for all humanity. The past is merely an unfortunate vagary of the time-line. Man can and WILL control the future; he will ultimately make the Universe God's country for God's children. Thus the science-fictionist.

These characteristics, of course, form a variant of the visions of Wells, Haldane, and Stapledon. But some of their ideas, of course, did not cross the Atlantic nearly so well: in particular, the suspicion of democracy and American capitalism, the infatuation with the Soviet Union, and the vision of humans as part of a single collective consciousness in which the individual counts for little—all these did not sit well with American individualism and the frontier spirit.

Robert Heinlein (1907–1988) was a central figure—perhaps *the* central figure—of science fiction's golden age. One of his earliest works that helped establish his fame was *Methuselah's Children,* serialized in *Astounding Science Fiction* in 1941 and published in reworked form in 1958. The novel's focus is the problems associated with human longevity. The story centers on a family of extremely long-lived individuals fleeing from the oppression of an envious society that falsely believes they owe their longevity to some technique or drug that they are keeping secret from the rest of humanity. (Actually, their longevity appears to be genetic, and they have no clue as to its nature.) The novel explicitly rejects *collective consciousness* for humanity as being incompatible with its individualistic nature. The leader of the family, the effectively immortal Lazarus Long, would reappear as a character in other Heinlein stories and as the central character in several of his later novels, notably *Time Enough for Love.*

In 1942, there followed Heinlein's novel *Beyond This Horizon,* serialized in *Astounding* and issued in book form in 1948: regarded by most critics as one of Heinlein's best, the novel was devoted almost entirely to a commentary on the views of the biological visionaries and the presentation of an alternative view. Heinlein's book is an attempt to portray a eugenic utopia that (unlike *Brave New World*) maintains human dignity, individualism, and freedom of choice.

Genetic changes weeding out "unfit" traits (negative eugenics) are only gradually and voluntarily introduced, studied with the help of voluntary "control naturals," and effected by techniques helping to select from a parental pair the best of their available eggs and sperm. There is also a public treasury of the best human genetic material ("Star lines"), which can serve as the basis for positive eugenics, but again, only with the fully informed permission and consent of the donor. (Indeed, the plot of the novel revolves around Hamilton Felix, a member of the Star line, who sees no reason to cooperate and needs to be convinced.) All genetic practitioners abide by a "Mendelian Oath," modeled on the Hippocratic Oath, a "Convenant in the Name of Life Immortal." Their only power in this free eugenic republic is genetic counseling.

From published letters, we know that Heinlein made himself very familiar with the developments of genetics in general and the ideas of Haldane and Stapledon in particular. In *Beyond This Horizon*, Heinlein explicitly lambastes Haldane's program on both scientific and moral grounds. Ectogenesis comes up explicitly late in the novel and is dismissed as "contrasurvival in nature": "the race would be dependent on complex mechanical assistance to reproduce" and "the time might come when it wasn't available." Ectogenesis is just egg laying, says Heinlein: "We mammals have a better method" (Heinlein, 1948, p. 195). The biological engineering of humans is also brought up in an unfavorable light as beastly, immoral, fascist, and incompatible with human values. Some clandestine experiments conducted by a cell of elitist revolutionaries are aimed at creating humans suitable for other planetary environments, including babies with gill slits for Venus and stumpy low-gravity types for Jupiter and the outer planets. Upon hearing plans to sacrifice the "experimental material" when it is no longer useful, our hero laments those "consigned without their consent or knowledge to the oblivion of the laboratory or death"—and decides to cut off the perpetrator's ears "a bit at a time" (p. 112).

The novel ends curiously: through his own children, its protagonist discovers that both mind reading and reincarnation are human possibilities. It ends with a stirring call for science to turn its powers to solving the really interesting, big questions—Where have we come from? Where are we going? What is the full range of human potential? Is there a God?—echoing, in certain respects, Lewis's critique of the godlessness of the visionaries, albeit in scientistic form.

In his other works, Heinlein's suspicions of the repressive power of organized religion over free thought, his faith in the power of science to achieve human betterment, and his optimism about the future left him very much at odds with the worldview of Lewis. At the same time, as his work demonstrates, although Haldane, Wells, Stapledon, Huxley, and others had linked their visionary biology to a worldview that was sympathetic to socialism, devoted to world government, and suspicious of capitalist American democracy, that was largely an artifact of an interwar British squabble. The power of the new biology to transform human destiny for the better could be made compatible with other social values present in other times and places. It was not the ideas themselves, but the social and political uses to which they might be put by evil societies, that was the problem.

An even more complex viewpoint was expressed by Heinlein's younger British colleague, Arthur C. Clarke (1917–), who skyrocketed to prominence in science fiction in the early 1950s. Clarke fell under the spell of Stapledon early in his youth. In later years, he still remembered the exact location on the library shelf where he first discovered *Last and First Men*, and declared that no other book had a greater influence on his life. Active in British science fiction circles in the 1930s, he earned a degree after the war in physics and mathematics. Clarke's early rise to fame was associated with a series of books in popular science and science fiction in the late 1940s and early 1950s heralding and detailing the coming age of space. Alongside the author of these hard-headed works about the near future, however, is another Clarke very much in the grand tradition of Stapledon.

The Stapledon influence is reflected in his most renowned science fiction, notably the short story "The Nine Billion Names of God" and his novels *Childhood's End* (1953), *The City and the Stars* (1956), and *2001: A Space Odyssey* (1968), based on his and Stanley Kubrick's screenplay for the movie, for which he was a 1969 Oscar nominee. These works contemplate ultimate human destiny in the breathtaking time spans of the earlier visionaries, and entertain the possibility of humans entering into higher nonmaterial forms of mentality and spirit in the universe, but they do so in a way that is much more religion-friendly. In the postwar years, Haldane followed the works of Clarke, who was his favorite science fiction author. In one of his last letters to Clarke, Haldane wrote, with his characteristic wit: "I would like to see you awarded a prize for theology, as you are one of the very few living persons who has written anything original about God. You have in fact, written several mutually incompatible things. . . . If you had stuck to one theological hypothesis you might be a serious public danger" (Clarke, 1999, p. 35). Indeed, as Clarke quipped at the time *2001* was being made, "MGM doesn't know it yet, but they've footed the bill for the first $10,500,000 religious film" (Agel, 1970, p. 10). The National Catholic Office for Motion Pictures apparently agreed, giving the film their 1968 award.

In *The City and the Stars* (1956), Clarke presents his fullest fictional treatment of the possibilities for human immortality and one of the most original ideas for achieving it. The novel is set 1 billion years in the future, when the Earth has become barren except for two remaining centers of advanced human culture. One is Lys, a pastoral society in which humans have fully developed the sciences of life, as well as the capacity for mind reading and communal mental links with both humans and animals, and have molded living forms to maintain a natural oasis; the other is Diaspar, an enclosed utopian city run by a central computer established by its founders. Although the citizens of Lys have achieved remarkable control over life and are long-lived, they die in natural ways as part of the natural cycle. By contrast, the citizens of Diaspar are immortal. They lead long lives, then sort through their memories and go into oblivion—but all the information that represents who they are is stored in the central computer, which re-creates them at some future time, when they slowly grow to maturity, at which point they regain only those memories of their earlier lives that they themselves had preselected.

Clarke was well ahead of his time in understanding the vast potential consequences of computers and information science. Indeed, he was the first to come up with the idea of geosynchronous earth communication satellites (in 1945) and to predict that this would lead to instantaneous worldwide access to information. His realization of the implications of the discovery of the structure of DNA (in 1953), combined with earth satellites and the concepts of cybernetics and information, led him to contemplate a new possibility for future human immortality free of the drawbacks of most earlier conceptions. Nonetheless, as the novel makes clear, Clarke fears that such immortality would have stultifying effects and produce a self-satisfied, isolated, timid, and self-indulgent society denied its true destiny of finding its place in the universe by exploring the stars. Thus his hero, who forces humanity out of its stagnation, is a "Unique," an individual programmed by the founders to appear at some point for the first time.

In his nonfictional book *Profiles of the Future* (1963), Clarke reprises his earlier ideas on immortality. The book is a tour de force. It begins with a historical evaluation of those in the past who tried to foresee the future and where they went wrong. On this corrective basis, he then dares his own prognostications based on the trends of modern science. In one chapter, he takes up the question of the human life span. Human life can be lengthened a bit by the substitution of mechanical or nonliving parts for defective or diseased parts, he grants, since the brain is the part that really counts. In the longer run, he foresees the possibility of extending human life further, although the burden of overlaid memories, he feels, would eventually become prohibitive, estimating that "as a good round figure, a thousand years would seem to be about the ultimate limit for continuous human existence—though suspended animation might spread this millennium across far longer vistas of time" (p. 209). He then reprises the possibility of immortality in the form he had developed it in Diaspar some seven years earlier, concluding: "Is this fantasy? I do not know; but I suspect that the truths of the far future will be stranger still" (p. 211).

But the most tantalizing part of the book is a chart at the end surveying developments in transportation, communication and information, materials and manufacturing, biology and chemistry, and physics from 1800 until 1960 (the present) and projecting future developments through 2100. Looking at his chart from the vantage point of 2004—40 years after it was drafted—one is impressed with how optimistic he was about some developments (e.g., colonizing other planets by 1980 or weather control by 2010) and how prescient in others (personal radio, artificial intelligence, a global library, telesensory devices, logical languages, and robots, all before 2020). Of most interest here are his biological forecasts: control of heredity by 2020, bioengineering by 2030, suspended animation by 2040, artificial life by 2060, and, by 2100 . . . immortality. Given Clarke's predictive track record, it is a prospect we cannot dismiss—especially in light of *Clarke's Law*, an aphorism he derived from his historical study of past predictions: "When a distinguished . . . scientist states that something is possible, he is almost certainly right. When he states that something is impossible, he is very probably wrong" (p. 14).

Final Thoughts

Here we have merely begun to sample the rich legacy of the biological visionaries, their critics, and their successors. Yet, even so, several features of this ongoing discourse are worthy of note.

First, one cannot help but be struck by the degree to which the exciting new prospects of biotechnology, as well as their human and moral dimensions, had already been anticipated and explored by a wide variety of thinkers more than a half century ago. Of course, such thinkers did not anticipate the details of current biotechnological developments, the techniques employed, or the exact timeline of discovery. But what they *were* certain about is that some techniques or other would become available, in the not too distant future, through the developments of experimental biology, to achieve breakthroughs in controlling human life and longevity. Such was the hopeful promise of the new experimental biology from its very inception; such was the conviction of its followers and practitioners. In this, surely, their prescience is in the process of being vindicated.

Second, we may note that human prolongevity was never treated as an isolated, separable problem. The prospects and problems of human immortality have always been nested in broader issues—whether long-term human evolution, or the relation of science to religion, or prospects for the fulfillment of human potential or destiny. Whether as a part of the general enthusiasm for the powers of the new biology, or as a violation of the natural religious order, or as an intriguing prediction about future science, prolongevity was always considered within quite particular philosophical worldviews and took on its meaning and implications in that context. Those worldviews, in turn, were characteristic of quite particular times and places, and indeed of particular generational cohorts. In addition, when public debates erupted, the opposing sides often represented those alternate worldviews, dealing with many issues then current, and issues concerning human prolongevity thereby became linked with other matters with which they had no necessary logical connection. What immortality meant was culture-specific in both the broadest and the narrowest sense.

Third, one cannot help but wonder to what degree current discussions and controversies have been colored by the legacies of these earlier discussions. As Haldane had anticipated, religious and moral misgivings about the use of human reproductive interventions and techniques, as well as the scientific experimentation necessary to develop them, would prove a major source of resistance to the development and deployment of these new scientific possibilities. But if Haldane had anticipated as much, he had also played his role in bringing such resistance to the fore: couching his projections in the context of an "in your face" broadside against established religion, an active endorsement of the communist experiment, and an explicit attempt to bring forth an alternative mythic credo more suitable to the scientific age, his polemics would call forth precisely the kind of critique from the likes of Lewis and Tolkien that he had predicted. In the context of the great intellectual and ideological battles sweeping the interwar years, it could hardly have been otherwise. Yet, need it continue to be so? The linkage of manipulative human experimental biology and longevity research with an explicitly antireligious credo was a product of those times; but are those times not long since past? Other thinkers, in different traditions, at other places and times, have explored possibilities for the new human biology more respectful of individual freedom and more accommodating to religious and spiritual human dimensions. Realizing the contingent historical roots of current, apparently intractable conflicts may help us, it is hoped, to get beyond them.

Fourth, we should note that, remarkably, despite their differences, the diverse works of visionaries, critics, and their successors alike share a consensus about one important point: there is a tension between the interests of the individual and those of the human race as a whole—immortality for the individual may undermine the prospects for the immortality of the human species. For Wells, this is because evolution works best through selective death, the sorting of variants to preserve the best types. Haldane, Huxley, and Stapledon grant that we may be able to greatly improve and lengthen human life, but this is secondary and subordinate to the far more important task of working toward the survival and immortality of humankind. For Lewis and Tolkien, the tension is a moral one: manipulative scientistic fiddling with the human life span violates the natural moral order of things of which the human race is a part and can lead to great evil. Clarke is able to portray the most plausible and benign scenario for human immortality—and yet, in the end, he rejects it as leading to stultification, thus denying humans their true collective destiny in the universe. Perhaps Heinlein put the matter most pithily: "Easy times for individuals are bad times for the race" (Heinlein, 1948, p. 32).

In the end, all seem to agree, the ultimate test of a life and its best claim to immortality is not an individual's life span, but his or her contribution to a higher purpose—whether as part of divine plan, a furthering of human progress, a contribution to the survival of the human race, or a gradual merging into some higher spiritual level.

Finally, one cannot help but be impressed by the vast range of social, political, and moral possibilities and problems arising from human biology that have been explored and weighed by earlier thinkers. These possibilities captivated and occupied some of the best minds of that age, members of remarkable generations now gone. What they have left us, however—in their works and writings and essays and fictions—is a rich legacy of considered possibility, a breathtaking panoply of thought experiments that have already surveyed in detail the intellectual and social terrain we are just now beginning to traverse. As we plot our future course, their rich legacy is worthy of due consideration, for their thinking may help us to avoid pitfalls, see new possibilities, and broaden our own narrow perspectives beyond the constraints of our own quite peculiar time and place.

References

Adams, M.B. (1990). (Ed.). *The Wellborn Science: Eugenics in Germany, France, Brazil, and Russia.* New York: Oxford University Press.

Adams, M.B. (2000). Last Judgment: The visionary biology of J.B.S. Haldane. *Journal of the History of Biology* 33:457–491.

Agel, J. (1970). (Ed.). *The Making of Kubrick's 2001.* New York: Signet.

Bergonzi, B. (1961). *The Early H.G. Wells.* Manchester: Manchester University Press.

Burchfield, J.D. (1975). *Lord Kelvin and the Age of the Earth.* New York: Science History Publications.

Carpenter, H. (1977). *Tolkien: A Biography.* London: George Allen & Unwin.

Clarke, A.C. (1956). *The City and the Stars.* New York: Harcourt, Brace.

Clarke, A.C. (1963). *Profiles of the Future: An Inquiry Into the Limits of the Possible.* New York: Harper & Row.

Clarke, A.C. (1999). *Greetings, Carbon-Based Bipeds! Collected Essays 1934–1998.* New York: St. Martin's Press.

Crossley, R. (1994). *Olaf Stapledon: Speaking for the Future.* Syracuse, NY: Syracuse University Press.

Dronamraju, K.R. (1995). (Ed.). *Haldane's Daedalus Revisited.* New York: Oxford University Press.

Fiedler, L.A. (1983). *Olaf Stapledon: A Man Divided.* Oxford: Oxford University Press.

Green, R.L. and Hooper, W. (1974). *C.S. Lewis: A Biography.* New York: Harcourt, Brace.

Haldane, J.B.S. (1924). *Daedalus, or Science and the Future: A Paper Read to the Heretics, Cambridge on February 4th, 1923.* London: Kegan Paul, Trench, Trubner & Co.

Haldane, J.B.S. (1927). The last judgment. In: Haldane, J.B.S. *Possible Worlds and Other Essays.* London: Chatto & Windus, pp. 287–312.

Haldane, J.B.S. (1946). Auld Hornie, F.R.S. *The Modern Quarterly*, N.S., 1(4), 32.

Heinlein, R.A. (1941). Methuselah's children. *Astounding Science-Fiction*, July, August, and September.

Heinlein, R.A. (1942). Beyond this horizon. *Astounding Science-Fiction*, April and May. (Originally published under the pseudonym "Anson MacDonald.")

Heinlein, R.A. (1948). *Beyond This Horizon.* Reading, PA: Fantasy Press.

Heinlein, R.A. (1958). *Methuselah's Children.* Hicksville, NY: Gnome Press.

Hillegas, M.R. (1969). (Ed.). *Shadows of Imagination: The Fantasies of C.S. Lewis, J.R.R. Tolkien, and Charles Williams.* Carbondale: Southern Illinois University Press.

Huxley, A. (1932). *Brave New World.* New York: Harper & Row.

Huxley, A. (1939). *After Many a Summer Dies the Swan.* New York: Harper.

Huxley, J. (1927). The tissue culture king. *Amazing Stories*, August. (Reprinted in Conklin, G., ed. *Great Science Fiction by Scientists*, New York: Collier, 1962, pp. 145–170.)

Huxley, J. (1957). *Religion without Revelation*, 2nd ed. New York: Harper. (1st ed. 1927.)

Huxley, J. (1960). The evolutionary vision. In: Tax, S. and Collender, C., eds. *Issues in Evolution: The University of Chicago Centennial Discussions*, vol. 3, *Evolution After Darwin* (Chicago: University of Chicago Press, 1960), pp. 249–261.

Huxley, J. (1970). *Memories.* New York: Harper & Row.

Jackson, P., Walsh, F., and Boyens, P. (2001). *The Lord of the Rings: The Fellowship of the Ring.* Special Extended DVD Edition. New Line Home Entertainment.

Lewis, C.S. (1938). *Out of the Silent Planet.* London: John Lane.

Lewis, C.S. (1943). *Perelandra.* London: John Lane.

Lewis, C.S. (1945). *That Hideous Strength.* London: John Lane.

Lewis, C.S. (1966). *Of Other Worlds: Essays and Stories.* Hooper, W., ed. New York: Harcourt Brace Jovanovich.

Metchnikoff, Él. (1908). *The Prolongation of Life.* London: Putnam.

Pauly, P.J. (1987). *Controlling Life: Jacques Loeb and the Engineering Ideal in Biology.* New York: Oxford University Press.

Réal, J. (2001). *Voronoff.* Paris: Stock.

Russell, B. (1924). *Icarus, or The Future of Science.* New York: E.P. Dutton.

Russell, B. and Whitehead A.M. (1910–1913). *Principia Mathematica*, 3 vols. Cambridge: Cambridge University Press.

Shaw, G.B. (1901). *Man and Superman, A Comedy and a Philosophy: Definitive Text.* New York and London: Penguin, 1982.

Shaw, G.B. (1921). *Back to Methuselah: A Metabiological Pentateuch.* Definitive Text: New York and London: Penguin, 1983.

Stapledon, O. (1930). *Last and First Men: A Story of the Near and Far Future.* London: Methuen.

Stapledon, O. (1932). *Last Men in London.* London: Methuen.

Stapledon, O. (1937). *Star Maker.* London: Methuen.

Tolkien, J.R.R. (1954–1955). *The Lord of the Rings.* 3 vols. vol. 1, *The Fellowship of the Ring* (1954); vol. 2, *The Two Towers* (1954); vol. 3, *The Return of the King* (1955). London: Allen & Unwin.

Voronoff, S. (1926). *Étude sur la vieillesse et le rajeunissement par la greffe.* Reissue: Paris: Éditions SenS, Chilly Mazarin, 1999.

Walsh, C. (1979). *The Literary Legacy of C.S. Lewis.* Harcourt Brace Jovanovich. San Diego, CA.

Wells, H.G. (1895). *The Time Machine: An Invention.* London: Heinemann.

Wells, H.G. (1905). *A Modern Utopia.* London: Chapman and Hall.

Wells, H.G. (1920). *The Outline of History.* 2 vols. London: Macmillan.

Wells, H.G., Huxley, J.S., and Wells, G.P. (1934). *The Science of Life.* New York: The Literary Guild. (Originally published in several volumes 1929–1930; reprinted 1930, 1931, 1934.)

Werskey, P.G. (1978). *The Visible College: The Collective Biography of British Scientific Socialists of the 1930s.* New York: Holt, Rinehart & Winston.

3

Decelerated Aging: Should I Drink from a Fountain of Youth?

Stephen G. Post

eon R. Kass, Chairman of the President's Council on Bioethics, prepared a discussion paper for the Council members prior to their meeting on January 16–17, 2003. Entitled "Beyond Therapy: Biotechnology and the Pursuit of Human Development," it established the Council's future agenda (Kass, 2003). Much of this paper is devoted to anti-aging research and the moral perils of anti-aging treatments to decelerate aging. If these emerge in the decades ahead, as Kass anticipates, should we implement them?

The anti-aging focus of Kass's concern is timely (Binstock, 2003). A reasonably clear statement on the current status of anti-aging science emerged from Robert N. Butler, M.D., and historian David Rothman, who co-chaired an International Longevity Center consensus panel entitled "Is There an 'Anti-aging' Medicine?" A balanced set of participants (including those who think that decelerated aging can be achieved) concluded that there currently is no "anti-aging medicine." Yet they also concluded that caloric restriction qualifies as "a true anti-aging intervention" because it has extended the life spans of primates by as much as a third (International Longevity Center, 2001). This is not a serious option for most humans, who presumably do not wish to live out their lives in a state of semistarvation. The panel recognized as well that genetic advances have resulted in increased animal life expectancy. They list respected researchers who have discovered 15 different genetic manipulations that produce life extension in yeast, nematodes, fruit flies, and mice (International Longevity Center, 2001, p. 5). Although the mechanisms for increased longevity are poorly understood, the Butler-Rothman panel understood that these studies "demonstrate that a single gene can regulate life expectancy and the timing of both cellular and extracellular senescence in a mammal" (p. 6). Here too, however, this nascent science cannot yet be applied to humans, in whom the genetics of the aging process is much more complex. The panel, after rightly excoriating the frivolous claims of anti-aging charlatans, argued for high-quality basic science research in three promising areas: stem cells, caloric restriction, and genetic intervention.

With biogerontologists, one of whom is affiliated with the National Institute on Aging, writing of "The Serious Search for an Anti-Aging Pill" that would mimic the effects of caloric restriction as an approach to the eradication of disease (Lane et al., 2002), there is reason to take this emerging science of anti-aging seriously. I remain somewhat impressed by the goal of deceleration. This is because, in an aging society beset by devastating chronic illnesses for which old age is the dominant risk factor, the best way to prevent such debilitation is to alleviate aging. The removal of this risk is not obviously contrary to human dignity, although in other respects anti-aging treatments may lead to "undignified" outcomes. Nevertheless, we would all, I hope, agree that removing the major risk factor for diseases such as Alzheimer's disease or osteoporosis would do quite a bit for the preservation of human dignity, for the control of health-care costs, and for the alleviation of sometimes overwhelming adult filial duties (Post, 2000).

While decelerated aging is potentially highly therapeutic in the above-mentioned sense, it must be recognized that the implications of altering the course of human aging are in almost all other respects questionable. The life span (the longest that any known member of the species has lived) in humans would eventually surpass the current limit of roughly 120 years, and surely life expectancy (the average length of life of a species) in humans would increase considerably beyond current levels. These possibilities present us with a true moral dilemma in the sense that deceleration might eradicate the terrible diseases of old age while simultaneously violating the transitional turnover from one generation to the next. Equally thoughtful persons may disagree on the ethics of such a pursuit, as they have perennially. The debate, which was once based on alchemical fantasies, now takes on new meaning as significant scientific research uncovers the nature of the aging process and thereby opens up the possibility for its modification.

My thoughts regarding this debate focus mostly on the existential question "Should I drink from the Fountain of Youth?" Wider concerns with justice, a common humanity, and commitment to future generations may be considered by individuals answering the question for themselves. Yet the individual prospects for a relatively youthful and therefore much healthier old age may in the end be determinative for some (Cole and Thompson, 2001–2002).

In considering the ethics of a controversial biomedical goal, several comments with regard to framework are warranted at the outset. Of the anti-aging paradigms delineated in the Introduction to this volume, I use the decelerated aging paradigm because only a few would be critical of the compression of morbidity paradigm, none would espouse prolonged senescence, and arrested aging is at this time a much less likely future scenario than is deceleration. The reader will also discover the use of the terms *posthumanism* and *anti-posthumanism*, referring to two perennial schools of thought. The posthumanists view human dignity in large part as a matter of seizing the opportunity to modify and "improve" human nature in fundamental ways, including the deceleration or arresting of aging, while the anti-posthumanists caution us to accept the existing contours of human nature as the gift of evolutionary or divine wisdom. The discussion of our existential query also inevitably involves some attention to the ways in which religion has functioned traditionally to soften the decline of embodied aging-toward-death with the hope for otherworldly immortality, although there is no obvious resistance within Judaism and Christianity to the idea of prolongevity, as evidenced by the emergence of anti-aging science within a broadly Judeo-Christian Western cultural context. Since religion is generally concerned with questions of finitude and immortality, it has an objective place in any complete discussion.

The dilemma with which we deal is not new. Nearly 40 years ago, historian Gerald Gruman, writing in *Transactions of the American Philosophical Society* (1966), created the term *prolongevity* to encompass the multiple goals of anti-aging interventions over the centuries. He defined it as significant extension of the human life span and/or average life expectancy, without suffering and infirmity. Although human beings have striven to achieve prolongevity, they have been more or less powerless in the face of biological aging, but this situation may be changing. Although in many industrialized countries life expectancy has expanded to the late 70s when measured from birth, this is the result of small increments of expansion secondary to the conquering of disease, the availability of antibiotics, public health measures, and especially the reduction of infant mortality. Could current and future research into the basic science of aging result in treatments that would actually slow the underlying biological process of aging, creating a dramatic increase in life expectancy and perhaps even breaking through the maximum human life span limit of approximately 120 years? And would the subsequent travail of individual, demographic, and social adjustment be justified by a potentially dramatic alleviation of the debilitating burdens of chronic conditions in older adults and the elimination of correlative caregiving demands in family and professional contexts?

While I do not think that aging is a disease, it is a process that creates so much susceptibility to disease that it can be approached by researchers with therapeutic intent (Post, 2000). Here therapy and enhancement merge, and become one and the same thing. While I will attend to the debate between posthumanists and anti-posthumanists below, this is followed by the equally important conversation that must be had between the anti-posthumanists and those who wish to erase the age-related illnesses that are our modern scourge. It is especially this latter conversation that is complex (Partridge and Gems, 2002).

argument: is aging a disease?

The Anti-Posthumanist Appeal

Should the individual, viewing his or her own prospects for deceleration of aging, pursue such anti-aging treatments when and if they actually become available? Perhaps yes, if this assures one that diseases for which old age is the overwhelmingly significant risk factor can be avoided. But there is an important school of thought that cautions against the development of treatments to slow aging.

The individual, when confronted with the availability of deceleration, ought to reflect carefully about the choice at hand, raising every question of relevance to self and to humanity. One of the wiser persons of the past century, Hans Jonas (d. 1993), an intellectual inspiration for today's anti-posthumanists, articulated these questions quite thoroughly. He wrote in 1984 that "a practical hope is held out by certain advances in cell biology to prolong, perhaps indefinitely extend, the span of life by counteracting biochemical processes of aging" (Jonas, 1985, p. 18). How desirable would this power to slow or arrest aging be for the individual and for the species? Do we want to tamper with the delicate biological "balance of death and procreation" (p. 18) and preempt the place of youth? Would the species gain or lose? Jonas, by merely raising these questions, meant to cast significant doubt on the anti-aging enterprise. "Perhaps," he wrote, "a nonnegotiable limit to our expected time is necessary for each of us as the incentive to number our days and make them count" (p. 19). Jonas's later essays raising many of these same questions were published posthumously (Jonas, 1996).

Many of these questions are developed further in the writings of Leon Kass. Kass for the most part accepts biotechnological progress within a therapeutic mode; his issue is chiefly with efforts to enhance and improve upon the givenness of human nature. He draws on the technological dystopians, such as Aldous Huxley, as well as on the writings of C.S. Lewis. An early anti-posthumanist, Oxford's Lewis wrote *The Abolition of Man* in 1944 (Lewis, 1944/1966). Lewis defended a natural law tradition: what is is good, and we should live within our God-given limits. He cautioned against a world in which one class of enhanced human beings would dominate and oppress the other. We might ask, then, if those freed from the decline of aging would become the superior and elite humans, while those who age would be deemed inferior.

Kass, with a rhetorically powerful style, calls us back to much deeper thinking than that of the card-carrying utilitarian. He urges us to think deeply before we leap into the unknown. His leadership role on President George W. Bush's Bioethics Council gave wide public attention to the need to reconsider the goals of medicine in the name of "a more natural science" (Kass, 1985). In a creative essay, "*L'Chaim* and Its Limits: Why Not Immortality?" (see Chapter 14), Kass provides arguments against prolongevity. He asserts, for example, that the gradual descent into aged frailty weans us from attachment to life and renders death more acceptable; that our numbered days encourage a creative depth in our humanity—a depth that escaped so many of the immortal Greek gods and goddesses, whose often debauched and purposeless behavior made Plato wish to ban them from the ideal Republic; that a preoccupation with the continuance of our lives is a distraction from that which is best for us; that in a world transformed by anti-aging research, youth will be displaced rather than elevated, and the parental investment in the young will give way to "my" perpetuation; and that in such a new world we will grow bored and tired of life, having "been there" and "done that." These assertions are all thoughtful, creative, and appropriately cautionary, for the implications of slowing or arresting aging itself are obviously monumental and mixed. Thus, I am by no means unappreciative of the ideas Kass eloquently presents.

Jonas and Kass touch on significant existential themes. There is arguably a tone of solipsism in grasping at extended life rather than accepting old age and celebrating rejuvenation in the lives of our offspring. Whatever capacities for compassionate love we possess emerged evolutionarily on the parent-child axis, and on this axis we generally achieve our higher degrees of self-forgetfulness and love—even if *selfish genes* provide a hidden substrate. It is impossible to imagine our capacities for kindness and benevolence evolving without a dominating investment in the young rather than in ourselves. Responsibility to future generations precludes a clinging to our own youthfulness. There is wisdom in simply accepting the fact that we evolved for reproductive success rather than for long lives. Without such wisdom, will we lose sight of our deepest creative motives? Possibly.

And so it is written, "teach us to number our days that we may get a heart of wisdom" (Psalm 90). However, wisdom may be born not so much from the existential acceptance of aging as from the accumulation of learning experiences over the years. We do, after all, for the most part have to learn from our mistakes. Presumably the longer one lives the wiser one becomes.

Another leading anti-posthumanist, Francis Fukuyama, has also served as a member of President Bush's Council on Bioethics and is the author of the widely reviewed and somewhat controversial book *Our Posthuman Future: Consequences of the Biotechnology Revolution* (2002). Fukuyama challenges those who would march us into a posthuman future, characterized by cybernetics, nanotechnology, genetic enhancement, reproductive cloning, life span extension, and new forms of behavior control. Undoubtedly the ambitions of posthumanists to create a new posthuman who is no longer human are arrogant, pretentious, and lacking in fundamental appreciation for natural human dignity.

Fukuyama is also drawn to the dystopian genre and sees much more bad than good in efforts to significantly modify human nature. He argues powerfully that the anti-aging technologies of the future will disrupt all the delicate demographic balances between the young and the old, and exacerbate the gap between the haves and the have nots. The concerns raised by a political scientist such as Fukuyama are ones that the individual decision maker ought certainly to have in mind.

The anti-posthumanists often appeal to nature and character as morally valuable categories. They understand the proper human attitude toward our evolved nature as one of humility, awe, and appreciation. Clearly, the emerging technological power to control nature does not always constitute progress. Reproductive cloning, for example, is both fraught with risks and offers no obvious improvement over natural procreation. The possibility of fundamentally modifying the rate of human aging and thereby altering the perennial process of generational transition could prove destructive of all the human propensities to nurture and elevate the young. Human nature, the gift of millennia of evolutionary selection, should be approached with respect rather than with disregard. Our attitude should be one of working with our human nature to get the best out of it, rather than one of cavalier dominion in an effort to re-create what is already good. Better to accept natural limits—or so, anyway, is the spirit of anti-posthumanism. Moreover, it is argued that the perfectibility of humankind lies not in modifying the human vessel but in developing the treasures within, such as compassion, virtue, and dignity.

Only with time constraints on life do we ask "What should I do with what I have?" If you could live to 200, how much of that time would you waste? The brevity of life makes it worth living; only allotted time makes time precious. We dread death, but as the existentialists write, this forces us to examine our lives. Did I achieve meaningful goals? Was my life in some sense justified?

The future will be different from the present, but by how much? And how much will biological power over longevity lead us away from the wisdom of nature and human nature toward a dystopia in which the species is divided into the elite, for whom the technology of radical life extension is affordable, and those for whom such technology is not? Will we see, on the one hand, a world of wealthy youthful people living radically extended lives and enjoying the world's longest beach parties and, on the other hand, the frail poor subjected to the natural ravages of aging, looked down upon as an inferior sub-species? The future will be complicated by the libertarian and entrepreneurial interests that would make such enhancement available according to one's ability to pay. There are these and then other questions to add. What is more important, "my" breaking though life span limits or my coming to a greater appreciation and manifestation of the capacities for compassionate love that exist within us? Am I already an immortal soul anyway, and therefore ageless?

In summary, the natural law traditions represented by anti-posthumanists exhort us to live more or less according to nature, and warn that our efforts to depart from what we are will result in new evils that are more perilous than old ones. To use an analogy, we are like the sailor who climbs as high on the mast as he can in order to rise high above the waters of nature, but only to see the boat capsize under his weight, tipping the mast into the waves below. How can we presume that the brave new world will be a better world? Should not the burden of proof be on the proponents of radical change? Who are we today to impose our arbitrary images of human enhancement on future generations?

Thus are anti-posthumanist thinkers critical of biogerontology to the extent that it seeks to slow the aging process. Our focus, argue the anti-posthumanists, should be on the acceptance of aging rather than on its scientific modification. The intergenerational thrust of evolution, by which we are inclined toward parental and social investment in the hope, energy, and vitality of youth, provides the basis for a natural law ethic that requires us all to relinquish youthfulness. Thus, anti-aging research and its disseminators have spawned a major reconsideration of the goals of biomedical science by a group of conservative intellectuals and politicians, both secular and religious, who invoke natural law and human dignity as reasons against prolongevity (Kristol and Cohen, 2002).

I agree with the anti-posthumanists that a decision for or against decelerated aging based on superficial thinking and a commitment to individual freedom is a formula for the easy destruction of what is good in being human. They are right to place an emphasis on

Aristotelian *final causes* and human goods. Unless we are radical relativists, it can and must be asked whether any scientific aspiration contributes to the human condition or detracts from it.

In addition, religious thought in many ways cautions against our efforts to solve the problem of aging. *First,* theology might affirm that we humans are not the ones to create everlasting life, which is already a gift rooted in the saving creativity of God. *Second,* we humans tend toward solipsism—that is, we each see ourselves as the center of the universe and find worth in other species only as they promote our interests and contribute to our agendas. But each of us is only one center in a universe of centers, and ontologically, others are emphatically not in orbit around "me, myself, and I." We lack ontological humility, and it is the reality of finitude that frees us from the illusion of centrality. Aging and death encourage within us an *ontological humility.* In the medieval and Renaissance periods, the *ars moriendi* (art of dying) writings of the theologians emphasized the achievement of love for others in the context of dying. Religion sees mortality as a source of spiritual creativity. *Third,* as the Hindus say, life is a bondage. Even Faust grew bored and lost his zest. Embodied life finally cannot fulfill our aspirations.

Anti-posthumanists are by no means all religious thinkers. Many are secular. But all are reacting to a genre of posthumanist thinking that is immature and disconnected from the narrative of human experience and values. Thus, I turn now to the posthumanist genre, which I too find distasteful—although decelerated aging presented outside of this context might still be elevated to a level of moral plausibility.

Posthumanism and the Religion of Technology

One reason anti-posthumanism has an immediate appeal is that many of the major defenders of posthumanism do sound extreme, irresponsible, and less than fully thoughtful about the implications of their ideas (see, e.g., www.betterhumans.com, www.transhumanism. org, www.forsight.org). Websites reflect the enthusiasm of the adolescent convert to some brand new image of the human creature, yet one who has little or no insight into the human condition. Off with biological constraints! Transcend humanness by technology!

The posthumanist embraces decelerated and even arrested aging, but only as a small part of a larger vision to reengineer human

nature, and thereby to create biologically and technologically superior human beings (Hayles, 1999). Posthumans are the much more
advanced models that we humans today will design for tomorrow. As
such, posthumans are no longer humans. Genetics, nanotechnology,
cybernetics, and computer technologies are all part of the posthuman vision, including the downloading of synaptic connections in
the brain to form a computerized human mind freed of mortal flesh
and thereby immortalized (Noble, 1997, pp. 143–171). This last scenario of immortalized minds liberated from any biological substrate
makes the biomedical goal of prolongevity appear conservative!

Posthumanists do not believe that biology is in any sense destiny,
and they seek a superman for whom human nature has been more
or less overcome (Hook, 2003). They urge us to take human nature
into our own re-creative hands as the next great step in evolution,
achieving a kind of postmodern morphological freedom. Their appeal
lies in the fact that, within the boundaries of technology, humans
have been reinventing themselves anyway through applied technologies for millennia. What is natural and what is unnatural, anyway?
Where do we draw lines? As Freeman Dyson writes, "the artificial
improvement of human beings will come, one way or another, whether
we like it or not," as scientific understanding increases, for after all,
such improvement has always been viewed as a "liberation from past
constraints" (1997). We long ago embarked on the human phase of
evolution through our technological prowess, and before us lies nothing less monumental than, to use Walt Whitman's language, a "Song
of the Open Road." After all, there was a time when the very idea of
human beings trying to fly was deemed heretical hubris in the light of
eternity—*sub specie aeternitatis.* Now, are the posthumanists to be
deemed the new heretics in the light of evolution—*sub specie evolu-
tionis?* Or shall we set aside trepidation and with confidence rethink
ourselves in the light of human creativity? The postmodernists have
paved the way by purportedly demonstrating that there is no essential
aspect to human nature, and *vive le difference.* So it is that Gregory
Stock writes a book entitled *Redesigning Humans: Our Inevitable Genetic
Future* (2002), in which he introduces the idea of *superbiology* as we
take full control of our own biology in turning toward perfectability.

As David F. Noble (1997) has demonstrated, the roots of this
posthumanist project lie in Western religion, and especially in the
ninth century, when the *useful arts* came to be associated with the
concept of human redemption. As a result, we have a *religion of tech-*

nology that gives rise to an uncritical and irrational affirmation of unregulated technological advance. In essence, technological advance is always deemed good. Noble hopes that we can free ourselves from the religion of technology, from which we seek deliverance, by learning to think and act rationally toward humane goals (1997, p. 6). Is Noble right about these religious roots? In general terms, he is. As Gruman pointed out in his definitive entry in the *Dictionary of the History of Ideas* (1973), the modern concern with enhancing longevity "stems from the decline since the Renaissance of faith in supernatural salvation from death; concern with the worth of individual identity and experience shifted from an otherworldly realm to the 'here and now,' with intensification of earthly expectations" (p. 88).

With the transition to a this-worldly millennialist human horizon, a powerful current of thought emerged in which the goal of significantly extending the length of human life through biomedical science was affirmed. Gruman (1966, 1973) termed the concept *prolongevity* as "a subsidiary variant of meliorism, the belief that human effort should be applied to improving the world" (1973, p. 89). Carl L. Becker, in his classic work *The Heavenly City of the Eighteenth-Century Philosophers* (1932), had similarly interpreted the great ideas of the Enlightenment and the merging goals of science as based on a secularization of the medieval idea of otherworldly salvation, resulting in an advance toward a heaven on earth. Thus did George Bernard Shaw, in his remarkable *Back to Methuselah* (1921), take up the variations in life spans between species such as parrots and dogs, or turtles and wasps, and ask that science rise to the redemptive occasion by vastly increasing human longevity.

Indeed, Francis Bacon, a founder of the scientific method, in his millennialist and utopian essay "The New Atlantis" (1627), set in motion a biological mandate for boldness that included both the making of new species or *chimeras*, organ replacement, and the *Water of Paradise* that would allow the possibility to "indeed live very long" (Bacon, 1996). Three centuries before Francis Bacon, the English theologian Roger Bacon argued that in the future, the 900-year-long lives of the antediluvian patriarchs would be restored alchemically. Like many Western religious thinkers, both Bacons saw death as the unnatural result of Adam's fall into sin. These Western dreams of embodied near-immortality could only emerge against a theological background that more or less endorsed them. There are various other cultural and historical influences at work besides religion, but the initial conceptual context for a scientific assault on aging itself is a religious one (Barash, 1983).

The modern goals of anti-aging research and technology, then, are historically emergent from a premodern religious drama of hope and salvation (Benecke, 2002). Longings for immortality within a religious context are understandable in light of existential anxiety over finitude and mortality, and the powerful biotech movement in molecular genetics is more or less shaped by such passions. Renaissance science transferred the task of achieving immortality from heaven to earth in the spirit of millennial hopes. The economy of salvation presented by Dante was replaced by the here and now. There is a vibrant millennialist enthusiasm in the responsible biogerontologists, for they have proclaimed aging itself to be surmountable to some degree through human ingenuity.

Yet this replacement of eternity with the immortal here and now was always a subtext in Western theology. The Russian Orthodox existentialist Nicholas Berdyaev wrote, "Death is the evil result of sin. A sinless life would be immortal and eternal" (1939, p. 252). Stanley and Harakas likewise note that "Theologically, Eastern Christianity viewed death as an enemy, a consequence of Adamic sin, and therefore a condition to be struggled against" (1986, p. 157). Augustine put it well in the fourth century C.E.: "For no sooner do we begin to live in this dying body, than we begin to move ceaselessly towards death"—but only, he argued, because our minds have lost control of our bodies (1950, p. 419). All Christians agree, he argued, that aging and death issue not from the "law of nature, by which God ordained no death for man, but by His righteous infliction on account of sin; for God, taking vengence on sin, said to the man, in whom we all then were, 'Dust thou art, and unto dust shall thou return' " (p. 423). Thomas Aquinas (*Summa Theologica* I, question 97, article 1) asked, "Whether in the State of Innocence Man Would Have Been Immortal?" He responded by citing St. Paul (Romans 5:12: "By sin death came into the world") and asserted that before sin the body was "incorruptable," that is, immortal. Specifically, "For man's body was indissoluble not by reason of any intrinsic vigor of immortality, but by reason of a supernatural force given by God to the soul, by which it was enabled to preserve the body from all corruption so long as it remained itself subject to God." Had Adam and Eve obeyed God, the corruption of aging and death would not have affected them. According to the Hebrew Bible, Adam lived to be a ripe old 930 years of age and was 130 when his third son, Seth, was born. Protestant theologians too saw death as the result of sin and drew on God's condemnation immediately after the trespass: "You are dust and to dust you will return" (Genesis 3:17–19). As Reinhold Niebuhr wrote, "The doctrine that death is a consequence of sin is of course variously stated; but it remains a consistent doctrine of Christian orthodoxy" (1941, p. 176).

It is true that modern theological liberalism has departed from the above orthodoxy. The idea of aging and death as natural, of course, makes eminent sense. My only point here is to underscore that for 1800 years Western culture, insofar as it was dominated by a religious worldview, did not accept the naturalistic view. Aging and death had to be eliminated by salvation, and when science began to view itself as a shaping force in the drama of salvation, anti-aging utopianism as a matter of technical progress was inevitable. I cannot image Bacon writing of his Waters of Paradise against the cultural backdrop of a religious culture in which aging and death were deemed good, natural, and unrelated to the mythic fall.

If aging is associated with human failure against the background of disobedience, one would expect that, while it might be construed as an unalterable part of the divine retributive economy, it might equally well be viewed as a problem to be overcome in a process of millennial restoration because it is not really a part of the economy of nature.

Judaism can assess the prospects of restoration in many ways. Rabbi Neil Gillman (see Chapter 14) presents *one* Jewish perspective that is surely provocative. Gillman contrasts Judaism with a Christian neoplatonic substance dualism, which asserts a nonmaterial soul destined for immortality. Without an immortal soul, he argues, we are not immortal. According to Judaism, there is nothing good or redemptive in death, which really is the enemy of life. Embodied life is inherently good and precious in God's eyes. Death is a chaotic force, argues Gillman, that must be banished either now or eschatologically through bodily resurrection. God chooses to have us in eternity just as we are here in an embodied resurrection. He concludes that Judaism will affirm efforts to immortalize our bodily lives. After all, do we not permit organ transplants already? Life in the world as we know it is valuable, and we strive to preserve it. There is truth in

Rabbi Gillman's assertion that "I am my body and it is my incarnation. Where my body is, I am." This embodied life may be the whole story, but should not Gillman still assert some limits on *L'Chaim*?

At the end of "The New Atlantis," to which I have already alluded, Bacon lists more specifically among the goals of science "the prolongation of life, the restitution of youth to some degree, the retardation of age," along with "making of new species, transplanting of one species into another" (1996, p. 481). This Baconian goal of "the retardation of age" is taken very seriously by today's biogerontologists who create scientific breakthroughs with fruit flies, round worms, rodents, and monkeys, but with an eye toward the alleviation of senility in an already aging society plagued by chronic age-related diseases. If this rings of utopian religious millennialism, the origins of Western science have been properly detected (Noble, 1997). Numerous biologists believe that death is not inevitable for humans, that the process by which cells are programmed to age and die is a contingent accident that can potentially be reversed, and that this process might begin with the regenerative capacity of stem cells.

Decelerated Aging as the Imperative Next Step in an Already Aging Society?

In the context of posthumanism, the religion of technology, and scientific hubris, efforts to slow or arrest human aging appear morally ambiguous at best. But if we bracket out this ancient debate between the natural law and its detractors, there is another context that is as immediate. The stark reality of our already aging societies is that, factoring out infant mortality, people can expect to live into their 80s. Many will experience chronic illnesses for which old age is the dominant risk factor, ranging from Alzheimer's and Parkinson's diseases to osteoporosis and vascular disease. Our demographic transition to a greatly increased life expectancy through means that do not involve the deceleration of aging has resulted in a scenario that is clearly not idyllic, and the solution may rest with advances in the basic science of aging that would achieve even greater prolongevity but without the perils of massive debilitation. In other words, to resolve the problems of senility and dementia, brought on chiefly by enhanced life expectancy absent anti-aging interventions, we could now develop those interventions or suffer the immense negative consequences. Among those consequences are future generations of young people extremely burdened with the direct and indirect support of tens of millions of citizens who require demanding, complex, constant, and expensive care.

When one considers the goal of decelerated aging in this context, it begins to appear rational, salutary, and necessary. No longer the bizarre dream of superficial technology zealots, decelerated aging appears to be a more reasonable aspiration. Indeed, the biogerontologists hard at work in serious research are much less the children of posthumanism than they are of a will to benefit a common humanity regrettably caught between the old world of a relatively short, "natural" life expectancy and the future world of the nonfrail and nonsenile.

So, the individual confronted with the possibility of decelerating his or her aging process may not question the dignity of human nature as we know it, or whether we humans are wise enough to control our future development. Instead, he or she may reflect on loved ones who have struggled with a syndrome that strips away memory and self-identity, such as dementia, and quickly declare that his or her true dignity lies in decelerated aging consistent with the retention of cognitive temporal glue between past, present, and future.

But will this next step, if it ever becomes available, really work? This raises the Swiftian caution. Jonathan Swift published *Gulliver's Travels* in 1727 while the rector of St. Patrick's Cathedral, Dublin. Recall the remarkable voyage of Gulliver, in which he encounters the Luggnaggians, a people among whom is occasionally born a baby with a red circular spot on its forehead above the left eyebrow. This is the mark of the Immortals or, in the language of this people, the struldbrugs. The spot grows over time and changes color, until, at age 40, it is coal black and the size of an English shilling. These are rare births, but they are not uncommon. Gulliver is entirely enthusiastic when he hears about these immortal embodied beings, and even envious:

> I cried out as in rapture: Happy nation where every child hath at least a chance for being immortal! Happy people who enjoy so many living examples of ancient virtue, and have masters ready to instruct them in the wisdom of all former ages! But happiest beyond all comparison are those excellent *struldbrugs*, who being born exempt from that universal calamity of human nature, have their minds free and disengaged, without the

weight and depression of spirits caused by the continual apprehension of death.

(1945, p. 210)

Gulliver imagines how, were he an Immortal, he would become the
wealthiest man in the kingdom by long-term thrift, and the most
learned by applying himself to the arts and sciences from youth on.
He would become "a living treasury of knowledge and wisdom, and
certainly become the oracle of the nation" (p. 212).

But Swift was, of course, mocking the Baconian hubris of
embodied life immortal. In fact, the Immortals, lacking the wisdom
that comes from accepting aging and death, are "peevish, covetous,
morose, vain, talkative," and the like (p. 214). They are altogether
superficial and lacking in wisdom or insight. As they age, they
become increasingly demented: "The least miserable among them
appear to be those who turn to dotage, and entirely lose their memories" (p. 215). By age 90, all "forget the common appellation of
things, and the names of persons, even of those who are their nearest
friends and relations" (p. 215). Suffering with what we would now
call progressive dementia, they are "despised and hated by all sorts of
people; when one of them is born, it is reckoned ominous" (p. 216).
Moreover, "They were the most mortifying sight I even beheld, and
the women more horrible than the men. Besides the usual deformi-
ties in extreme old age, they acquired an additional ghastliness in
proportion to their number of years, which is not to be described"
(p. 216). The king of the Luggnaggians wished Gulliver to bring a
couple of these creatures back to his own country, "to arm our people against the fear of death" (p. 216).

Dean Swift's satire of Baconian utopianism remains relevant.
While his dystopian alternative is purely imaginative, it raises all the
right questions regarding efforts at embodied near-immortality. Will
we live in world where everyone outlives his or her brain? Where
dementias of the Alzheimer's type are even more plentiful than is
already the case in our aging society? Will we have life span extension
in the absence of the compression of morbidity? Perhaps we should
set some immediate goals associated with the concept of quality of
life. Few people would welcome the onset of Alzheimer's disease as
the price for extended life (Post, 2000).

Yet, it may well be that the only real progress we will see in ridding the world of such debilitating diseases as Alzheimer's is through

slowing the process of aging because old age is by far the most significant risk factor. Currently there is no reason for optimism about scientific breakthroughs to cure this disease, or to stabilize its symptoms in the long term, although there are some compounds in use to ameliorate some symptoms for a limited period. Thus, basic scientific advances in the area of aging itself could, if successful, significantly reduce the incidence of diseases associated with old age that are too complex to be eliminated on their own. It is then unfair to responsible anti-aging researchers to suggest that they are engaged in an effort that will only radically protract the lives of the most deeply forgetful, that is create near-Immmortals. Maybe greatly enhanced prolongevity is not all bad if a number of conditions can be met regarding preserved memory and other dimensions of health and vigor. It might also be that, given the realities of the old-age boom, anti-aging research will prove curative where all else has failed.

Will anti-aging researchers provide the solution? Two respected researchers from the University of London conclude in *Nature* that ultimately we will find the human life span to be quite plastic, and scientific progress in this area "may allow us to reduce the impact of ageing-related diseases as the limits on the human lifespan recede" (Partridge and Gems, 2002). Yet such optimistic voices too easily ignore the Kassian cautions.

Conclusion: The Need for Balance

Throughout this chapter I have tried to convey the richness of the dialectic between posthumanism and anti-posthumanism, while also underscoring that anti-aging research is much less driven by the desire to carelessly modify human nature than by the salutary wish to eradicate the age-related diseases that plague our already established demographic transition to an aged society. The essence of human nature has always been freedom over human nature. Freedom causes us to break the harmonies of nature and establish new harmonies. In exercising freedom, the restraint of reason is imperative, as anti-posthumanists caution. Yet anti-aging interventions with the goal of eradicating our modern epidemic of chronic illnesses, which grows more extensive and costly with every elevation in average life expectancy, will not be easily restrained in the name of anti-posthumanism. It may well be that, in the process of decelerating aging with the intent of ameliorating chronic diseases, the human life span will be extended.

Kass rejects the goal of decelerated aging (and even the compression of morbidity) on a variety of grounds, and yet he appears *relatively attentive* to the possibility that such treatments could save many of us from severe cognitive and physical disabilities. He believes that "the finitude of human life is a blessing for every human individual, whether he or she knows it or not" (Chapter 14) and that "to covet a prolonged life span [he seems to mean *increased average life expectancy*] for ourselves is both a sign and a cause of our failure to open ourselves to . . . any higher . . . purpose" (Kass, 1985, p. 316). Kass argues that even if the human life span (read *life expectancy*) were increased by only 20 years, we would lose the benefits that finitude confers: (*1*) interest and engagement in life; (*2*) seriousness and aspiration; (*3*) beauty and love; and (*4*) virtue and moral excellence (Chapter 14). Perhaps, and perhaps not. As for the compression of morbidity that decelerated aging might bring, Kass rejects it because it will deny individuals the blessings of anticipated mortality: "it is highly likely that even a modest prolongation of life with vigor or even only a preservation of youthfulness with no increase in longevity would make death less acceptable and exacerbate the desire to keep pushing it away" (Chapter 14). Here I think Kass may be argued with, for a potential solution to the widespread problem of the death of the mind before the death of the body may rest with the anti-aging technologies of the future.

Responsible biogerontologists sense the therapeutic promise as well as the perils of their craft. Human beings have been more or less powerless in the face of biological aging, but this situation may be changing. We do not easily accept the dictates of a biological process that leads ultimately to frailty, and therefore a growing number of significant scientists are leading the way in a war against aging that some call progressive, some ageist, and some contrary to the law of nature. A number of these scientists convened in 1999, under the auspices of the National Institute on Aging, for a conference entitled "Caloric Restriction's Effects on Aging: Opportunities for Research on Human Implications," where they charted a bold new therapeutic research agenda focused on slowing or "retarding" the aging process, which implies the extension of the life span (Masoro, 2001). The driving motivations expressed, however, were focused on slowing aging in order to prevent the many diseases for which old age puts people at risk. This scholarly meeting sparked no significant public debate, although few things could be more deserving of critical reflection on human aspirations than this. A principal topic was the research to develop a treatment to prolong life and youthful vigor by imitating the remarkable effects of caloric restriction, which for more than 60 years has been documented for its dramatic ability to slow aging in nonhuman mammals and significantly extend life their spans (Lane et al., 2002).

I surmise that more research on the basic science of aging will eventually give rise to the ability to decelerate this natural process. People will be attracted to this technology because they know how burdensome are the diseases to which old age makes us all susceptible. Should they wish to select this medical option as a way of ensuring a better quality of life for themselves and for those loved ones who would otherwise have to provide long-term care, few would condemn them unless the Swiftian problem of prolonged senescence arises. We simply cannot predict the future, but over the past century we have seen a dramatic rise in life expectancy, and it is hard to imagine that the addition of more healthy years would be widely deemed contrary to human dignity.

But there is reason to urge extreme caution. The technology to slow the aging process may be coming closer to reality, yet the goal of prolongevity has not been carefully considered (Juengst et al., 2003). At a time when biotechnology is allowing the reconstruction of both nature and human nature, all thoughtful citizens must ponder the implications of potentially dramatic change. Of the many possible biotechnological goals on the horizon, which ones are likely to enhance the human condition and which ones are likely to diminish human dignity? We think of the provocative developments in therapeutic cloning, in fertility and reproduction, in organ procurement and transplantation, in genetic testing and therapy, or in the treatment of myriad illnesses, and our collective breath is taken away by the pace of change. But we are also rightly haunted by the reality that while biotechnological powers grow, human nature has in no obvious way progressed with regard to unselfish behavior, humility, peace, and equality. Thus, we raise the question of the very nature of goodness, and whether some biotechnological developments divert us from growth in virtue or even tempt us to create a new class of an ageless elite that inevitably begins to look down upon the ordinary older adult as a misfit. ~~Should we move forward in the twenty-first century as bold new cocreators of our somewhat malleable human nature, or should we accept a more humble approach that endorses a caring and just stewardship over human nature more or less as it is, seeking therapies rather than transformations?~~ At least in the area of decelerated aging, where therapy and enhancement merge, we will probably move forward, but not without moral risk.

References

Augustine. (1950). *The City of God.* Trans. M. Dods. New York: Modern Library.

Bacon, F. (1996). The new atlantis. In: Vickers, B., ed. *Francis Bacon: A Critical Edition of the Major Works.* Oxford: Oxford University Press, pp. 457–489.

Barash, D.P. (1983). *Aging: An Exploration.* Seattle: University of Washington Press.

Becker, C.L. (1932). *The Heavenly City of the Eighteenth-Century Philosophers.*

Benecke, M. (2002). *The Dream of Eternal Life: Biomedicine, Aging, and Immortality.* Trans. R. Rubenstein. New York: Columbia University Press.

Berdyaev, N. (1939). *The Destiny of Man.* Trans. N. Duddington. London: Geoffrey Bles.

Binstock, R.H. (2003). The war on "anti-aging medicine." *The Gerontologist,* 43, 4–14.

Cole, T.R., and Thompson, B. (Eds.). (Winter 2001–2002). *Anti-Aging: Are You For It or Against It? Generations: The Journal of the American Society on Aging* (special volume).

Dyson, F.J. (1997). *Imagined Worlds.* Cambridge, MA: Harvard University Press.

Fukuyama, F. (2002). *Our Posthuman Future: Consequences of the Biotechnology Revolution.* Baltimore: Johns Hopkins University Press.

Gruman, G.J. (1966). A history of ideas about the prolongation of life: The evolution of prolongevity hypotheses to 1800. *Transactions of the American Philosophical Society,* 56(Part 9), Philadelphia, PA: American Philosophical Association.

Gruman, G.L. (1973). Longevity. *Dictionary of the History of Ideas,* vol. 3. New York: Charles Scribner's Sons, pp. 88–93.

Harris, J. (2000). Intimations of immortality. *Science,* 288 (5463), 59.

Hayflick, L. (1994). *How and Why We Age.* New York: Ballantine Books.

Hayles, N.K. (1999). *How We Become Posthuman: Virtual Bodies in Cybernetics, Literature and Informatics.* Chicago: University of Chicago Press.

Hook, C.C. (2003). Transhumanism and posthumanism. In: Post, S.G., ed. *The Encyclopedia of Bioethics,* 3rd ed., 5 vols. New York: Macmillan Reference (in press).

International Longevity Center. (2001). *Is There an "Anti-Aging Medicine?* New York: International Longevity Center-USA.

Jonas, H. (1985). *The Imperative of Responsibility: In Search of an Ethics for the Technological Age.* Chicago: University of Chicago Press.

Jonas, H. (1996). *Mortality and Morality: A Search for the Good After Auschwitz.* Vogel, L., ed. Evanston, IL: Northwestern University Press.

Juengst, E.T., Binstock, R.H., Mehlman, M., and Post, S.G. (2003). The social implications of genuine anti-aging interventions: The need for public dialogue. *Science,* 299, p. 1323.

Kass, L.R. (1985). *Toward a More Natural Science: Biology and Human Affairs.* New York: Free Press.

Kass, L.R. (2003). Retrieved March 12, 2003, from Beyond therapy: Biotechnology and the Pursuit of Human Development http://www.bioethics.gov/material/kasspaper.html

Kristol, W., and Cohen, E. (Eds.). (2002). *The Future Is Now: America Confronts the New Genetics.* New York: Rowman & Littlefield.

Kurzweil, R. (1999). *The Age of Spiritual Machines: When Computers Exceed Human Intelligence.* New York: Viking.

Lane, M.A., Ingram, D.K., and Roth, G.S. (2002). The serious search for an anti-aging pill. *Scientific American,* 287, 36–41.

Lewis, C.S. (1944/1996). *The Abolition of Man.* New York: Simon & Schuster.

Masoro, E.J. (2001). Caloric restriction's effects on aging: Opportunities for research on human implications. *Journal of Gerontology, Series A,* 56A (Special Issue 1).

Miller, R.A. (2002). Extending life: Scientific prospects and political obstacles. *The Milbank Quarterly,* 80, 155–174.

National Institute on Aging. (2001). *Action Plan for Aging Research: Strategic Plan for Fiscal Years 2001–2005.* Washington, DC: U.S. Department of Health and Human Services.

Niebuhr, R. (1941). *The Nature and Destiny of Man,* vol. 1. New York: Charles Scribner's Sons.

Noble, D.F. (1997). *The Religion of Technology: The Divinity of Man and the Spirit of Invention.* New York: Penguin.

Olshansky, S.J. and Carnes, B.A. (2001). *The Quest for Immortality: Science at the Frontiers of Aging.* New York: W.W. Norton.

Olshansky, S.J., Hayflick, L., and Carnes, B.A. (2002). No truth to the fountain of youth. *Scientific American,* 286, 92–95.

Partridge, L. and Gems, D. (2002). A lethal side-effect. *Nature,* 418, 921.

Post, S.G. (2000). *The Moral Challenge of Alzheimer Disease: Ethical Issues from Diagnosis to Dying.* Baltimore: Johns Hopkins University Press.

Post, S.G. (Ed.). (2003). *The Encyclopedia of Bioethics,* 3rd ed., 5 vols. New York: Macmillan Reference (in press).

Stanley, S. and Harakas, S.S. (1986). The Eastern Orthodox tradition. In: Numbers, R.L. and Amundsen, D.W., eds. *Caring and Curing: Health and Medicine in the Western Religious* Traditions. New York: Macmillan, pp. 146–172.

Shaw, G.B. (1921). *Back to Methuselah: A Metabiological Pentateuch* NY, London: Penguin.

Stock, G. (2002). *Redesigning Humans: Our Inevitable Genetic Future.* Boston: Houghton Mifflin.

Swift, J. (1727/1945). *Gulliver's Travels.* Garden City, NY: Doubleday.

4

A Jewish Theology of
Death and the Afterlife

Neil Gillman

*I*n a book-length study of the doctrines of bodily resurrection and spiritual immortality in Judaism (1997), this author defended a number of claims, among which were the following:

1. With the exception of three brief passages (Isaiah 25:8, Isaiah 26:19, and Daniel 12)—all relatively late in the biblical corpus— the Bible denies any form of life after death other than some shadowy form of persistence in what is termed *sheol,* a realm in the bowels of the earth, where the dead are cut off from God and from relations with other dead people, and from which there is no return to life on earth;[1]

2. In the early postbiblical period (roughly from the late second century B.C.E to the first century C.E.), two doctrines of life after death become progressively more prominent in rabbinic and apocryphal texts: the resurrection of the body and the immortality of the soul;

3. Somewhat later, in rabbinic texts, these two doctrines become conflated. This conflated doctrine teaches that at the end of life on earth, the soul separates from the body, the body disintegrates in the earth, and the soul journeys to be with God. At the end of days, the body and the soul will be reunited and the

individual human being, reconstituted as during life on earth, will come before God in judgment. Allowing for various reinterpretations in medieval Jewish philosophy and mysticism, this conflated doctrine remained canonical in Judaism until the rise of the Jewish Enlightenment near the close of the eighteenth century when, in liberal Jewish circles, bodily resurrection was dismissed as a primitive superstition and spiritual immortality was affirmed as a more lofty expression of enlightened Judaism.

The net effect of these three claims is that though the Hebrew Scriptures affirm both the reality of death and its finality, the post-biblical tradition denies both: the doctrine of resurrection denies the finality of death, and the doctrine of immortality denies its reality. Though it is not rare to find the rabbinic tradition circumventing or even overturning biblical doctrines, there is no underestimating the revolutionary character of this transformation. At a certain point in Jewish history, the scriptural denial of the very possibility of life after death was clearly perceived as no longer tenable and was replaced by two doctrines that affirmed the very opposite.

In my earlier work, I make a cursory attempt to account for this reversal. Other attempts have drawn on methodologies such as the historical-critical analysis of texts, anthropology, and the sociology of religion (for one notable recent contribution, see Setzer, 2001). Despite these efforts, the factors that impelled it remain obscure; we know relatively little about the period under question or about the motivations of the authors of our representative texts. This chapter constitutes an attempt to pursue that inquiry in a more thorough fashion. My approach here will be less historical and text-based and more phenomenological, psychological, and theological. I will attempt to speculate about the mindset of the Jewish community in that elusive period to discover what dissatisfactions with the biblical tradition might have contributed to the transformation.

Theological Issues

The theological issues at the heart of the turnabout are the easiest to uncover and the most fruitful place to begin. The biblical insistence on both the reality and the finality of death raises two central theological problems: first, the justice, and second, the sovereignty of the monotheistic God.

The classic biblical justification for human suffering is to view it as God's punishment for sin. That obedience and loyalty to God will bring about divine blessing, and that disobedience will lead to famine, drought, military defeat, exile, and death, is omnipresent in the Pentateuch and informs prophetic historiography. If we highlight Deuteronomy 11:13–21 as a classic statement of that doctrine, it is only because this text is recited twice daily by the worshiping Jew, in the morning and in the evening, at the very heart of the prescribed liturgy.[2] In Judaism, as in the Credo of the Roman Catholic Mass, it is the liturgy that articulates the central doctrines of the faith community. Beyond this, one of the conventional understandings for the etiology of death in the Bible is the interpretation of Genesis 3:17–19, according to which Adam and Eve are punished for having eaten of the forbidden fruit by, among other punishments, death.[3] In prophetic and, later, rabbinic historiography, the destruction of the two Temples, in 586 B.C.E. by Babylonia and in 70 C.E. by Rome, was understood as punishment for the sins of the community.

There is no underestimating the power of this doctrine. Clifford Geertz's classic study of the way religion accounts for the eruption of chaos in God's ordered world suggests that it must meet three challenges: (*1*) an intellectual challenge: that is, it must explain, in an intellectually acceptable way, why the chaos emerged; (*2*) an emotional challenge: that is, it must provide the means for coping with the suffering that ensues; and (*3*) a moral challenge: that is, it must justify or vindicate the divine judgment that caused the pain (the enterprise of theodicy—literally, the vindication of God's judgment) (1973, pp. 100ff). The biblical account meets all three of these challenges. It provides an intellectual accounting for why the suffering occurs—namely, as punishment for sin; it provides a way to cope with the suffering by providing the means for reversing the punishment— namely, repentance and return to God; and finally, it vindicates God's moral standing. God's justice remains inviolate.

As testimony to the enduring power of this doctrine, we need simply note that to this day, in certain traditionalist Jewish circles, the Nazi Holocaust is justified by viewing it as God's punishment for the sins of European Jewry, "sins" such as the Enlightenment, Zionism, and the emergence of liberal forms of Jewish religious expression. Most contemporary Jews view this position with a sense of horror, but the fact remains that it is still staunchly upheld in these right-wing circles.[4]

Restricting ourselves to the biblical version of that doctrine, it raises multiple problems, preeminently the fact that though it might account for communal suffering, it seems to fail to account for the suffering of individuals; famine and military defeat do not discriminate between sinners and individuals who might well have remained righteous. Beyond this, it was patently clear to the authors of the Bible that many righteous human beings suffer terribly for reasons that are beyond human understanding. That failure is accentuated in at least one central biblical text, the Book of Job, which deals precisely with the suffering of an individual and explicitly rejects the doctrine. Job was a righteous man who suffered terribly simply because God had to respond to Satan's challenge that Job's righteousness had never been tested. God frees Satan to injure Job, which he does, but Job never denounces God. Job's consolers advance the traditional explanation that Job's suffering must be divine punishment for Job's sins, but Job refuses to accept this account; he insists that he has never sinned, or certainly never sinned enough to justify this kind of suffering. At the very end of the book (42:7–10), God confirms that Job had been thoroughly righteous and that his suffering was never intended to be punishment. God denounces the consolers and their traditional doctrine and adds that if Job will intercede on their behalf, God will forgive them.[5]

Job leaves us with a frightful dilemma. The traditional doctrine of suffering as punishment is rejected, but nothing is left in its place. God never really tells Job why he suffered, apart from the sublime speeches out of the whirlwind (Job 38–41), which are a paean to the complexity and majesty of God's creation and to the fact that no human being can even hope to understand how God relates to God's creatures. At the end, Job himself seems to have achieved a measure of closure, but the reader can only remain bewildered. Effectively, all three of Geertz's challenges remain unanswered; Job never understands why he suffered, he is left with no resources to cope with his suffering, and God's justice remains a mystery.

Of the three biblical texts that do affirm some form of life after death, Daniel 12 is the only one that can be dated with some accuracy.[6] Scholars agree that Daniel 10–12 was composed shortly before the death of Antiochus IV, that is, about 166–165 B.C.E. Antiochus IV was the Syrian monarch who is recalled to this day as one of the more memorable villains in Jewish history. During his reign, the Temple was desecrated, Mosaic law was prohibited, and Jews were coerced to perform pagan ritual practices or be killed. These persecutions eventually led to the Maccabean uprising, in the course of which the Syrians and their Jewish sympathizers were defeated, the Temple was cleansed of its impurities, and the Jews won their independence under the Hasmonean dynasty.[7] That victory is celebrated to this day through the festival of Hanukkah. But in the course of these persecutions, multitudes of righteous Jews were martyred because they refused to worship a pagan god. Here was a community that embodied Job's paradox: righteous Jews were dying precisely because of their loyalty to God.

Against this background, the author of Daniel 10–12, clearly identified with the Maccabean cause, offers what is nothing less than a theological motivation for martyrdom, and thus implicitly a recruitment pamphlet for the Maccabees. The core of his argument is that the community is facing a crisis "the like of which has never been since the nation came into being. At that time, your people will be rescued, all who are found inscribed in the book." And then, "Many of those that sleep in the dust of the earth will awake, some to eternal life, others to reproaches, to everlasting abhorrence" (Daniel 12:1–2). This passage, arguably one of the most discussed verses in the entire Hebrew Scriptures, answers the questions. "Why should Jews accept martyrdom? Why indeed, if their death will mark the absolute end, not only of life but also of any further relationship with God? How could their suffering be justified?" The traditional doctrine of suffering as punishment did not apply to these pious Jews, nor did the Book of Job provide any alternative explanation apart from suggesting that a capricious God makes innocent people suffer to win a wager with Satan. Why not simply join those Jews who were abandoning God?

Daniel's answer is to broaden the frame of God's dealing with humanity. God's justice may not be fully manifest during the course of a natural human life on earth, but if we posit an afterlife, then eventually the righteous will be rewarded and the evildoers will be punished. Martyrdom now becomes a justifiable expression of faith.

We shall claim, below, that theology never arises in a vacuum. Theological revolutions invariably emerge out of an existential crisis. On a purely theological level, then, the emergence of Daniel's denial of the finality of death met a profound existential need. The dating of the Book of Job is uncertain, though it is conventionally assigned to the fifth to fourth centuries B.C.E. Daniel 10–12 can be clearly dated from the mid-second century B.C.E. The notion that at some point in the near future dead bodies will rise from the earth—and that is the only way we can understand the statement that "those who sleep in the dust of the earth will awake"—must be understood as the answer to the quandary posed by the conclusion of the Book of Job. Eschatology becomes theodicy. Geertz's challenges are now met once again; believers could understand why they suffered, for after all, human beings sometimes do terrible things to one another; but they now had the means to cope with their martyrdom, namely, the assurance that they would soon live again; and above all, God's justice remained inviolate, for the righteous will earn eternal life and the evildoers eternal abomination.[8]

Daniel's promise of a life after death applies only to a limited portion of the community, only to the righteous and the evildoers of the author's immediate community. It says nothing about those members of the community who were neither righteous nor evil, nor does it hold out any promise for the countless dead of generations past.

But within two centuries, those qualifications disappear. Again, it is the liturgy that most explicitly reflects the expansion of the doctrine. At the heart of the *Tefillah,* another central portion of the daily liturgy, this one of rabbinic origin, there lies a benediction called *Gevurot,* literally a celebration of "God's mighty acts." The dating of this passage is a matter of scholarly controversy. It is assumed that the passage developed over time and that the precise wording of the text varied. But scholars agree that the current version of the passage, the one that is recited three times daily to this very day, was probably extant by the middle of the first century C.E.[9] This passage praises God's power, which is manifest in God's healing the sick, supporting the fallen, and releasing the confined. Six separate times in the course of this passage, the single one of God's mighty acts that is repeated again and again is God's giving life to the dead.

Two points must be made about this passage. First, the frame has widened. It is not only Daniel's contemporaries who will be brought to life again. Now, it is all the dead, from the beginning of time to the end of time. The claim is not rooted in a specific historical context, as it is in Daniel; it has now broadened. One dimension of God's sovereign power is the ability to give life to the dead. Second, the theological claim no longer addresses the issue of God's justice, but rather God's power. The ability to overcome death is now a statement about God's unfettered power. The entire passage ties God's power to the theme of reversal. God has the power to reverse the natural course of events by, for example, healing the sick. One of these reversals is God's power to conquer death.

It is not at all clear why the earlier biblical tradition denied that God had this power to overcome death. It might have reflected a wish to avoid blurring the distinction between God and human beings—human beings die, but God is eternal—and/or, it might have reflected the biblical preoccupation with avoiding the pagan practice of necromancy. The Bible explicitly prohibits this practice, for which it prescribes death (Leviticus 20:27), as one of a number of pagan cultic rites that it finds abhorrent (Deuteronomy 18:10–11). The preoccupation is to establish a clear distinction between Israelite religion and paganism.

But by the end of the biblical age, both of these factors paled in the light of other, more pressing theological demands: the need to vindicate God's justice in the wake of a traumatic historical experience in which pious Jews were being martyred precisely because of their loyalty to God, and thereby the need to proclaim God's sovereign power as total and unqualified. If God's power to affect the destiny of human beings ceased with the death of the person, then it could be claimed that death was more powerful than God. Then, in fact, death was the ultimate power in the world, and then death should be worshipped. That possibility was simply inconceivable. It then became necessary to affirm that God's power extends beyond the grave. God now has the power to renew life for all the dead from time immemorial.

From here, it is but a short step to the final affirmation that at the end of days, not only will the dead arise again, but death itself will die. That final step is most explicit in a hymn composed by an anonymous author during the Late Middle Ages and designed to be sung as the concluding hymn of the home celebration of the Passover festival. The hymn, called "Had Gadya," literally "One Goat," is composed on the model of familiar nursery rhymes where each stanza builds on and then repeats the earlier ones in reverse order. My father bought a goat, the cat bit the goat, the dog bit the cat that bit the goat that my father bought, and so on. At the end, the slaughterer slaughters the cow, then the angel of death slaughters the slaughterer, and finally, to our surprise, come the words with which both the entire liturgy and the evening end: "Then came the Holy Blessed One who slaughtered the angel of death." This final stanza marks a formidable leap in the imagination of the poet. He did personally see all of the other links of the chain. He did see cats biting goats, dogs biting cats, and slaughterers slaughtering cows. He even saw slaughterers die. But what he never saw was the death of the angel of death. That final link in the chain of mortality is reserved for the eschatological age, the age of the ultimate redemption, the redemption from death. It thus forms a most fitting close for the festival that celebrates redemption. The death of the angel of death at the hands of God signifies what a teacher of mine once called the final step in the triumphant march of the monotheistic idea.[10]

Spiritual Immortality

It is not totally clear what the liturgists who composed the passage praising God for "resurrecting the dead" understood by that phrase. When the author of Daniel 12 prophesied that "those who sleep in the dust of the earth will awaken," he could only have meant bodily resurrection; what sleeps in the dust of the earth can only be the body. The liturgical phrase then does include bodily resurrection, but it may also mean what we referred to earlier as the conflated doctrine, whereby at the end of days, God will resurrect the body and reunite it with the individual's immortal soul, which never died but left the body at death, so that the individual person, reconstituted as during life on earth, comes before God in judgment. In other words, along with a reference to bodily resurrection, it may also include a reference to the doctrine of the immortality of the soul.

That the human being is composed of two distinct elements, body and soul, is nowhere to be found in the Bible. The Hebrew words *nefesh* and *neshamah*, which, in postbiblical texts are commonly used for the English word *soul*, in the Bible, mean "a living person," a material body that is animated by a divine "breath" that itself has no independent existence outside the body. The Bible knows nothing of a Cartesian-style dualism. The human person is one entity: animated matter. The textual basis for that view is Genesis 2:7, which describes how God "formed man from the dust of the earth" and "blew into his nostrils the breath of life," whereby man "became a living being." This "breath of life" does not come from anywhere, nor upon death does it go anywhere. It is simply extinguished.

Whether the doctrine of bodily resurrection was borrowed from some neighboring culture—possibly Persian Zoroastrianism—or whether it represents an internal development within biblical religion is not clear. But there is no dispute that the doctrine of the immortality of the soul entered into Judaism from Greek philosophy. It is omnipresent in Plato. It has no biblical source, but it can be found in the apocryphal Wisdom of Solomon, believed to have been written by a hellenized Jew in Alexandria about the middle of the first century C.E.[11] Later, it appears throughout rabbinic sources,[12] as does what we have referred to as the conflated doctrine.[13] In these Jewish sources, the doctrine is never as radical as it appears, for example, in Plato's *Phaedo.* Jewish sources never claim that the soul represents the real person, nor is there the sharp disparagement of the body that we find in the Greek sources. But that the body and the soul are independent entities, that at death the soul departs the body to be with God, and that it will be reunited with the body at the end of days—this complex doctrine become normative in Jewish sources until the Jewish Enlightenment.[14] That the doctrine has in fact become quasi-canonical is confirmed by this statement in Mishnah *Sanhedrin* 10:1: "All Israelites have a share in the age to come. . . . And these are they that have no share in the age to come: He who says that there is no [mention of] resurrection of the dead in the Torah." The Mishnah, conventionally understood to have been formulated about 200 C.E., is a code of law; the presence of a theological doctrine in a text of this kind is quite unusual. But this doctrine is present.[15]

By the dawn of the third century C.E., then, the Jewish denial of both the finality and even the reality of death is an accomplished fact. The doctrine of bodily resurrection denies the finality of death, while the doctrine of spiritual immortality denies its reality. Ultimately, rabbinic eschatology proclaims the very death of death itself. These traditions could not possibly envision the indefinite extension of life on earth as we moderns do. But it did claim the next best thing: to use a rabbinic metaphor, life here on earth is but a vestibule before the Age to Come[16] (Mishnah *Avot* 4:16), and the life that we will enjoy in the Age to Come will be eternal.

The Existential Context

Theological revolutions of the kind that we are studying here can only emerge out of a profound existential crisis. The issue is nothing less than the fact that human beings must die or, speaking as a true existentialist, the fact that I must die. The issue is not death in the abstract but the reality of *my* death. For one who worships the monotheistic God, the question acquires an even sharper edge: Why does God require or tolerate the death of human beings? Why does God require or tolerate my death? Why does a God who creates life in the first place, who is, as the Jewish tradition claims, a "living" God, require or tolerate that we must die? Why does this God who has Jews pray, each High Holiday season, that we be remembered unto life,[17] at the same time require that we must die? Or tolerate the fact that we must die?

These questions raise an even prior question: the Jewish account of the origin of death. Did God create us to die? Or did God create us to be immortal, with death entering the world as a result of some human, presumably rebellious, act, as the conventional interpretation of the story of the Garden of Eden in Genesis 3 suggests?[18] The answer to that question depends on our interpretation of obscure biblical texts and is the subject of considerable scholarly inquiry; that inquiry is beyond the scope of this chapter. However we answer that prior question, the fact remains that beginning with Genesis, throughout the Bible and thereafter, every human being (with the exception of Enoch, as related in Genesis 5:21–24 and, later, Elijah, in II Kings 2:11–12—both of whom mysteriously disappear from the earth without our being told explicitly that they died) dies.

Is Death a Blessing?

That death itself—not only an "easy" death, not only the death that brings relief from severe pain, but the simple reality of death—is a blessing is a claim that is given an eloquent defense in Dr. Sherwin B. Nuland's National Book Award–winning *How We Die* (1994). For Nuland, death is the thoroughly natural and desirable end of everything that lives. We die so that others may live. For "plants and animals," he writes, "renewal requires that death precede it so that the weary may be replaced by the vigorous" (p. 58). Death is the invariable and ultimately welcome result of the natural cycle. We die in order to maintain the balance of nature. Nuland even proposes his own version of the afterlife: we live on as part of the broader ecosystem.

Dr. Nuland's understanding of death reflects his personal values. It is shaped by his myth, by his personal way of making sense of the world and of his own existence. It is a singularly powerful myth, possibly even the reigning myth of our scientific/technological civilization, but it remains a myth. By the term *myth* here, I mean not a fiction, as the term is popularly used, but rather the more academic sense of the term as an imaginative way of shaping complex data into a structure of meaning.[19] Myths of this kind can neither be verified nor falsified. They can only be challenged by an alternative myth, and they can be testified against.

There is no more explicit alternative to Nuland's myth than the one that is provided by the Jewish tradition. To trace the contours of that alternative way of making sense of human existence is a singularly complex task. Jewish teachings are collected in multiple texts, authored over at least three millennia in a wide range of cultures and civilizations. Particularly in this modern age, Jewish teachings reflect a good deal of disagreement between the more traditionalist and the more liberal wings of the community. To isolate or define a normative understanding of what Judaism has to say on any single topic is an inherently suspect enterprise. But at least on this issue, there is a surprising degree of unanimity.

To put it succinctly, Judaism views every human life as a gift from God. That proposition leads to a series of conclusions that, as with every theoretical teaching in Judaism, eventually become codified in law. These legal statements have won a surprisingly wide range of acceptance in contemporary rabbinic circles. For example, Jewish law forbids the taking of a life by suicide, with or without the assistance of a physician. Some contemporary rabbinic authorities debate the distinction between passive and active euthanasia, but that distinction remains blurred: doing nothing can be a very aggressive way of doing something. There is also a large measure of agreement that the prolongation of life should not be qualified by *quality-of-life* factors. That elusive phrase remains singularly difficult to define. The most hotly debated issues revolve around withholding or withdrawing hydration, nutrition, or medication when death is immanent. On this issue, the more traditionalist authorities would forbid, and the more liberal would permit, a measure of both, but always under the most careful medical and rabbinic supervision.[20] To put all of this in more positive terms, the aggressive treatment of the sick and the prolongation of life are divine commands. One of the more common metaphors for God in the liturgy is "healer of the sick." One is permitted to violate every single divine command in order to avoid injury or to promote healing.

The choice between opposing myths is a singularly subjective enterprise. It is an existential decision in the most technical sense of that term: a decision that does not claim to be rational or logical, that has little objective basis, that is neither objectively true nor false, but rather represents an individual's conscious and deliberately responsible choice, and for which one is prepared to risk one's life and destiny.

For this writer, this decision is clear. Writing as a believing Jew, I cannot but view my death as an absurdity, an eruption of chaos in God's ordered world. My problem with Dr. Nuland's myth is that it may work for plants and animals but it does not work for that class of animals that is aware of itself as being human. The difference is awareness. Not only must I die, but I know that I must die. Plants and other animals don't. That difference is not insignificant. I live my entire life with a looming awareness, growing steadily the older I get, that I will die. That double burden shapes my every waking moment. I view my death as an enemy to be resisted as long as possible. Even more, I want my physicians to share that view. My fear is that Dr. Nuland's myth, in some subtle, even barely conscious way, may inform clinical decisions that may have to be made as my death approaches. I confess that, thankfully, I have not yet had to face that moment, and I fully realize that I may feel very differently when that moment does approach. But all I can do at this point in my life is to voice my feelings as candidly as I possibly can.

The fact remains that I will eventually die. My myth enables me to face my death with the certainty that at the end of days, I will live again, reconstituted as I was during my years here on earth. I hasten to add that this faith is by no means a biological or scientific claim. The reality is that I, no more than any other human being, know with certainty what will happen to me after I die. But what I *believe* will happen to me after I die makes an enormous difference in the way I live today. In that sense, my belief is a mythic claim, less a statement about the future than a statement about the present, about the way I make sense of my existence today.

However we understand the biblical view of the etiology of death and of God's role in introducing or tolerating the reality of death in historical time, Judaism soon came to proclaim the eschatological defeat of death. In historical time, God is not yet fully God. Until then, we can only wait—and we can hope. Hope may be the most precious resource we have. Hope is an act of defiance against the inroads of despair, of scientific positivism, or of an easy reliance on the technological/scientific temper of the age. Hope, particularly what has been called *hope against hope,* the hope that surges within us when the tests are all positive, when the statistics are all stacked against us, when the prognostications are all gloomy, is not simply denial or resistance. This kind of hope does not deny the value of the critical impulse; it simply challenges its imperialism. Without that kind of hope, how is it possible to live?

Notes

1. The solitary exception is Samuel, as narrated in I Samuel 28, who returned to earth at Saul's command for a singularly brief sojourn. Other biblical references to some form of resurrection are either one-time miracles (as with Elisha in II Kings 4) or a metaphor for political revival (the vision of the dry bones in Ezekiel 37). Neither of these speaks of a generalized resurrection of the dead, as in our three texts.

2. A more extended and vivid expression of the doctrine is in Deuteronomy 28 and, in prophetic literature, in Isaiah 1.

3. That death is understood to be God's punishment is enshrined in the Christian doctrine of original sin. For alternative interpretations of the Garden of Eden story that avoid the notion of divine punishment, see Gillman (1997, Ch. 2).

4. For an eloquent rebuttal of that position by a prominent traditionalist thinker, himself a survivor of the Holocaust, see David Weiss Halivni, "Prayer in the Shoah," *Judaism,* 50:3, Summer 2001. Halivni's note 6, p. 289f, documents the various arguments in support of the position and cites sources.

5. On the theology of the Book of Job, see "Reflections on Job's Theology," in Moshe Greenberg, *Studies in the Bible and Jewish Thought,* JPS Scholars of Distinction Series, (Philadelphia: The Jewish Publication Society, 1995), pp. 327ff.

6. On the dating and interpretation of Daniel 12, see inter alia, the volume in the Anchor Bible, Introduction and Commentary on Chapters 10–12 by Alexander A. Di Lella, O.F.M. (Garden City, NY: Doubleday, 1978), pp. 255ff; John, J. Collins, *A Commentary on the Book of Daniel* (Minneapolis, Fortress Press, 1993), pp. 361ff; and George W.E. Nickelsburg, Jr., *Resurrection, Immortality and Eternal Life in Intertestamental Judaism* (Cambridge, MA: Harvard University Press, 1972).

7. On the persecutions of Antiochus IV and the Maccabean revolt, see Elias Bickerman, *From Ezra to the Last of the Maccabees* (New York: Schocken Books, 1967).

8. Of the three biblical texts that seem to affirm unambiguously some form of afterlife, I have concentrated here exclusively on Daniel 12 because

it is the only one of the three that can be dated with some certainty, and therefore where the historical context in which the text was composed seems to be reasonably clear. The two Isaiah texts are found in what is called the Isaiah Apocalypse (Isaiah 24–27), which scholars date anywhere from the seventh to the second centuries B.C.E. There is a general consensus, however, that Daniel postdates the Isaiah texts and builds upon them. See my discussion in Gillman (1997, pp. 90–93).

9. For an exhaustive discussion of the issues involved in dating the Jewish liturgy, see Ismar Elbogen, *Jewish Liturgy: A Comprehensive History*, trans. Raymond P. Scheindlin (Philadelphia: Jewish Publication Society, 1993). On our passage, see pp. 24–53.

10. The song can be found in any edition of the Passover Haggadah. On its origins and its varied interpretations, see *Encylcopedia Judaica*, vol. 7 (NY: Macmillan, 1972), pp. 1048–1050.

11. *The Wisdom of Solomon*, A New Translation, with Introduction and Commentary by David Winston, The Anchor Bible (New York: Doubleday, 1979). Dating of the text is discussed on p. 3, the doctrine of the immortality of the soul on pp. 25ff, and a representative statement of the doctrine in 2:22–3:12 together with Winston's commentary on pp. 125–129.

12. See my discussion of representative liturgical and rabbinic sources on spiritual immortality and on the conflated doctrine in Gillman (1997, pp. 134ff).

13. The most explicit statement of what we have called the conflated doctrine is the parable of the blind and lame guardians of the orchard in B. Talmud, *Sanhedrin*, 91a–91b. See Gillman (1997, pp. 139–140).

14. The most notable postbiblical champion for the preeminence of the doctrine of spiritual immortality is Maimonides. See my discussion of the convoluted history of his treatment of the doctrine in Gillman (1997, Ch. 6). The parallel treatment of the doctrine in Jewish mystical texts is discussed in Chapter 7.

15. In some versions, the phrase *in the Torah* is omitted. If by *Torah* the reference is to the Pentateuch, then as we have noted, there is no textual basis for the doctrine, though ingenious rabbinic exegesis does succeed in locating it there. The issue then is whether the doctrine itself has become canonical or its Pentateuchal basis. The latter version would seem to postdate the former.

16. The Hebrew phrase for the eschaton is *Olam Haba*, which is variously translated as "World to Come" or "Age to Come," in contrast to *Olam Hazeh*, literally "this world," the age of history. In biblical Hebrew, *olam* can have both a spatial and a temporal referent. I prefer the latter translation because the primary location of the eschaton is temporal.

17. The High Holiday insertion into the liturgy reads, "Remember us unto life, God who loves life, and inscribe us in the Book of Life, for Your sake, O living God."

18. The notion that Adam's sin brought death into the world can also be found in rabbinic teachings. See the discussion in George Foot Moore,

Judaism in the First Centuries of the Christian Era, vol. 1 (Cambridge, MA: Harvard University Press, 1950), pp. 474ff.

19. See my more extended discussion of this use of the term *myth* in Gillman (1997, p. 25).

20. For a masterful overview of these issues from the perspective of Jewish law, see Aaron L. Mackler (ed.), *Life and Death Responsibilities in Jewish Biomedical Ethics*, Part III (New York: Louis Finkelstein Institute, Jewish Theological Seminary of America, 2000). The positions expressed here largely reflect the position of the Conservative (i.e. the center) movement in contemporary Jewish life, but they include manifold references to both the more traditionalist and liberal options.

References

Geertz, C. (1973). Religion as a cultural system. In Geertz, C., *The Interpretation of Cultures*. New York: Basic Books, Ch. 4.

Gillman, N. (1997). *The Death of Death: Resurrection and Immortality in Jewish Thought*. Woodstock, VT: Jewish Lights.

Nuland, S.B. (1994). *How We Die: Reflections on Life's Final Chapter*. New York: Alfred A. Knopf.

Setzer, C. (2001). Resurrection of the dead as symbol and strategy. *Journal of the American Academy of Religion*, 69(1), 65–101.

5

In Defense of Immortality

Carol G. Zaleski

*I*n 1904, less than 6 years before his death, William James made a
revealing statement in response to a questionnaire circulated by his
former student James Pratt. To the question "Do you believe in personal immortality?" James answered, "Never keenly, but more strongly
as I grow older." "If so, why?" "Because I am just getting fit to live."

Not a ringing endorsement perhaps, but James was sure of one
thing: that the common arguments against immortality need not
deter us. In his 1898 Ingersoll Lecture on the Immortality of Man,
James set out with his usual relish to kick over the obstacles to belief.
Chief among those obstacles was a general climate of learned doubt.

Our situation today is not so different. Although social surveys
indicate that roughly 80% of Americans believe in life after death, it
is a belief cherished against the grain of perceived official skepticism.
Therefore it is a belief riddled with anxiety and doubt. While our
ancestors worried about their fate at the seat of judgment and hun-
gered for assurance that their sins would be dissolved, we moderns
worry about our fate at the hands of death and hunger for assurance
that our personalities will remain intact. To this worry and this
hunger one can attribute much of the current fascination not only
with life extension but also with personal transcendence of death.

Among academically trained religious thinkers, one finds a
greater measure of skepticism about life after death, and other unseen

things, than in the population at large. This is not necessarily a sign that academics are better at critical thinking. For many, immortality is not a matter for reasoned debate but is simply ruled out of play, along with guardian angels and statues that weep. It is taken for granted, as if it were a premise accepted by all reasonable people, that no one seriously believes in heaven, hell, or purgatory, the life of the soul, the resurrection of the body, or the personality of God as the concrete realities they were once imagined to be.

One thinks especially of Rudolf Bultmann, who made it a cornerstone of his New Testament hermeneutics that the three-story structure of the cosmos (heaven above, earth in the middle, hell below) is over, finished; it cannot be "repristinated." Similarly, Jürgen Moltmann began his 1967 Ingersoll Lecture by observing that the old ways of thinking about the future life "have dried up like fish in a drained pond."[1]

More than any particular objections, it is this practice of taking it for granted that the traditional *mythos* can no longer speak to us that weighs heavily against belief in immortality. The burden of proof thus shifts from the skeptic to the believer, and the believer finds that not only his or her reasons but also his or her motives are under suspicion. Belief in immortality begins to look shabby and self-serving, like something we fall back on in weak moments but rise above when we are at our best.

The specific objections to immortality are secondary and can be briefly stated. Belief in immortality is criticized on moral grounds as self-aggrandizing, on psychological grounds as self-deceiving, and on philosophical grounds as dualistic. Concern for the soul is faulted for making us disregard the body, neglect our responsibilities to the earth, and deny our kinship with other life forms. We share 90% of our genes with mice. Even the lowliest bacterium is our cousin. Why do we persist in imagining that there is some fifth essence in us that sets us apart?

What shall we say to these objections? First of all, we can say that there is no correlation between narcissism and belief in personal immortality. We feel the need for immortality most acutely when we are made sensible of the inexhaustible value of another person or of the tragedy of a human life cut short, not when we are looking for gratification. None of the developed conceptions of immortality fosters self-absorption. Every religious tradition insists that immortality costs us a death, both of the body and of the narrow ego-self. What are our images of eternal life if not ways of picturing a wider sphere of existence, a more generous personal life, less closed in upon ourselves, less fearful and grasping, more real in every respect? It is by contrast to the real persons we hope to be in heaven that we realize what pale, self-absorbed ghosts we are most of the time here below.

Recently a colleague said to me, "I'm all for eternal values, but I don't need eternity for my little self." One may as well say, "I'm all for joy, but I don't need for it my little self"—when in fact joy is what overcomes our little self; and immortality is its other name.

As for dualism, much has been said of the violence it does to our unity as psycho-physical creatures; but this is questionable. Multiplicity and disunity are as strong features of our existence as is psychosomatic unity. We are legion, as the demons say. It is a marvel that all of our different parts work together. At best, we are a symphony; but the second violins have quarreled with the wind section, and as we age these quarrels increase. Why should it surprise us if at death the soul separates from the body? Separating is the order of our lives as we tend toward death. If a man's jowls can sink down while his brow stays up, why can't his soul rise up when his body sinks down? All of our flesh is being pulled downward by the gravity of the grave; every day our skin is sloughing off cell by cell, like a great river; at each stage of life we slough off the skin of a previous stage; and at death we lose what was left of those skins. Perhaps that will be the chance to emerge as the person one was meant to be.

Against the charge that soul talk is superfluous, there is the common witness of humanity that some language of this sort is necessary to capture the full range of human experience. The human genome has been mapped, and the neurophysiology of awareness and cognition is beginning to be well understood, yet we have more reason than ever to stand in awe before the mysteries of consciousness and selfhood. We may be made in the image and likeness of a mouse, genetically speaking, but our kinship with the mouse is a kinship with life that is perishing. There remains an irreducible quality to our experience that tells us that we are not perishing with it, that we are also made in the image and likeness of Another, whose code is transcendent.

But if dualism troubles you—as it sometimes troubles me—there are nondualistic ways of thinking about life after death. If you have studied classical Buddhist literature, you know that one need not be committed to a substantial soul in order to affirm the reality of persons, their identity over time, or their capacity for transcendence. Consciousness may be understood as an emergent phenomenon that, upon coming forth from its neural matrix, has the capacity to generate ever more complex structures of awareness, including an autobiographical sense of self.[2] The theist can leave it to God to decide whether the self that emerges from this matrix shall endure after its neural basis is destroyed. And once God is in the picture, the emergence of consciousness begins to look foreordained, as in the words to Jeremiah: "Before I formed you in the womb I knew you, and before you were born I consecrated you" (Jeremiah 1:5).

The more serious challenge to belief in immortality is an internal one, coming from biblical theology, from the varieties of liberation theology that have captured the flag of eschatology for this-worldly aims, and from existentialist religious thought with its emphasis on human finitude.

The biblical case against immortality language is plain enough. Like other ancient Near Eastern cultures, ancient Israel bisects reality into two overarching realms—the heavens and the earth—and two kinds of beings—mortals and immortals. As the Psalmist says, "The heavens are the LORD's heavens, but the earth he has given to the sons of men. The dead do not praise the LORD, nor do any that go down into silence" (Psalm 115:16–17). To speak of human beings as immortal, to venerate them after death, or to conjure them by magic is to slide down the slippery slope toward the polytheism of Israel's neighbors. God's cult is the cult of the living, not of the dead.

It must be remembered, however, that biblical realism about death has very little in common with a modern skeptic's realism about death. Like most ancient cultures, Israel at first envisaged a shadowy half-life after death. The official religion of Israel never denied that the dead persist in some form; it simply deprived them of their glamour, reserving the glory for God.

Where intimations of eternal life do appear in the Hebrew Bible, they are driven by the same passion for monotheism and longing for communion with God that, at an earlier stage, had to exert itself against preoccupation (especially of a cultic sort) with the dead. To confine God's power to the realm of the living began to seem like an arbitrary limitation. Is it right that there should be any realm where God's power is not felt? Is it not fitting that the martyrs who die in God's cause should be raised from the dust and regain their youthful splendor? Is it not proper that wise observance of the law should confer an enduring relationship to the maker of that law? These are but implications of the promise that God's righteousness will be vindicated, even in the face of suffering and death. They may not amount to a fully realized teaching on life after death, but they certainly can be viewed as preparation for such a teaching.

Step into the intertestamental period, however, and the picture begins to change dramatically.[3] One encounters a stunning array of images of angelic metamorphosis, astral immortality, even apotheosis. What is impressive is not just the clear evidence of belief in a beatific afterlife for the just, but the giddy profusion of different ways to imagine that afterlife. Echoes of astral and angelomorphic immortality persist in the New Testament, rabbinic literature, early patristic writings, and Jewish mysticism, whence they enter the full stream of Jewish and Christian thought.

Some theologians have seen this rich array of images for eternal life as cause for alarm. In his 1955 Ingersoll Lecture, Oscar Cullman convinced his hearers, and a generation of theologians and pastors, that the language of immortality was unbiblical and sub-Christian (1965). Taking up the familiar distinction between immortality of the soul and resurrection of the dead, he sharpened it into a disjunctive contrast.[4] After the manner of an allegorical type drama, Cullman juxtaposed the serene death of Socrates to the anguished death of Jesus. In a didactic tour de force, Cullman set these two figures before us and said, "You must choose." If you affirm immortality of the soul, you make Easter superfluous. If your hope is in the resurrection, you should abstain from all talk of immortality.

Cullman's argument was electrifying.[5] So striking was the contrast he drew that it was easy to miss his own efforts to qualify it. In fact, he qualified it significantly, acknowledging that the post-Easter consciousness of the early Church resembled, at least in its effects, a confident faith in immortality. This might be no more than a battle over semantics, were it not for one very real stumbling block: the interim period between the death of individuals and the general resurrection of the dead. Where are the dead? What are they doing? According to St. Paul they are with Christ, and the Holy Spirit is their pledge of continued existence in God's hands. To convey this sense of continuity, the New Testament and early Christian sources use a rich array of images, all of Jewish origin: the dead sleep or wake; they are in Sheol or in a place of heavenly refreshment, light, and peace; they are gathered to the fathers or resting in the bosom of Abraham; they are sheltered under the altar or hidden under the throne of God awaiting the final redemption. Cullman, following Luther, would have us select from this rich array only the single image of sleep. It's a tidy way to dispose of the doctrine of purgatory and to downplay, if not completely efface, the cult of the saints.

Of course, Cullman's Ingersoll Lecture was just the tip of the iceberg. If there was any common agenda for the twentieth-century biblical theology movement, it was to sort out Greek from Hebraic, individualistic from communal, dualistic from holistic, and other-worldly from this-worldly elements in biblical thought. Marked as it was by the compelling presence of Karl Barth, biblical theology could not ignore Barth's insistence on the finality of death; it could not desert the theology of the cross for the allure of a theology of glory.

The revival of eschatology during the 1960s intensified the polemic. Theologians like Jürgen Moltmann, Johan Baptist Metz, and Eberhard Jüngel, who envisioned eschatological hope as embodied in social and political praxis, were calling on Christians to close their ears to the siren song of immortality language. Rejecting the medieval "four last things" model, which it judged to be individualistic, static, hierarchical, juridical, and hieratic, the eschatology movement emphasized the communal, dynamic, immanent, holistic, and future-oriented aspects of Christian hope. A similar impulse guided the implementation of the liturgical changes mandated for Catholics by Vatican II. Liturgical reformers sought to downplay individualistic, penitential, sacrificial, and otherworldly themes in favor of an ecclesiology of communion. Venerable ideas like the angelic presence at the liturgy and the Eucharist as medicine of immortality began to be an embarrassment. The lovely word *anima*, with all its bridal associations and evocations of mystical and ascetic life, was suppressed; and its vernacular counterpart (*soul*) largely disappeared from translations of the Roman rite.

As is often the case with intellectual revolutions, these movements were splendidly right in what they affirmed but dangerously wrong in what they denied. The eschatology movement recovered the Christological basis for hope, indeed brilliantly so in the case of Moltmann.[6] Yet that recovery was undermined by those who would reduce it to political hope, or would empty out its concrete meaning with evasions like *resurrection in death*. The liturgical reforms recovered the ideal of the whole church as the body of Christ, but tended too often to reduce that ideal to a this-worldly model of egalitarian fellowship.

The result was to flatten the symbolic cosmos in which the Christian imagination dwells, distancing modern believers from the great tradition of Christian literature, liturgy, and art. No longer could one read the Church fathers, the monastic tradition, the Anglican divines, indeed most of the spiritual classics of the Christian heritage without making mental reservations: "I must not allow myself to think along these lines; this is too Platonic, too dualistic."

Even more serious—if consistently applied, the veto on immortality language cuts off the community of the living from the community of the dead. It shakes the foundation of funeral and mourning customs. It makes the practice of praying for one's dead kin or praying to one's favorite saints lose its rationale. It renders absurd the innocent resolve of St. Thérèse of Lisieux: "I want to spend my heaven doing good on earth." This places theologians in the unenviable position of working to deny hope.

During the 1960s and 1970s, however, many eminent theologians were of the opinion that the ordinary folk in the pews no longer cared about life after death. We were finally done with such pie-in-the-sky considerations, they thought. Yet in 1975—midway through a long stretch in which no Ingersoll Lectures were given—Raymond Moody's book *Life After Life* appeared, soared to the top of the best-seller lists, and spawned a succession of immensely popular books on near-death experiences, all promising to offer evidence for the immortality of the soul.[7] The public hunger for this material was seemingly inexhaustible, and it shows no sign of abating.

How should we view this discrepancy between learned religious opinion and popular enthusiasm? Should we chalk it up to the narcissism of our culture or should we consider the possibility that something has been missing from contemporary theology, that a fundamental and legitimate need has been going unmet? People are not satisfied by an eschatology that focuses exclusively on social justice; they are not convinced that individualism is the root of all evil; they are starved for transcendence, hungry for miracles, and sure of only one thing: if life is to be truly meaningful, death must not be allowed to have the last word. Under these conditions, to suppress immortality language is indeed to deny hope.

Models of Immortality

The good news is that recent scholarship has progressed beyond the campaign to deplatonize eschatology, and a more nuanced interpretation has come into view. Without denying the advances made in the past few decades, we are now in a position to reclaim the language of immortality. It is a good moment to rethink what immortality might mean, and a little reflection reveals that it can mean many things. Suppose we arrange these meanings on a scale. Several distinct types will emerge.

One model—let's call it *Alpha immortality*—is immortality in its primary and obvious sense: physical invulnerability to death. In all cultures of the world, Alpha immortality has been attributed only to exceptional people. One thinks of Utnapishtim, the flood hero of the Gilgamesh epic, or al-Khidr, the mysterious green man of Sufi lore.

Alpha immortals are set apart and in some respects are inhuman. They seem to lack the defining characteristic that makes *mortal* a synonym for man and an antonym for god. Yet they are not gods, and what they achieve may be more properly called *everlasting longevity* rather than *eternal life*. The Taoist immortals attain their perpetual youth, power of flight, and immunity to physical harm by means of yogic practices and alchemical arts. They embody the ordinary human aspirations for longevity, prosperity, and posterity sanctioned by Taoist naturalism, yet they achieve their preternatural longevity only by being translated to a state of purity and unity that is strictly outside the human condition.

For an ordinary human being, however, Alpha immortality is a prison sentence: as for Dracula's victims, so for the Wandering Jew of invidious legend. To be given everlasting longevity without being remade for eternal life is to live under a curse. This drawback of Alpha immortality is endlessly described in science fiction novels that speculate about the possibility of uploading our memories and consciousness onto cosmic databanks; but somehow it has escaped the notice of our new alchemists, the biotechnologists who predict that cellular immortality is just around the corner.

For computer game developers the lesson is clear: while it's easy enough to give your characters immortality, it can ruin the game. Ernest W. Adams, a seasoned game developer, found that this got him to thinking about the practical difficulties extreme longevity would entail, including socioeconomic catastrophes, stagnation in the world of work and culture, the end of family life as we know it ("if you have spent 18 years in the company of your parents and another 500 without them, it's unlikely that you will really have much in common any more"), and, worse yet, no end to in-laws (1998, 1999). No wonder that the most original computer role-playing game whose protagonist is immortal is a hellish creation called Planescape: Torment. In this Advanced Dungeons and Dragons game, vintage 1998, immortality is associated with amnesia: "You awake on a cold stone slab in the Mortuary of the City of Sigil. You have no idea how you got there, who you are, or any of your past identity(s). You must escape and explore the strange world to uncover the secret of your death and rebirth. Each time you take enough damage to kill a standard mortal, you fall into a deep coma, eventually to reawaken ready for more."[8]

It is Alpha immortality that Gilgamesh seeks in vain and Odysseus wisely rejects. It is Alpha immortality that Paul Tillich condemns, in his 1962 Ingersoll Lecture and elsewhere, when he declares that immortality conceived as unending temporal existence is his definition of hell. It is Alpha immortality that the elves in J.R.R. Tolkien's myth possess: immortal without being eternal, they eventually grow weary of time and envy humans the gift of death.[9] One can reject Alpha immortality without disparaging either the natural goodness of long life or the supernatural grace of eternal life.

Another type, *Beta immortality*, is immortality of the soul understood as the soul's intrinsic invulnerability to death, an idea we associate with Plato and with classical Hindu thought. The soul is immortal because it is essentially perfect, or at least perfect after its own kind, self-sufficient, impassible, simple, with no beginning, and beyond time. Your true self is already immortal; you have only to realize it. Yet this realization requires intense philosophical self-scrutiny or yogic self-mastery. The body may be disparaged as a hindrance, but more often it is prized as a vehicle for the program of spiritual discipline by which one awakens to Beta immortality. The world of appearances may be devalued as illusory, but more often it is prized as the bottom rung of the ladder by which one ascends to Beta immortality.

If the paradigmatic practice for Alpha immortality is alchemy, the paradigmatic practice for Beta immortality is philosophy conceived as spiritual discipline. And the practice of this discipline, or yoga, furnishes in itself direct evidence of the soul's sovereign immortality. Hence, among the classic arguments for immortality, Beta immortality favors the argument from the inherent nature of the soul. It is Beta immortality that Cullman believes has been smuggled into Christianity from Greek philosophy.

Gamma immortality is a variant of Beta immortality in which the attainment of immortality is a particularly strenuous project, requiring heroic spiritual exertion, specialized knowledge, or magical skills. It is a path open only to initiates, whose practices can be gleaned from records like the Greek magical papyri or the Orphic gold leaves with their spells, charms, and passwords for ascending to heaven. In Gamma immortality, one learns to outwit the cosmic powers, forge a new adamantine body for oneself, and storm the gates of heaven. The twentieth-century movement known as the *Gurdjieff work* offers a Gamma immortality path. The paradigmatic practice for Gamma immortals is esoteric initiation.

Delta immortality is the variant of Beta immortality that belongs to the Enlightenment religion of reason. It is dualistic but antiesoteric. What is eternal in us, according to Delta immortality, is our capacity for moral reasoning. The pledge of our survival of death resides in the integrity and universality of our values. The elixir of immortality is a liberal education made universally available or philosophy conceived as the awakening of our powers of critical reasoning. Among the classic arguments for immortality, Delta immortality favors the moral argument.

The first Ingersoll Lecture ("Immortality and the New Theodicy"), delivered in 1896 by George Gordon, minister of the Old South Church in Boston, is a good example of Delta immortality as it plays out in nineteenth-century liberal theology. The lecture is awash with noble sentiments of a religiously generic kind. "Why," Gordon asks us, "should the believer not trust these high feelings . . . these surges from the eternal deep that carry upon their white crests and toss upon their glorious spray the verdict of the Infinite in favor of the life everlasting?" (1897, pp. 113–114). Gordon's purpose was to proclaim a gospel of universal immortality and universal salvation to New England congregations still shackled, in his view, to a hidebound and censorious traditional theology (1893, 1916).

Delta immortality was also the position taken early on by American Reform Judaism, as expressed in this official statement from the 1885 Pittsburgh platform:

> We assert the doctrine of Judaism that the soul is immortal, founding this belief on the divine nature of the human spirit,

which forever finds bliss in righteousness and misery in wickedness. We reject as ideas not rooted in Judaism, the beliefs both in bodily resurrection and in Gehenna and Eden as abodes for everlasting punishments and rewards.

(Quoted in Olan, 1971, p. 96)

In retrospect, it is easy to see why a softening of the demands of traditional eschatology was bound to fail. When the thorns are removed, a lot of the sap runs out with them. Immortality and resurrection, though distinct, have become so intertwined in Jewish and Christian thought as to be indecipherable apart from each other. When a Jew or Christian rejects belief in the resurrection, what remains is an abstraction that resembles Beta immortality only superficially, for it is without *mythos*, without *askēsis*, without the rigors of yogic discipline, without the juiciness of Orphic, Platonic, or Gnostic mystagogy. It is reduced to a metaphor for the transcendent value of our animating ideals.

But Delta immortality still has its champions. Its chief appeal today is that it solves the problem of pluralism. Its chief weakness, and a sign of its Enlightenment pedigree, is its disregard for the divergent claims of the historic religious traditions.

Epsilon immortality is yet another variant of Beta immortality found in modern theosophy and spiritualism. It has many points in common with Delta immortality, but it is monistic rather than dualistic. Spirit is rarefied matter; energy, electricity, and magnetism are the key metaphors. The translation to eternity, or at least to the next world after this one, occurs by way of an emanated subtle body that carries with it in replica nearly everything to which we are attached: our personalities, our familiar appearance, our clothing, even our pets. When Sir Oliver Lodge contacted his deceased son Raymond through a medium, he learned how the spirits get their clothes: "My suit I expect was made from decayed worsted on your side" (1916, p. 199).

The paradigmatic practice is trance mediumship and, for the intelligentsia, psychical research. Epsilon immortality borrows notions of the subtle body, rebirth, and transmigration from Asian religious cultures, but adapts them to an optimistic harmonial philosophy of unending progression to ever higher planes of existence, a kind of *samsāra* on nitrous oxide, that is very much at odds with classical Hinduism and Buddhism. Among the classic arguments for immortality,

Epsilon immortality favors the argument from experience, especially of the paranormal kind.

Zeta immortality, which combines features of Delta and Epsilon immortality, conceives of the future life as an archetypal or imaginal world along the lines suggested by Carl Jung, Henry Corbin, and other advocates of the mantic character of the religious imagination. At death each person experiences the ultimate mystery in the form he or she most deeply desires and expects. On an imaginalist reading, all otherworld visions are true. But are they true enough? What we want from immortality is reality. As the Brhadāranyaka Upanishad puts it,

> From the unreal
>   lead me to the real!
> From the darkness
>   lead me to the light!
> From death
>   lead me to immortality!
>
> (1.3.28; Olivelle, 1998, p. 13)

For classical Hinduism as for classical Greece, for Buddhists and Taoists as for Muslims, Christians, and Jews, immortality means awakening from the world of shadows to reality unalloyed. If death is to be the doorway to an imaginal realm of dream palaces and docetic theophanies, then it hardly seems worth the trouble of dying.

At the far end of the scale, skipping over other variations that will undoubtedly occur to you, we arrive at *Omega immortality*, the central insight of Jewish and Christian eschatologies. It has two main premises: that human beings are creatures, composite of dust and God's animating breath; and that they are created in the image and likeness of God, with a destiny—a royal dignity—that overtakes their finite status. They hope to see God, not because of their merit or strength, but because he has made them and stamped them with his image. To be immortal, then, is to be a mortal who has a share in God's immortality (1 Tim. 6:16); conversely, to be estranged from God is death—or *second death*, which is either annihilation or a particularly wretched form of Alpha immortality.

The keynote of Omega immortality, for both Jews and Christians, is that it is a sheer gift. Adam and Eve may or may not have possessed immortality before their exile from the Garden, but if they did possess it, it was by grace and not by right. The immortality of which

Hellenistic Jewish wisdom literature speaks belongs first to God and then only by participation to the wise man who observes God's law.[10] Similarly, when Christian theologians like Gregory of Nyssa, Gregory the Great, and Thomas Aquinas affirm the soul's natural immortality, they do so from within the horizon of Omega immortality. Our nature itself is a gift; it's a gift all the way down.

In Christian terms, the gift of Omega immortality is the perfecting of the divine image and likeness in humanity, known as *theōsis* in the East. This perfecting, coming as it does from a higher power, differs significantly from the Beta immortality ideal of self-mastery even though it bears some of the same marks of tranquility and freedom from passions. When Antony the Great comes forth from his 20-year seclusion, looking for all the world like a Cynic or Stoic sage, in perfect equilibrium and health, what radiates from him is the reflected light of Christ, not a brilliance of his own making; he is an Omega immortal.

Of the classic arguments for immortality, the one most suited to Omega immortality is the argument from desire. God has created human beings with spiritual and moral capacities, and therefore with good desires, that will be left unfulfilled if death is the end. Our reason and our piety are offended by such waste. Hence it seems only fitting that the God who uttered the spell of creation would reverse the spell that binds us to death.

Another kind of evidence for immortality can be found in the lives of the saints, whose deification or sanctification by the Holy Spirit is the beginning of the great work that God will complete with the resurrection of the dead (Sherry, 1983). In St. Paul's words, the activity of the Holy Spirit in this life is the first installment of immortality.[11] Omega immortality is the life of the world to come, already partially realized in the communion of saints both living and dead. Its effects are not confined to a circle of illuminati orbiting the divine throne, but spill over to all souls, both living and dead, who are—like William James—"just getting fit to live."

Omega immortality is a universal vocation but not a settled fact. It always has a dimension of longing and expectancy. The anthropology proper to Omega immortality is an ecstatic one. It is shaped like the Triune God, self-giving rather than self-contained. When monastic writers speak of the soul as a cloister or cell, what they describe is not an inner chamber enclosed upon itself but a cloister that opens out to a cathedral, a cell that turns into a bridal chamber, a bridal chamber that will one day be a banquet hall. This was also Augustine's great insight: my self exceeds itself; I become myself only when I give myself away. The best use I can make of myself is to offer myself as a sacrifice, in life and in death; at death I go up to the altar of God, and it is God who renews my youth.

The contrast between the two poles of the immortality scale could not be more stark. Alpha immortality is pride. Omega immortality is humility. Yet it is Omega immortality that, in the face of death, truly honors the dignity and worth of the human creature.

Death is real for Omega immortality. At death, "we are like water spilt on the ground, which cannot be gathered again" (2 Samuel 14:14). Or rather, we are like water spilt on an altar stone, like a sacrificial libation poured into God's hands. The pledge of survival of death resides not in the integrity of our personality or our memory, nor in any other ontological glue. Therefore, we need not feel threatened by reductionist accounts of the human person or by the paradoxes of identity and memory that dog philosophical doctrines of immortality. Of course we will disintegrate at death, just as we have been disintegrating all our lives. At death we will descend into the land of the shades but will find that God is already there. He has kept our memories for us and waits to restore them to us, now purified and made real. He holds the secret of our identity, which we misplaced at the age of 3. How will I know it is the same me if I have no subjective certainty of continuity and no external guarantees? I will know it is the same me because I will see the same Him.

This point has been illustrated for me by a game my 4-year-old is always playing with me. He pretends to be a baby animal, but he never remains the same baby animal for long. He always uses the same words to introduce this game: "You're a person, and I'm your baby velociraptor." A moment later, it's "You're a person and I'm your baby porcupine" or "You're a person and I'm your baby mouse." Andy can change identities at will, but I must always be the "person," the maternal polestar who remains fixed so that he can change.

For Christianity, that polestar is Christ, the archetypal person, the mirror in which the full extent of human possibility can be seen. Omega immortals do not possess their own immortality but are possessed by it as it radiates from the risen Christ. They experience their beatitude on loan, so to speak, from the fullness of eternity that will be theirs only with the resurrection to glory. Their immortality is not timeless, like Beta immortality, but comes stamped with a date, a certain Sabbath, Holy Saturday, when Christ invaded the realm of death and rescued Adam and Eve. The effects of Holy Saturday flow backward to beginning times and outward beyond the inner circle of the saints toward the larger company of mortal pilgrims and strangers. Its scope is universal, in that sense one calls it *natural* even though it is sheer gift.

The classical Christian view, expressed in countless catechisms and confessions, is that upon death the souls of the blessed enter immediately into the divine presence, where they enjoy the unmediated vision of God, join in the angelic liturgy, and attend to the needs of the living who turn to them for intercession. In restful industry and industrious rest, they await the return of Christ, the resurrection of the dead, and the renewal of all creation. Their bliss is perfect after its kind; but until the soul regains its body and the whole body of Christ is complete in all its members, this perfection is, paradoxically, an unfinished work.

An analogy may be found in the Mahāyāna Buddhist bodhisattva ideal. If we take our cue from the *Vimalakīrtinirdeśa Sūtra*, the bodhisattva is a fully awakened being for whom it is an implication of his perfect enlightenment (rather than a postponement of it) that he remain in solidarity with all who are afflicted by illness and ignorance, birth and death. Similarly, the beatitude of the Christian saint entails the altruistic wish that all may be saved, death vanquished, hell emptied. For the locus of Omega immortality is not the individual soul per se, but the complete society created by God's love, in which individuality is realized in fellowship.[12]

In this respect, all fully developed teachings about immortality gravitate toward the Omega end of the scale. Plato locates beatitude in the *polis* rather than in a private interior realm, and in their mature form all religions tell us that ultimate fulfillment shall be found not in self-sufficiency but in fellowship. From this perspective, we can appreciate the nearly universal idea that the dead may benefit from having the merit of others transferred to their own account: salvation is corporate.

The special genius of Omega immortality is that it never lets us forget that beatitude must be both individual and social, both theocentric and anthropocentric at once.[13] We learn this from the famous scene in the *Confessions*, where Augustine and his mother anticipate the joys of the blessed in heaven. As they lean against a window overlooking a garden in Ostia, the conversation of mother and son becomes so exalted that they begin to ascend toward "that Wisdom by which all things are made" and then "for one instant attain to touch it." This is no flight of the alone to the Alone; it has to be recounted in the first person plural. Comrades in rapture, Monica and Augustine have experienced something like a foretaste of the beatific vision as enjoyed in the communion of saints.

The tenth-century Irish Vision of Adamnan portrays the beatific vision with a curious image that captures its sociable nature. Adamnan discovers that the company of saints who encircle the divine throne have acquired the power to face in all directions at once: "None turns back nor side to other, but the unspeakable power of God has set and keeps them face to face, in ranks and lofty coronels, all round the throne, circling it in brightness and bliss, their faces all toward God."[14]

How does one rehearse for such a vision? We have seen that the paradigmatic practice for Alpha immortality is alchemy, for Beta immortality philosophy, for Gamma immortality initiation, and for Delta immortality liberal education. In the case of Omega immortality the paradigmatic practice is liturgical adoration, which recapitulates the vision of God in the Temple and anticipates the vision of God on his Throne. The Psalms are full of hints about this. The presence of God in the sanctuary establishes a relationship against which death cannot prevail; hence it is logical that when notions of a beatific after-life eventually begin to develop, they should take a liturgical shape.

The liturgy gives us our best and most complete picture of heaven, portraying the life of the blessed as a choral and complex affair in which solitary and communal elements are fused. One joins in adoration with angels and saints, with the dental hygienist and the mailman, daring to borrow from the seraphim the chant Isaiah over-heard: "holy, holy, holy." The divine liturgy on earth mirrors the cosmic liturgy in heaven even as it recapitulates sacred history. If ever there was realized eschatology, it is here.

Therefore, if we wish to decide whether Omega immortality is an intelligible idea, we have only to ask ourselves whether perpetual adoration is an intelligible ideal. Is our chief end to glorify God and enjoy Him forever, as the old catechisms say? Is G.K. Chesterton right when he says that "all human beings, without any exception whatever, were specially made, were shaped and pointed like shining arrows, for the end of hitting the mark of Beatitude" (1929, p. 26; quoted by Fagerberg, 2000, p. 24)?

On this view, our inclination to adore God is constitutive; it is written into our whole being. It is not merely a subjective need, but rather a need so completely interwoven throughout our rational, moral, spiritual, and sensible nature that if it is illusory, then we are comprehensively false, we are creatures of *mauvaise foi*.

One can imagine an *argument from adoration* for immortality. The object of adoration who made us to adore him: can his will be utterly frustrated by death? Can his justice be thwarted by death? Can his love be defeated by death? Must we understand the details before we can believe that he will vanquish death?

Our ancestors were afraid of hell; we are afraid of heaven. We think it will be boring. But adoration cannot be boring, for one is gazing at the face of the beloved, and the face of the beloved is inexhaustible.[15] We find it hard to imagine the kind of happiness that might flow from a condition of perfection. The very idea of perfection has become alien to us. We prefer to speak of *human flourishing*, an open-ended ideal that incorporates change and imposes no absolute standards. As an ideal, perfection produces anorexics and martinets, we think; only the *spirituality of imperfection* can promote human flourishing. But this is to confuse perfection with perfectionism; *true* perfection is evergreen and alive, including within itself everything that we value about change.

A further stumbling block is that adoration entails submission, both to the object of adoration and to the tradition that leads us to it. Submission is not a popular idea, especially where Christianity is concerned. A student told me that she had rejected her childhood Christian faith because of its emphasis on humility and self-abnegation; she then took up with a Buddhist group, where the practice involved making hundreds of prostrations. The prostrations felt good! Perhaps this is a clue that adoration—when the object is truly worthy—puts our powers to proper use. It is a self-emptying posture but also a stance filled with dignity and joy, the very opposite of groveling before a tyrant or an *idée fixe*.

If adoration is the chief end for which we were made, we would be well served by a tradition that helps us to picture that end, making it imaginatively plausible. Historically, both Judaism and Christianity have done just that, wisely tolerating a great variety of images for eternal life and requiring only that the nonnegotiables, the essential insights, are preserved. Some of these images originate with Alpha or Beta versions of immortality; but if so, they are altered by their new context. The imagery of esoteric initiation, ritual purgation, the flight of the alone to the Alone, alchemical elixirs, spells for ascending to heaven, and passwords for getting past the guardians of the planetary spheres all take their turn to express the mystery of entry into eternal life.

Similarly, Omega immortality is hospitable to diverse images for the resurrection of the dead, from the seed imagery of St. Paul to the exhumation imagery of medieval piety.[16] But this brings us to another aspect of Omega immortality that is, if not counterintuitive, then countercultural: its strangeness in association with the bodily resurrection. Admittedly it is bizarre to think of martyrs' bodies being regurgitated by the beasts that devoured them—but is it any more bizarre than birth, when compared to the more decorous view that finds babies under cabbage leaves? As Santayana says, the fact of being born is a bad augury for immortality. But it makes anything else seem possible! This was the apologists' main defense of the resurrection, and it is still a good one—that with God, all things are possible.

Concluding Thoughts

The plurality of images and conceptions of eternal life is a normal function of the religious imagination. In fully realized religious cultures, however, the religious imagination is not capricious. It obediently serves and unfolds the central insights; it is handmaiden to what is received by a community as the truths of its faith. It is subject to correction, but wise masters of discernment know when such correction is necessary and are very cautious about exercising it.

We may prefer to view images of life after death as metaphors for the transcendent dimension of human existence. This is right, but it is not enough. Talk of the transcendent dimension is effective only as long as it continues to have a purchase on a concrete and living myth of the other world, a *true myth*, to use Tolkien's expression. We can live by a vague creed only because our ancestors lived by a definite one; we can develop a second naivté only if we still have access to the first one. We have been living off the capital of a concretely supernaturalist worldview. Once that capital is spent, however, our abstractions will seem like thin fare.

The iconoclasts among us would like to limit the ration of images we may use to anticipate what Jonathan Edwards calls *God's ineffable manifestations of love*; yet there are times when even the most childish analogies can be of service. Take, for example, Elizabeth Stuart Phelps's novel *The Gates Ajar* (published in 1868, when she was only 24), which portrays a heaven of the most domestic and senti-mental kind. In one scene, a little girl named Faith is describing her vision of heaven to a friend: "'P'r'aps I'll have some strawberries too, and some ginger-snaps,—I'm not going to have any old bread and butter up there,—O, and some little gold apples, and a lot of play-things; nicer playthings—why, nicer than they have in the shops in Boston, Molly Bland! God's keeping 'em up there a purpose'" (1896, Ch. 10; reprinted in Zaleski and Zaleski, 2000, p. 144). A short while later, Faith's mother explains why she encourages such fancies: "I treat Faith just as the Bible treats us, by dealing in *pictures* of truth that she can understand. . . . if I told her that her heavenly ginger-snaps would not be made of molasses and flour, [she] would have a cry, for fear that she was not going to have any ginger-snaps at all; so, until she is older, I give her unqualified ginger-snaps" (2000, p. 145).

I have been trying to suggest that *qualified* ginger-snaps may be a better diet for us than no ginger-snaps at all.

Acknowledgments

A briefer version of "In Defense of Immortality" appeared in *First Things* 105 (September 2000), 36–42, and it is reprinted here by permission. It was adapted from the Ingersoll Lecture given at Harvard Divinity School on March 16, 2000. The Ingersoll series was inaugurated by Caroline Haskell Ingersoll in 1893, when she bequeathed to Harvard University $5000 to establish an annual lectureship in honor of her father, George Goldthwait Ingersoll, on the subject "the immortality of man." The series as a whole provides an index of changing attitudes toward immortality.

Notes

1. "[T]he Christian tradition of the resurrection hope as well as the idealist teaching of the immortality of the soul has been caught in the frus-trating situation of offering a heap of superfluous answers no one is inter-ested in the first place. The answers are not wrong. At least no one has proved them wrong thus far. But they have lost the character of open ques-tions. They have dried up like fish in a drained pond." Jürgen Moltmann, "Resurrection as hope," *Harvard Theological Review*, 61 (1968), 129.

2. This is the view advocated by cognitive neuroscientist Antonio Damasio in *The Feeling of What Happens: Body and Emotion in the Making of Consciousness* (New York: Harcourt Brace, 1999).

3. A landmark work on the subject is George W.E. Nickelsburg, Jr., *Res-urrection, Immortality, and Eternal Life in Intertestamental Judaism* (Cambridge, MA: Harvard University Press, 1972). The scholarly literature is vast; for ori-entation see the following by Alan F. Segal: "Some Observations about Mys-ticism and the Spread of Notions of Life After Death in Hebrew Thought,"

Society of Biblical Literature 1996 Seminar Papers (Atlanta: Scholars Press, 1996); and "Life after Death: the Social Sources," in *The Resurrection*, ed. Stephen T. Davis, Daniel Kendall, and Gerald O'Collins (Oxford and New York: Oxford University Press, 1997), pp. 90–125.

4. As Georges Florovsky pointed out in his 1951 Ingersoll Lecture, "The Resurrection of Life," *Harvard Divinity School Bulletin*, 17 (1951–1952), 5–26, the distinction between immortality and resurrection was widely recognized by the second-century apologists as well as by later Greek and Latin Church fathers; yet they continued to use both idioms. See the discussion by Joseph Ratzinger, *Death and Eternal Life*, trans. Michael Waldstein (Washington, DC: Catholic University of America Press, 1988), pp. 104–112.

5. For a recent example of New Testament interpretation along similar lines, see Stanley B. Marrow, "ΑθΑΝΑΣΙΑ/ΑΝΑΣΤΑΕΣΙΣ: The Road Not Taken," *New Testament Studies*, 45 (1999), 571–586.

6. Moltmann has now given definitive expression to his theology of hope with *Das Kommen Gottes: Christliche Eschatologie* (1995), published in English as *The Coming of God: Christian Eschatology*, trans. Margaret Kohl (Minneapolis: Fortress Press, 1996).

7. No Ingersoll Lectures were given in 1968, 1972–1976, and 1978–1980.

8. From the Planescape: Torment website at http://www. planescapetorment.com/nsfaq.html

9. The immortal nature of the elves is discussed at length in Christopher Tolkien, ed. *Morgoth's Ring: The Later Silmarillion*, part one, which is vol. 10 of *The History of Middle-Earth* (Boston: Houghton Mifflin, 1993).

10. Wisdom 3:2. See John J. Collins, "The Root of Immortality: Death in the Context of Jewish Wisdom," *Harvard Theological Review*, 71 (1978), 177–192. On immortality in apocalyptic literature, see John J. Collins, "Apocalyptic Eschatology as Transcendence of Death," *Catholic Biblical Quarterly*, 36 (1974), 21–43.

11. Romans 8:23, 1 Corinthians 1:22, 1 Corinthians 5:5, Ephesians 1:13–14.

12. This was the main theme of C.H. Dodd's 1935 Ingersoll Lecture, *The Communion of Saints* (Cambridge, MA: Harvard University Press, 1936).

13. The distinction between theocentric and anthropocentric conceptions of heaven is a central theme of Colleen McDannell and Bernhard Lang, *Heaven: A History* (New Haven, CT, and London: Yale University Press, 1988).

14. Fis Adamnáin, trans. by C.S. Boswell, *An Irish Precursor of Dante* (London: David Nutt, 1908), Ch. 12, p. 34. Reprinted in Carol Zaleski and Philip Zaleski, eds., *The Book of Heaven* (New York: Oxford University Press, 2000), p. 213. Jeffrey Burton Russell highlights this passage in *A History of Heaven: The Singing Silence* (Princeton, NJ: Princeton University Press, 1997), p. 105.

15. Jean-Luc Marion, in his 1998 Ingersoll Lecture, *The Face: An Endless Hermeneutics*, (adapted in *Harvard Divinity Bulletin*, 28[2/3][1999], 9–10), argued for immortality on the basis of Levinas's idea of the inexhaustibility of the human face.

16. Richly documented and interpreted by Caroline Walker Bynum in *The Resurrection of the Body in Western Christianity* (New York: Columbia University Press, 1995), pp. 200–1336, and in her 1989 Ingersoll Lecture.

References

Adams, E.W. (1998). *Some Practical Problems of Immortality.* Lecture given to the Game Developer's Conference Roadtrip, San Francisco (http://www.members.aol.com/ewadams/Lectures/Immortality/immortality.html).

Adams, E.W. (1999). Immortality for game developers. *Game Developer Magazine,* 6 (4).

Chesterton, G.K. (1929). Is humanism a religion? In: Chesterton, G.K. *The Thing.* London: Sheed & Ward, pp.

Cullman, O. (1965). Immortality of the soul or resurrection of the dead: The witness of the New Testament. In: Stendahl, K., ed. *Immortality and Resurrection; Four Essays by Oscar Cullmann, Harry A. Wolfson, Werner Jaeger, and Henry J. Cadbury,* (Ingersoll Lecture, 1955–1959). New York: Macmillan, pp. 9–53.

Fagerberg, D.W. (2000). The essential Chesterton. *First Things,* 101, 23–26.

Gordon, G.A. (1893). *The Witness to Immortality in Literature, Philosophy and Life.* Boston and New York: Houghton Mifflin.

Gordon, G.A. (1897). *Immortality and the New Theodicy.* Cambridge, MA: Riverside Press.

Gordon, G.A. (1916). *Aspects of the Infinite Mystery.* Boston and New York: Houghton Mifflin.

Lodge, O.S. (1916). *Raymond, or Life and Death: With Examples of the Evidence for Survival of Memory and Affection After Death.* New York: George H. Doran.

Olan, L.A. (1971). *Judaism and Immortality.* New York: Union of American Hebrew Congregations.

Olivelle, P. (Trans.). (1998). *Upaniṣads.* Oxford and New York: Oxford University Press.

Phelps, E.S. (1896). *The Gates Ajar.* Boston: Fields, Osgood, and Company.

Sherry, P. (1983). A neglected argument for immortality. *Religious Studies,* 19, 13–24.

Zaleski, C. and Zaleski, P. (Eds.). (2000). *The Book of Heaven.* New York: Oxford University Press.

II

THE SCIENCE OF PROLONGEVITY

6

In Search of the Holy Grail of Senescence

S. Jay Olshansky and Bruce A. Carnes

Why is the average duration of life 1000 days for most strains of mice, 5000 days for beagle dogs, and 29,000 days for humans? Why is the risk of death extraordinarily high at birth for most forms of life, followed by a notable decline in age-specific mortality until puberty and then an exponential increase from sexual maturity throughout most of the remaining life span? Why are the bodies that carry the immortal genetic instructions not themselves immortal? These and other related questions about life, death, and the duration of life have not only occupied the minds of the greatest thinkers of every era, but have led to countless efforts to combat aging and forestall death (Gruman, 1966).

One of the more interesting developments in the study of aging and mortality that formed the core of a heated debate among numerous scientists for nearly two centuries was a discovery in 1825 by the British actuary Benjamin Gompertz. He noted that human deaths tend to occur in a predictable age pattern (Gompertz, 1825)—a seemingly innocuous and now obvious finding that has done nothing less than shape the mathematics of death ever since. Gompertz believed he had discovered a law about the timing of death that was akin to Newton's law of gravity. Gompertz called his equation the *law of mortality*. So much attention was paid to Gompertz's law for more than a century that many scientists from a wide range of disciplines devoted their entire research careers to an attempt to understand why common age patterns of death should exist. Indeed, scientists were so convinced by the biological arguments for a law of mortality that they extended its applicability to all living things—suggesting that just as Newton's law was universal, so was the law of mortality. Thus began an intensive era of biological and demographic research to understand and quantify the temporal kinetics of senescence that has been as elusive as the fabled search for the holy grail.

Ironically, antecedents to a biological understanding of the timing of death and Gompertz's law of mortality existed well before Gompertz was born. Although there is certainly a literature on aging and death that extends as far back as Egyptian times (Gruman, 1966), one of the earliest related ideas was the belief based on the Old Testament that the life spans[1] of humans and other species are fixed by a supernatural power or by biological laws that apply to all living things. "My spirit will not contend [remain in] man forever, for he is mortal; his days will be a hundred and twenty years" (Genesis 6:3). The famous Italian noble and health "expert" of the sixteenth century Luigi Cornaro, in a now classic statement on this topic, suggested that even the weakest people had enough *vital principle* to live for 100 years, and those endowed with a stronger constitution could live to the biblical maximum of 120 years (Cornaro, 1903).

One of the more interesting theories about the timing of death was devised by the influential eighteenth-century zoologist Georges Buffon (1749). Buffon suggested that every person has the same allotment of time from birth to death, and that the duration of life depends not on our habits, customs, or quality of food, but rather on *physical laws* that regulate the number of our years. This belief was based on his observation that species possessed a suite of fixed biological attributes (e.g., gestation period, age patterns of growth, constant physical form). If all biological phenomena conform to fixed laws like those governing the timing of gestation and sexual maturity, Buffon reasoned, then duration of life must also be fixed. Buffon's interest in the life span was based on an extensive database of life history characteristics that he collected for a variety of species (e.g., dogs, cats, rabbits, humans; Buffon, 1747). Based on these data, Buffon reasoned that a species' life span was a product of interconnected chains of functional relationships between biological attributes. He envisioned a fixed duration of gestation giving rise to a fixed duration of growth, which, in turn, leads to a fixed duration of life. These data supported his hypothesis that the average life span of individuals within a population (i.e., life expectancy) should be proportional to the amount of time that is allocated to growth and development. Specifically, Buffon discovered that life expectancy was consistently six to seven times greater than the time required to reach puberty. As you will see, Buffon's observation was prophetic, although he made the common mistake of his time in assuming, much like Luigi Cornaro, that everyone had the potential to live the same length of time. In other words, the early thinkers in this area predicted that a fixed, biologically based limit to life existed and applied equally to everyone, while Gompertz discovered, to the contrary, that there is an age pattern of death, suggesting that not everyone shares the same chance of living to older ages.

A Universal Law of Mortality

Following in the footsteps of Gompertz, in a series of articles published in the late nineteenth century, the famous actuary William Makeham (1860, 1867, 1872, 1889, 1890) noted that some "diseases depending for their intensity solely upon the gradual diminution of the vital power" (1867, p. 335), a conclusion that fit the Gompertz equation far more closely than a mortality schedule based on all causes of death combined (i.e., total mortality). Even though medical science was not sufficiently advanced at that time to permit the partitioning of total mortality into its constituent elements (Makeham, 1867), he proposed a modification to the Gompertz equation by including a parameter that was intended to account for environmental forces of mortality that were unrelated to those associated with aging, as well as a parameter directly associated with aging itself. Makeham's refinement of the Gompertz equation and his quantitative development of what he called *partial forces of mortality* are the origins of what is called *competing risk theory* today. Ironically, although Makeham did not know it, his recognition of the importance of partitioning total mortality into its constituent elements would later prove to be an important element in clarifying Gompertz's law of mortality.

Early in the twentieth century, scientists began looking at patterns of mortality for species other than humans to determine whether they also conformed to Gompertz's law. Their goal was to test the universality of this law. Their assumption was that mortality differences among species were simply a function of scale—compressed within short time periods for some and expanded for others. For example, biologists Loeb and Northrop (1916, 1917a,b) theorized that a species' life span was determined either by the depletion of important biological substances or by the toxic buildup of damaging by-products of living. Biochemist Samuel Brody (1924) speculated on a biochemical basis for a law of mortality after demonstrating that several biological processes related to senescence could be described by an equation used to quantify changes in chemical reactions over time. These early researchers were among the first to suggest that growing old was an inherently biological phenomenon.

The first scientist to empirically assess the pattern of death for more than one species was biologist Raymond Pearl. Pearl (1921, 1922) and Pearl and Miner (1935) asserted that a fundamental biological law of mortality would be revealed if differences in life span were removed by superimposing two biologically comparable points within the life cycles of humans and *Drosophila* (fruit flies). After two decades of research using this scaling approach on an expanded repertoire of species, Pearl and Minor (1935) eventually declared that a universal law of mortality did not exist because the death curves for the animals studied remained different, even after adjusting for life span differences. Edward Deevey (1947, p. 47), the respected zoologist who encouraged ecologists to apply life table methodology to the comparison of mortality among natural populations of animals, noted that Pearl and Minor (1935) gave up their attempt to formulate a general theory of mortality when they realized that "the *environmental* determinants of life duration can not, at least as yet, be disentangled from such *biological* determinants as genetic constitution and rate of living."

After Pearl gave up his search in 1935, most scientists focused on seeking mathematical models that might improve upon the quantitative description of mortality provided by the Gompertz distribution (e.g., Weibull, 1951; Beard, 1959; Pollard and Streatfield, 1979; Heligman and Pollard, 1980; Economos, 1982, 1985; Pollard and Valkovics, 1992). In addition, advances were being made in developing biological explanations for why age patterns of mortality follow Gompertzian dynamics (Brues and Sacher, 1952; Mildvan and Strehler, 1960; Sacher and Trucco, 1962; Sacher, 1966). Strong statistical support for Gompertz also emerged when it was shown that the Extreme Value distribution applies to situations where the weakest link of a complex system (e.g., organisms) causes the entire system to fail (Gumbel, 1954). The significance of this finding becomes clear when it is realized that Gompertz is simply an alternative name for the special case where the Extreme Value distribution (truncated and normalized to unit area) is applied to failure times that cannot be negative—like those of living things (Elandt-Johnson and Johnson, 1980).

As can be seen from the prior discussion, research directed to understanding, quantifying, and comparing age patterns of mortality has a long and rich history of scholarship. Although biological implications and arguments are interwoven throughout this history, the most influential efforts to explain why individuals grow old, why they die, and why they die when they do have come from evolutionary biologists.

Evolutionary Theories of Senescence

One of the earliest evolutionary explanations of senescence dates back to a theory of aging proposed by August Weismann (1891). According to Weismann, an accumulation of physical injuries to the body caused by a constant barrage of unavoidable environmental insults is an inescapable reality of life. Since these accumulated injuries inevitably exceed the ability of the body to repair them, the survival of any species depends on the replacement of older individuals by younger ones. Although group selection (i.e., populations, species) arguments like this are no longer deemed scientifically acceptable, Weismann was one of the first scientists to make a connection between the need for reproduction and the inevitability of death. Within his conceptual framework, immortality is an unattainable goal in a world where the external forces of injury and death are ubiquitous and unavoidable.

The late Nobel laureate Sir Peter Medawar (1952) proposed one of the first and most influential modern evolutionary theories of aging. Like Weismann before him, Medawar also created a link between external forces of mortality and senescence. He declared that the biological consequences of senescence are rarely observed in nature because external forces of mortality kill most members of a population before they live long enough to experience them. Medawar's most remembered contribution to the field of aging was his mutation accumulation theory concerning the timing of gene expression and its consequences for senescence. Genes expressed early in life not only affect large numbers of individuals, but also have the potential to impact reproductive success. As alleles at polymorphic loci compete for representation in the gene pool of the next generation, those with deleterious effects on early survival and reproduction will be at a disadvantage. Thus, over time, alleles with beneficial effects will have age distributions of expression that occur earlier than those with less desirable effects. As Medawar described it, alleles with detrimental effects will be figuratively pushed into the later portions of the life span, where fewer individuals are affected and their reproductive consequences are far less profound. In this framework, senescence arises from the accumulation of alleles whose detrimental effects have been relegated to the postreproductive region of life (via selection for later expression), where they can do no evolutionary harm. Medawar not only referred to the postreproductive period of the life span as a *genetic dustbin,* but also considered senescence to be "something revealed and made manifest only by the most unnatural experiment of prolonging an animal's life by sheltering it from the hazards of its ordinary existence" (Medawar, 1952, p. 13)—in other words, an inadvertent by-product of extended survival.

The acclaimed evolutionary biologist George Williams (1957) also provided an important and influential addition to the modern theory of senescence. Williams used the well-known genetic concept of pleiotropy to explain how the frequency of alleles with detrimental effects could actually increase in the gene pool of a population. His innovative concept was to hypothesize the existence of genes whose effects are pleiotropic in time rather than function. Alleles with highly deleterious effects in the postreproductive period could not only persist but increase in frequency under selection pressure if they performed important functions early in life. For example, oncogenes are usually involved in normal growth and development pathways early in life. If they become dysregulated later in life, their inappropriate temporal expression can cause cancer (Cutler and Semsei, 1989). Williams described this presumed beneficial early gene expression and detrimental late expression as *antagonistic pleiotropy.* Despite continuous debate over their existence and relative importance, the mutation accumulation theory of Medawar and the antagonistic pleiotropy theory of Williams remain two of the dominant evolutionary theories of aging.

A more recent extension of the evolutionary theory of senescence appears in a series of articles published by Kirkwood and colleagues (Kirkwood, 1977; Kirkwood and Holiday, 1979; Kirkwood and Rose, 1991; Kirkwood, 1992). Kirkwood also emphasizes the important role that external forces of mortality play in determining the timing of senescence. Three key points emerge from his theory. First, external forces of mortality establish a probabilistic time frame of survival within which growth, maturation, and reproduction must occur. Second, the intensity of mortality within this probabilistic time frame dictates whether physiological resources should be invested in reproduction or somatic maintenance and repair. Third, the inevitability of premature (extrinsic) death makes the bodies (soma) of organisms disposable. Since every species is by definition a unique experiment in life, the temporal kinetics of aging and death will vary from species to species. As such, species experiencing high levels of extrinsic mortality would be expected to invest more physiological resources in rapid growth, early maturation, and high fertility and less in somatic maintenance and repair. Conversely, species under lower extrinsic mortality pressure (e.g., bats, many birds, humans, predators in general, tortoises) can afford to delay maturation (i.e., altricial young), have lower fertility, and invest more physiological resources in somatic maintenance and repair. Thus, species living under a low force of extrinsic mortality would be expected to live longer than ecologically similar species facing high levels of extrinsic mortality. Under the disposable soma theory, therefore, senescence is a product of accumulated damage to somatic cells that arises from trade-offs between investments in reproduction and/or maintenance and repair dictated by the intensity of extrinsic mortality and its probabilistic consequences for survival.

Evolutionary biology is based on the concept that natural selection alters the gene pool of a population through the differential reproductive success of individuals. The effectiveness of selection is time dependent; it should be greatest before reproduction has occurred (prereproductive period), progressively diminish over the course of the reproductive period as the cumulative reproductive output (propagation of genetic information) of individuals in the

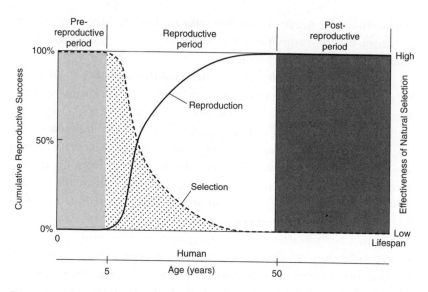

Figure 6.1. The decline in effectiveness of natural selection as the reproductive success of individuals is achieved, displayed within a potential life span partitioned into biologically meaningful age segments. *Source*: Carnes et al. (1996, p. 235), with permission.

population is achieved, and become weak or nonexistent once reproduction has ceased (postreproductive period) (Fig. 6.1). This age-dependent behavior of selection leads to a natural partition of the life span of organisms into biologically meaningful time periods—the prereproductive, reproductive, and postreproductive periods.

All modern evolutionary theories of senescence rely on the premise that selection is blind to the consequences of gene expression in the postreproductive period of the life span. This premise has numerous implications for aging, health, and longevity. First among these is that aging and death genes or programs cannot arise from the direct action of natural selection. Instead, senescence-related diseases and disorders observed in the postreproductive period are unintended by-products of selection acting upon genes participating in biological processes important earlier in the life span (e.g., growth, development, maintenance and repair, maturation, and reproduction). This view of senescence also implies that aging is not an unnatural disease, but is instead a natural by-product of survival extended into the postreproductive period of the life span. From a biodemographic perspective, it also means that bodies are not designed for indefinite survival. The biological warranty period implied by the certitude of death has important implications for limits on the life span of individuals and the life expectancy of populations (Carnes et al., 2003).

Continuing the Search for a Law of Mortality

Gompertz did several important things. He was astute enough to notice that the human populations he studied had a similar pattern of mortality, and he developed a mathematical model to describe this pattern that still bears his name. Then he did something very unusual for an actuary. He developed a biological explanation for the temporal behavior of his mathematical model. Gompertz was not a biologist, and all his work was accomplished in an intellectual environment that preceded Darwin's evolutionary treatise. He had a great idea, but the necessary knowledge base needed to give it more biomedical substance was not available.

Fortunately, an address to the Royal Society means that Gompertz's ideas were heard by some of the great thinkers of his time. One of those was William Makeham, one of the most influential actuaries in the history of the profession. Although Makeham called them *partial forces of mortality*, his competing risk theory and the mathematics he developed to support it have survived almost unchanged to this day. His motivation for distinguishing between partial forces of mortality (causes of death) was to improve Gompertz's law of mortality. Interestingly, the partial forces of mortality that Makeham believed would enable him to distinguish "the permanent and essential law from the temporary and accidental circumstances by which that law is obscured and modified" (Makeham, 1867, p. 333) were remarkably similar to those that would be proposed independently by researchers decades later.

Researchers from disciplines as diverse as actuarial science (Benjamin, 1959), demography (Bourgeois-Pichat, 1978), ecology (Bodenheimer, 1938; Deevey, 1947; Ricklefs and Scheuerlein, 2001), evolutionary biology (Stearns et al., 1998), medicine (Clarke, 1950), population biology (Caughley, 1966), public health (Pearl, 1921), radiation biology (Carnes et al., 1988), and statistics (de Finetti and Rossi, 1982) have independently recognized a need to distinguish between causes of death when performing mortality comparisons between populations. Although the terminology used to describe the mortality partitions differs (e.g., *biological mortality, endogenous mortality, intrinsic causes of death*), the common goal of these researchers was to identify a collection of causes of death that produce mortality schedules for populations that are consistent and persistent across time (calendar period) and space (geographic location).

In reviewing this history of scholarship, it is easy to see that *biodemography* (a melding of biology and demography) is a new term for an old and well-established concept that has been pursued within a variety of relatively independent disciplines that have had little communication with each other. Today there is far more communication and collaboration between disciplines, and biodemographic research has become far more interdisciplinary (Kessel et al., 2003). As a consequence, researchers have access to and an awareness of a vastly expanded knowledge base as they continue the historical search for why organisms die, and why they die when they do.

As described earlier, the lack of data on causes of death brought the search for a general theory of mortality to a halt early in the twentieth century. The search would probably have remained in this state had it not been for a unique database at Argonne National Laboratory (ANL) in Illinois. For over 50 years, Argonne has been recognized as one of the world's major research facilities for studying the biological consequences of exposure to radiation. Histological examination, pathological identification, and determination of the cause of death have always been standard elements of the long-term animal studies conducted at ANL. Carnes et al. (1996) recognized that the control populations of these studies provided a unique opportunity to resume the search for the law of mortality that had eluded researchers in the past.

The Argonne database contains detailed mortality information for a variety of mouse strains and the beagle dog. Control animals were protected from external sources of mortality and were permitted to live in controlled environments for the duration of their lives. As such, the principal mortality risks experienced by these animals should have been those associated with growing old. However, Carnes and colleagues recognized that an experiment occurred with these animals that was not planned by the original investigators. Over the nearly 50-year course of these studies, the science of animal husbandry continually improved. The principal benefit of this improvement was a progressive decline in deaths caused by infectious diseases. The presence of identifiable mortality risks from infectious diseases created the conditions needed to determine whether mortality schedules that are persistent (invariant) across time could be identified.

As with previous investigations, the initial step in this investigation was to distinguish between deaths caused by external factors (extrinsic mortality) and those judged to arise from the basic biology of the animals (intrinsic mortality). This partitioning was accomplished over a 3-year period by a group of board-certified veterinary pathologists who reviewed and discussed the pathology information on every control animal in the database. Once these diagnoses were made, they were not subject to modification by the research scientists. The mortality partition established the censoring definitions used in standard competing risk methodology (proportional hazard models) to test for differences in schedules of age-specific death rates (mortality signatures).

Six inbred and hybrid mouse strains were consistently used as experimental animals over the long history of the Argonne animal studies. When comparisons were based on all-cause mortality (i.e., the partition was ignored), mice living under the improved husbandry environments experienced significantly better survival than their counterparts raised in suboptimal environments (Fig. 6.2). Conversely, the mortality schedules for the two environments were visually and statistically indistinguishable when comparisons were based on intrinsic

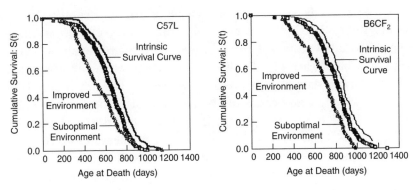

Figure 6.2. Plots for two strains of mice (one inbred and one hybrid) showing temporally separated populations with different patterns of total mortality but statistically indistinguishable patterns of intrinsic mortality. *Source*: Carnes et al. (1996, p. 247), with permission.

mortality. In other words, the intrinsic mortality signatures of these six mouse strains exhibit the stable behavior predicted by Gompertz and Makeham. Further, the stability of the intrinsic mortality signatures suggests that the underlying biology of the organisms that give rise to the signature is also stable across time.

Once the invariance of intrinsic mortality signatures between cohorts of the same mouse strain separated by time was established, the next step was to examine whether these signatures were similar across mouse strains. The most immediate problem is that the 12 mouse strains in the Argonne database used for this investigation have median life spans that differ by a factor of 3. This disparity in duration of life is exactly the same problem that confronted Raymond Pearl and his colleagues in their search for a universal law of mortality. Although researchers have developed several ingenious solutions to this problem, they invariably rely on the statistical concepts of location (central tendency) and scale (dispersion). In the interspecies context, location is a nuisance parameter. Of course, humans live longer than dogs and dogs live longer than mice. One solution is to normalize the time scales of the species being compared to a common measure of location (e.g., median survival time). The comparison task then reduces to determining whether the scaled failure times of the strains and/or species are similarly distributed around their common measure of location. When this comparison was done for the Argonne animal data, not only did strains of mice share a common intrinsic mortality signature, but the intrinsic mortality signatures of mice, beagles, and humans (presented here as survival curves) were also statistically indistinguishable (Carnes et al., 1996) (Fig. 6.3). An identical comparison based on all-cause mortality failed to reveal common age patterns of death, which is exactly what Pearl (1921) discovered when he made the same attempt using data on humans and *Drosophila*. The apparently (but not statistically significant) improved survival of humans at older ages (relative to the mice and dogs) was attributed to *manufactured survival time* (Olshansky et al., 1998)—medical interventions received by humans but not by the laboratory animals that delayed the age at death (i.e., extended life). To quote Makeham (1867, p. 333), our mortality partition enabled us to distinguish "the permanent and essential law from the temporary and accidental circumstances by which that law is obscured and modified."

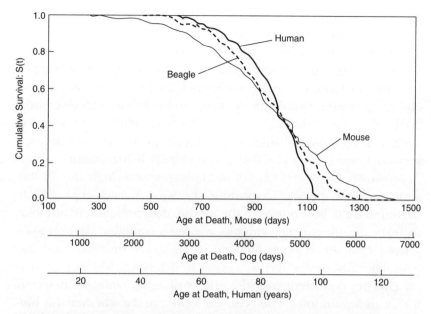

Figure 6.3. Comparison of cumulative survival curves for the mouse, beagle, and human populations plotted on the time scale for the B6CF1 mouse strain. Additional time axes are shown for the beagle and human to demonstrate the effect of scaling. *Source:* Carnes et al. (1996, p. 249), with permission.

What is the Biological Warranty Period on the Duration of Life?

Empirical evidence for the law of mortality implies not only that there is a characteristic age pattern of death for humans and other species, but also that there are biological forces that limit the duration of life of individuals and the populations they comprise. This does not mean that species and the individuals that comprise them have predetermined limits to the duration of life that are regulated by the equivalent of a biological clock with an alarm indicating when death should occur. Such a limit, if it existed, would require the presence of death genes driven by a genetic program *designed* by selection specifically for the purpose of causing organisms to age— an impossible scenario because selection does not operate in the post-reproductive region of the life span. Rather, we contend that the bodies of organisms are subject to biological warranty periods and limits on the duration of life much like automobiles that, in the absence of aging programs, also operate under warranty periods and a limited duration of use.

If most humans, on average, are biologically capable of living to 100 years or more (Oeppen and Vaupel, 2002), and if there are no biological reasons why death rates cannot decline to zero (Wilmoth, 2001), then there should be little evidence of significant functional decline or pathological anomaly among people living to the average survival times (75–80 years) that are already being attained today. According to Gompertz's law of mortality, the same logic should also apply to other species. To examine this issue, Carnes et al. (2003) partitioned the life courses of the mouse, dog, and human into biologically meaningful age windows and then compiled data on age–related changes in reproduction, physiological function, and the pathology observed at death in order to determine whether biological changes consistent with the effects of aging could be detected within these windows. The goal was to determine whether this biological evidence was more consistent with bodies capable of much longer survival than is currently observed, or with bodies that have approached or even surpassed (via medical interventions) the expiration date of their biological warranty periods.

The earliest age window examined was the reproductive period. For female mice the data demonstrate that indicators of physiological decline in reproduction (e.g., smaller litter sizes, lower pup survival, longer intervals between litters) were detectable at ages that were only one-third of the median age at death for the mouse strains examined (Fig. 6.4). Reproductive data for human females from a broad range of fertility and mortality backgrounds demonstrated that some girls as young as 9 years of age have given birth, and that by 35 years of age approximately 75% of the reproduction that will be accomplished by both women and men has been accomplished (Fig. 6.5). As with female mice, the reproductive age window for human females opens and closes at ages that are far younger than the life expectancy at birth currently achieved by women in low-mortality countries (80 years). In addition, this age pattern of female fertility is remarkably similar for high-mortality, low-mortality, and natural-fertility populations. These data suggest that, as with female mice, the reproductive biology of human females is well defined and follows a stable and highly predictable time course. If evolutionary theories of aging are correct, the temporal manifestations of aging

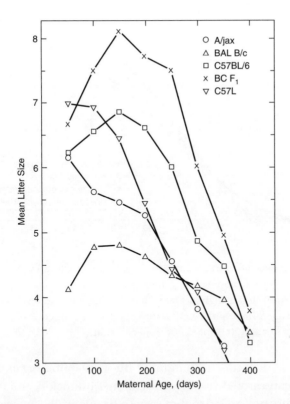

Figure 6.4. Mean litter size at birth plotted as a function of maternal age for four mouse strains (A/Jax, BALB/c, C57BL/6, C57L) and the hybrid (BCF₁) arising from a cross of the BALB/c and C57BL/6 strains. *Source:* Carnes et al. (2003, p. 35), with permission.

and the age distribution of death are intimately related to the reproductive biology of a species (Charlesworth, 1994; Holliday, 1996; Ellison, 2001). The largely immutable reproductive biology observed for female mice and humans and the predictable age patterns of their respective mortality are consistent with bodies that are subject to biological warranty periods.

The fertility data presented by Carnes et al. (2003) are for twentieth-century humans. Since many women today consciously delay their fertility, it is likely that the ages associated with specified levels of cumulative fertility for modern women are higher than those experienced by their ancestors. As such, the median age at death for humans from intrinsic causes estimated from the mouse model probably errs on the high side. Carnes et al. used intrinsic mortality as

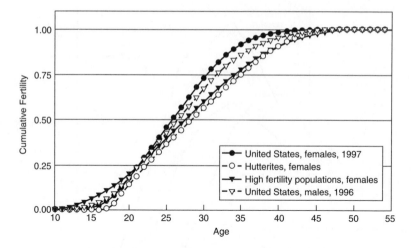

Figure 6.5. Age-specific fertility rates for U.S. males (1996) and females in a low-mortality/low-fertility population (United States, 1997), a natural-fertility population (Hutterites) and a high-mortality/high-fertility population (a composite of Mali, 1987; Niger, 1998; and Uganda, 1988) plotted as a function of age (in years). *Source*: Carnes et al. (2003, p. 37), with permission.

an endpoint in order to eliminate the contaminating influence of extrinsic causes of death (i.e., accidents, homicide, infectious and parasitic diseases, suicide) that vary so dramatically between populations (Shryock and Siegel, 1975). If humans adhere to the same relationship between reproduction and longevity as mice, then the predicted median age of death from intrinsic causes would be less than 100 years (see Table 6.1). Furthermore, because deaths from extrinsic causes can never be completely eliminated, a more realistic estimate of a biological warranty period (based on intrinsic mortality) for humans as predicted from the mouse model would be in the range of 85–95 years.

Next, Carnes et al. (2003) expanded the age window under examination to include the postreproductive period—a period of the life span that has typically been associated with a loss of functional integrity (Fries, 1980). For a wide range of physiological parameters derived from published studies of humans, it appears that approximately 80% of functional capacity is lost by age 80 (Harman et al., 2000). Significantly, this is an age that, when viewed in terms of life expectancy, has been achieved by only a few populations (i.e., among females in some parts of the world). Because there is no aging or death program, the age-dependent rate of loss of some but not all of

Table 6.1 Regression of Median Age at Death (MAD) for Intrinsic Causes of Death on Effective End of Reproduction (EER) Estimated from Mouse Data and Applied to Hypothetical Human Data

Human EER (years)	Human EER (days)	Human MAD (years)
32	11,680	81.8
34	12,410	86.9
36	13,140	92.0
38	13,870	97.0

MAD = 195 + 2.54 EER; R^2 = 0.44.
Source: Carnes et al. (2003, p. 37).

this functional capacity can be reduced with exercise, diet, and with medications (Bortz, 1982; Fiatarone and Evans, 1990). Nevertheless, the biological evidence is clear; the documented degradation of function (vital capacity) over time for numerous physiological parameters is consistent with bodies whose duration of functional existence is subject to biological warranty periods.

According to data on the species-specific pathology burdens observed at death from Carnes et al. (2003), there is incontrovertible evidence that age takes a severe toll on the bodies of mice, dogs, and humans. Laboratory animals surviving to the fourth quartile of the failure distribution (operationally defined as old age) experienced an increased burden of tumors that neither caused nor contributed to death, more pulmonary disease, and more frequent diseases of the skeleton. Using nothing more than this pathology profile, it was possible statistically to distinguish animals that died old from those that died young. Although death certificate data for humans are far less reliable than the pathology diagnoses available for laboratory animals, the pathology implications are no less conclusive. In humans dying over the age of 80, every organ system exhibits a greater burden of disease involvement (abnormal pathology) than is observed in humans dying before age 50. As with the reproductive and physiology data, humans have an age-related pathology burden that is consistent with bodies that are subject to biological warranty periods that limit the duration of life.

Empirical evidence suggests that biological warranty periods exist for the duration of life, even in the absence of biological programs that cause aging. Indeed, a program for aging is not even needed for aging to occur (Hayflick, 2002). What is required are biological programs for other attributes of the life spans of species that have, as an inadvertent by-product of their existence, imperfect mechanisms for maintaining and repairing the damage caused by the process of living. The presence of a warranty period for the duration of life represents the biological evidence that Gompertz and many other scientists in the past 170 years speculated must exist as the biological rationale supporting the presence of a law of mortality.

Projecting Life Expectancy Using Mathematical Models

Although demographers study populations, the results of their work are often used to make inferences about limits on the life spans of individuals. The basic logic is that if there is a limit to the life expectancy of a population, then limits must also exist for the life spans of the individuals who make up that population. Some researchers have argued that if low-mortality populations are approaching a limit to life expectancy, as claimed by some biodemographers (Olshansky et al., 1990, 2001; Carnes et al., 1996), then the approach to these limits should be reflected in the behavior of vital statistics. For example, populations approaching a limit should be characterized by a stagnation in the age trend of the oldest prevalent individual (Wilmoth, 1997). Critics of limit hypotheses also argue that limits imply that there must be an age beyond which there can be no survivors. Documented violations of both of these conditions have led some demographers to conclude that limits on human life expectancy either do not exist or are not yet in sight (Wilmoth, 1997; Oeppen and Vaupel, 2002).

Critics of a purely mathematical approach to the study of the human life span suggest that the validity of limit hypotheses cannot be ascertained without considering biological evidence on senescence (Carnes et al., 2003). Duration of life is an outcome variable for scientists in the demographic/actuarial sciences. However, from a biological perspective, duration of life is the product of a multidimensional process that involves behavioral, environmental, genetic, and random forces (Finch and Kirkwood, 2000; Carnes and Olshansky, 2001). As such, there is no defensible basis for the claim, based on purely mathematical models of mortality, that there are no biological or demographic reasons why death cannot decline to zero (Wilmoth, 2001) and that life expectancy at birth can rise to 100 years or more (Oeppen and Vaupel, 2002).

The regularity of the rise in human life expectancy during the twentieth century perceived by the advocates of mathematical extrapolation has led them to predict dramatic increases in life expectancy in the twenty-first century (Oeppen and Vaupel, 2002). However, the unprecedented life expectancy gains achieved during the twentieth century occurred primarily because of dramatic reductions in death rates among the young. Duplicating these gains in low-mortality populations is no longer possible because the lives of children can be saved only once. The advocates of mathematical extrapolation also ignore the biomedical significance of the profound shift that has occurred in the underlying causes of death. Historically, infectious and parasitic diseases (extrinsic mortality) caused the vast majority of deaths in humans. Heart disease, cancer, stroke, and diabetes (intrinsic mortality) dominate the mortality schedule today. Biologically, there is no reason to expect that these two fundamentally different categories of death should or would adhere to the same mortality trend.

Contrary to the perception of those advocating extrapolation methods for projecting life expectancy, the time frame from the past that has been used to predict the future is anything but representative of the historical mortality experience of humans. The quantum leap in life expectancy achieved over the past 100 years is an unprecedented anomaly in a human history better characterized by fluctuating (Olshansky and Carnes, 1997), stagnating, or slowly rising life expectancy (McNeill, 1976). Because the future course of mortality cannot possibly mimic such an episodic anomaly (characterized by declining early age mortality), this unusual time frame should not be used as the basis for predicting the future course of human life expectancy. The public policy implications of this recommendation are evident; it is essential that government agencies responsible for assessing the future solvency of their age-based programs incorporate biological reasoning into their long-term forecasts.

Death is a biological phenomenon of individuals, not a mathematical property of populations, and the biological evidence is undeniable. The pathology burden within individuals clearly exhibits an age dependence. Cancer and cardiovascular disease are symptoms of a complex underlying age-related pathogenesis that causes cells to lose functionality—a functionality that is necessary for the health and well-being of the individual. The molecular repair processes that maintain the functional integrity of cells also degrade over time. Managing the symptoms of age-related disease (geriatric medicine) is not the same as intervening in the underlying processes (biogerontology) that give rise to these manifestations (Hayflick, 2000; Carnes and Olshansky, 2001). Although evolution does not and cannot produce genetic programs for aging or death, forces of deterioration that exist at virtually all levels of biological organization (e.g., molecules, cells, tissues, organs) lead to the undeniable conclusion that there is a limit (expiration date) to how long (warranty period) an individual can live. Since every member of a population is operating under his or her own unique warranty period, it is equally impossible to deny that limits also exist for the life expectancy of populations.

Aging and death are predictable by-products of stable reproductive biologies that evolved under environments far less conducive to survival than those experienced today. Although it is likely that anticipated advances in biomedical technology and lifestyle modification will permit life expectancy to continue its slow rise over the short term, a repetition of the large, rapid gains in life expectancy observed during the twentieth century is extremely unlikely. Such gains would require an ability to slow the rate of aging (de Grey et al., 2002; Miller, 2002)—a technological capability that does not exist today and that, even if it did, would require implementation on a broad scale in order to have a measurable impact on the vital statistics of a population (Olshansky et al., 2001). As such, mathematical models that assume that the future course of life expectancy over the long term will continue the trend observed during the twentieth century are likely to fail because they ignore the underlying biology that influences the duration of life. Further, the predictions of extreme longevity (life expectancy of 100 years or more) produced by these models are not supported by the biological evidence.

The image of a biological warranty period for the duration of life has been used here to capture a universal and undeniable biological reality: indefinite survival is not possible, and the duration of life will remain limited by biological constraints even if every cause of premature death can be eliminated.

Conclusions

At its core, the fundamental biological explanation for why individuals senesce—which is the basic question asked by Gompertz in 1825 about the age pattern of death he observed for humans—is predicated on the importance of natural selection and its declining effectiveness relative to the timing and distribution of reproduction within the life spans of organisms. Applying these principles of evolutionary biology in order to explain age patterns of death among and between sexually reproducing species has come to be known as the *biodemography of aging*—a concept with historical roots in the search for a law of mortality (Loeb and Northrop, 1916; Brownlee, 1919; Pearl, 1921; Brody, 1924; Greenwood, 1928; Pearl and Minor, 1935; Deevey, 1947) and contemporary interdisciplinary research on aging (Carnes et al., 1992, 1996; Carnes and Olshansky, 1993; Olshansky and Carnes, 1994; Wachter and Finch, 1997). Although a vast number of genetically based biological processes that exist within organisms to sustain life and maintain functional integrity have been identified and characterized, senescence is not among them. A genetic program for aging is not required for animals to age, just as no program for aging is required for machines to experience degradation with time (Hayflick, 1994, 2000; Miller, 1999).

Although unknown to Buffon in the eighteenth century and to Gompertz in the nineteenth century, it is the underlying and invisible actions of genes that control and establish the predictability and temporal regularity of growth, development, reproduction, and physical form that led to their speculations on a fixed life span. After all, it does appear on the surface that life span is genetically programmed. Why else would mice tend to live 1000 days, dogs 5000 days, and humans 29,000 days. As it turns out, natural selection favored these life history traits and biological clocks as ways to ensure that genes, having acquired the property of immortality, are passed on through time (Dawkins, 1990). These biological phenomena were molded by the environments in which they arose. Their specific forms and functions were not actively designed in the same way that an engineer would draw the plans for creating a machine and then constructing it. Instead, the biological attributes of individuals that influence the duration of life are the product of a directionless and ongoing competition among preexisting genetic variants (alleles) whose "victors" are determined by their ability to propagate themselves.

From a biodemographic perspective, most of the rise in human life expectancy has come from saving children from infectious and parasitic diseases and reducing mortality in women during childbirth. These gains in life expectancy cannot be repeated in developed countries today because the reservoir of potential person-years associated with further declines in these causes of death has been nearly exhausted. Future gains in life expectancy will have to come from saving the lives of older people through the development and use of interventions that alter the fundamental processes of aging. Although this is not impossible, there are no interventions in existence today that have been demonstrated to modulate the rate of aging (Olshansky et al., 2002). Thus, if another quantum leap in human life expectancy is going to occur among today's population, future trends in mortality will have to be fundamentally different from those observed in the past.

Although Buffon and Gompertz lacked access to knowledge about evolution, Buffon's intuition that senescence and species-specific duration of life are related to a fixed period of growth and development, and Gompertz's prediction of a biological basis for a law of mortality, can now both be supported by evolutionary theory and biological evidence. This, in turn, establishes effective constraints on how long individuals can live and how high life expectancy and maximum life span can practically rise. Today, aging and death are viewed as the inadvertent but inevitable by-products of the degradation of biological structures and processes that evolved for growth, development, and reproduction rather than extended operation. These structural and functional constraints exist at every level of biological organization (cells, tissues, organs, and organ systems) within an individual, and it is their existence that imposes practical (i.e., probabilistic) limits on the life spans of individuals and the life expectancy of populations.

Acknowledgments

Funding for this work was provided by the National Institute on Aging (Grant Nos. AG-00894-01 and AG13698-01). Elements of this manuscript have been published in Carnes, B.A., Olshansky, S.J., and Grahn, D. (2003). Biological evidence for limits to the duration of life. *Biogerontology*, 4(1), 31–45; Olshansky, S.J., and Carnes, B.A. (2003). A journey through the interdisciplinary landscape of biodemography. In: Kessel, F., Rosenfeld, P., and Anderson, N., eds. *Expanding the Boundaries of Health and Social Science: Case Studies of Inter-disciplinary Innovation.* Oxford: Oxford University Press, pp. Olshansky, S.J.

(2003). From Michelangelo to Darwin: The evolution of human longevity. *Israel Medical Association Journal*, 52, 316–318, and Olshansky, S.J., Carnes, B.A., and Brody, J.A. (2002). A biodemographic interpretation of lifespan. *Population and Development Review*, 28(3) 501–513.

Note

1. The term *life span* was most often used in the historical literature as a single number intended to represent the expected duration of life of *every member of a species*. The concept of an average of individual life spans was antithetical, for it was believed that everyone had the same longevity potential, and that most people did not live up to their longevity potential because of poor lifestyles or accidental mortality. Thus, throughout history, the concepts of life span and maximum life span were identical.

References

Beard, R.E. (1959). Note on some mathematical mortality models. In: Wolstenholme, G.E.W. and O'Connor, M., eds. *The Lifespan of Animals*. CIBA Foundation Colloquia on Ageing, vol. 5. Boston: Little, Brown, pp. 302–311.

Benjamin, B. (1959). Actuarial aspects of human lifespans. In: Wolstenholme, G.E.W. and O'Connor, M., eds. *The Lifespan of Animals*. CIBA Foundation Colloquia on Ageing, vol. 5. Boston: Little, Brown, pp. 2–19.

Bodenheimer, F.S. (1938). *Problems of Animal Ecology*. Oxford: Oxford University Press.

Bortz, W.M. (1982). Disuse and aging. *Journal of the American Medical Association*, 248(10), 1203–1208.

Bourgeois-Pichat, J. (1978). Future outlook for mortality decline in the world. *Population Bulletin of the United Nations*, 11, 12–41.

Brody, S. (1924). The kinetics of senescence. *Journal of General Physiology*, 6, 245–257.

Brownlee, J. (1919). Notes on the biology of a life-table. *Journal of the Royal Statistical Society*, 82, 34–77.

Brues, A.M. and Sacher, G.A. (1952). Analysis of mammalian radiation injury and lethality. In: Nickson, J.J., ed. *Symposium on Radiobiology: The Basic Aspects of Radiation Effects on Living Systems*. New York: Wiley; London: Chapman & Hall, pp.

Buffon, G.L.L. (1749). *Histoire Naturelle, Générale et Particulière*. Paris: Imprimerie Nationale.

Carnes, B.A. and Olshansky, S.J. (1993). Evolutionary perspectives on human senescence. *Population and Development Review*, 19(4), 793–806.

Carnes, B.A. and Olshansky, S.J. (2001). Heterogeneity and its biodemographic implications for longevity and mortality. *Experimental Gerontology*, 36, 419–430.

Carnes, B.A., Olshansky, S.J., and Grahn, D. (1996). Continuing the search for a law of mortality. *Population and Development Review*, 22(2), 231–264.

Carnes, B.A., Olshansky, S.L., and Grahn, D. (1988). An interspecies prediction of the risk of radiation-induced mortality. *Radiation Research*, 149, 487–492.

Carnes, B.A., Olshansky S.J., and Grahn, D. (2003). Biological evidence for limits to the duration of life. *Biogerontology*, 4(1), 31–45.

Caughley, G. (1966). Mortality patterns in mammals. *Ecology*, 47(6), 906–918.

Charlesworth, B. (1994). *Evolution in Age-Structured Populations*, 2nd ed. New York: Cambridge University Press.

Clarke, R.D. (1950). A bio-actuarial approach to forecasting rates of mortality. *Proceedings of the Centenary Assembly of the Institute of Actuaries*, 2, 12–27.

Cornaro, L. (1903). Discourses on the temperate life. In: Butler, W., ed. *The Art of Living Long*. Milwaukee: W.F.Butler, pp. 77–90.

Cutler, R.G. and Semsei, I. (1989). Development, cancer and aging: Possible common mechanisms of action and regulation. *Journal of Gerontology: Biological Sciences*, 44(6), 25–34.

Dawkins, R (1990). *The Selfish Gene* Oxford, UK: Oxford University Press.

de Grey, A.D.N.J., Ames, B.N., Andersen, J.K., Bartke, A., Campisi, J., Heward, C.B., McCarter, R.J.M., and Stock, G. (2002). Time to talk SENS: Critiquing the immutability of human aging. *Annals of the New York Academy of Sciences*, 959, 452–462.

de Finetti, B. and Rossi, C. (1982). Bio-mathematical models of mortality. In: Preston, S.H., ed. *Biological and Social Aspects of Mortality and Length of Life*. Liege (Belgium): Ordina Editions, pp. 315–327.

Deevey, E.S., Jr. (1947). Life tables for natural populations of animals. *Quarterly Review of Biology*, 22, 283–314.

Economos, A. (1982). Rate of aging, rate of dying and the mechanism of mortality. *Archives of Gerontology and Geriatrics*, 1, 3–27.

Economos, A.C. (1985). Rate of aging, rate of dying and non-Gompertzian mortality-encore . . . *Gerontology*, 31, 106–111.

Elandt-Johnson, R.C. and Johnson, N.L. (1980). *Survival Models and Data Analysis*. New York: Wiley.

Ellison, P.T. (2001). *On Fertile Ground: A Natural History of Human Reproduction*. Cambridge, MA: Harvard University Press.

Fiatarone, M.A. and Evans, W.J. (1990). Exercise in the oldest old. *Topics Geriatric Rehabilitation*, 5(2), 63–77.

Finch, C.E. and Kirkwood, T.B.L. (2000). *Chance, Development, and Aging*. Oxford: Oxford University Press.

Fries, J.F. (1980). Aging, natural death, and the compression of morbidity. *New England Journal of Medicine*, 303, 130–135.

Gompertz, B. (1825). On the nature of the function expressive of the law of human mortality and on a new mode of determining life contingencies. *Philosophical Transactions of the Royal Society of London*, 115, 513–585.

Greenwood, M. (1928). Laws of mortality from the biological point of view. *Journal of Hygiene*, 28, 267–294.

Gruman, G.J. (1966). A history of ideas about the prolongation of life. *Transactions of the American Philosophical Society*, 56(9), 1–102.

Gumbel, E.J. (1954). Statistical theory of extreme values and some practical applications: A series of lectures. *National Bureau of Standards Applied Mathematics Series*, 33, 1–51.

Hamilton, W.D. (1966). The moulding of senescence by natural selection. *Journal of Theoretical Biology*, 12, 12–45.

Harman, S.M., Metter, E.J., Tobin, J.D., Pearson, J., and Blackman, M.R. (2000). Longitudinal effects of aging on serum total and free testosterone levels in healthy men. *Journal of Clinical Endocrinology and Metabolism*, 86(2), 724–731.

Hayflick, L. (1994). *How and Why We Age*. New York: Ballantine Books.

Hayflick, L. (2000). The future of ageing. *Nature*, 408, 267–270.

Heligman, L. and Pollard, J.H. (1980). The age pattern of mortality. *Journal of the Institute of Actuaries*, 107, 49–80.

Holiday, R. (1996). Endless quest. *Bioessays*, 18(1), 3–5.

Kessel, F., Rosenfeld, P., and Anderson, N. (2003). *Expanding the Boundaries of Health and Social Science: Case Studies of Inter-Disciplinary Innovation*. Oxford: Oxford University Press.

Kirkwood, T.B.L. (1977). Evolution of aging, *Nature*, 270, 301–304.

Kirkwood, T.B.L. (1992). Comparative life-spans of species: Why do species have the life spans they do? *American Journal of Clinical Nutrition*, 55, 1191S–1195S.

Kirkwood, T.B.L. and Holliday, R. (1979). The evolution of ageing and longevity. *Proceedings of the Royal Society of London B: Biological Sciences*, 205, 531–546.

Kirkwood, T.B.L. and Rose, M. (1991). Evolution of senescence: Late survival sacrificed for reproduction. *Philosophical Transactions of the Royal Society of London B: Biological Sciences*, 332, 15–24.

Loeb, J. and Northrop, J.H. (1916). Is there a temperature coefficient for the duration of life? *Proceedings of the National Academy of Sciences*, 2, 456–457.

Loeb, J. and Northrop, J.H. (1917a). What determines the duration of life in Metazoa? *Proceedings of the National Academy of Sciences*, 3, 382–386.

Loeb, J. and Northrop, J.H. (1917b). On the influence of food and temperature upon the duration of life. *Journal of Biological Chemistry*, 32, 102–121.

Makeham, W.M. (1860). On the law of mortality and the construction of annvity Tables. *Journal of the Institute of Actuaries*, 13, 325–358.

Makeham, W.M. (1867). On the law of mortality. *Journal of the Institute of Actuaries*, 13, 325–358.

Makeham, W.M. (1872). Explanation and example of a method constructing mortality tables with imperfect data; and of the extension of Gompertz's theory to the entire period of life. *Journal of the Institute of Actuaries*, 16, 344–354.

Makeham, W.M. (1889). On the further development of Gompertz's Law. *Journal of the Institute of Actuaries*, 28, 152–160, 185–192.

Makeham, W.M. (1890). On the further development of Gompertz's Law. *Journal of the Institute of Actuaries*, 28, 316–332.

McNeill, W.H. (1976). *Plagues and Peoples*. Garden City, NY: Anchor.

Medawar, P.B. (1952). *An Unsolved Problem of Biology*. London: Lewis.

Mildvan, A., and Strehler, B.L. (1960). A critique of theories of immortality. In: Strehler, B.L., Ebert, J.D., Glass, H.B., and Shock, N.W., eds. *The Biology of Aging*. Washington, DC: American Institute of Biological Sciences, Pub. No. 6, pp. 216–235.

Miller, R.A. (2002). Extending life: Scientific prospects and political obstacles. *The Milbank Quarterly*, 80(1), 155–174.

Miller, R.A. (1999). Kleemeier award lecture: Are there genes for aging? *Journal of Gerontology A, Biological Sciences*, 54(7), B 297–307.

Oeppen, J. and Vaupel, J. (2002). Broken limits to life expectancy. *Science*, 296(5570), 1029–1031.

Olshansky, S.J. (1988). On forecasting mortality. *The Milbank Quarterly*, 66(3), 482–530.

Olshansky, S.J., and Carnes, B.A. (1997). Prospects for extended survival: A critical review of the biological evidence. In: Caselli, F., and Lopez, A., eds. *Health and Mortality Among Elderly Populations*. Oxford, UK: Oxford University Press, pp. 39–58.

Olshansky, S.J. (2003). From Michelangelo to Darwin: The evolution of human longevity. *Israel Medical Association Journal*, 52, 316–318.

Olshansky, S.J. and Carnes, B.A. (1994). Demographic perspectives on human senescence. *Population and Development Review*, 20(1), 57–80.

Olshansky, S.J., Carnes, B.A., and Cassel, C. (1990). In search of Methuselah: Estimating the upper limits to human longevity. *Science*, 250, 634–640.

Olshansky, S.J., Carnes, B.A., and Désesquelles, A. (2001). Prospects for human longevity. *Science*, 291(5508), 1491–1492.

Olshansky, S.J., Carnes, B.A., and Grahn, D. (1998). Confronting the boundaries of human longevity. *American Scientist*, 86, 52–61.

Olshansky, S.J., Hayflick, L., Carnes, B.A., et al. (2002). Position statement on human aging. *Scientific American* (June), http://www.sciam.com/explorations/2002/051302aging/html. Also published in the *Journal of Gerontology: Biological Sciences*, 57A(8) (2002), B1–B6.

Pearl, R. (1921). A biological classification of the causes of death. *Metron*, 1, 92–99.

Pearl, R. (1922). A comparison of the laws of mortality in *Drosophila* and in man. *The American Naturalist*, 56, 398–405.

Pearl, R. and Miner, J.R. (1935). Experimental studies on the duration of life. XIV. The comparative mortality of certain lower organisms. *Quarterly Review of Biology*, 10, 60–79.

Pollard, J.H. and Streatfield, K. (1979). Factors affecting mortality and the length of life. Presented at the Joint Convention of the Institute of Actuaries of Australia, Christchurch, New Zealand.

Pollard, J.H. and Valkovics, E. (1992). The Gompertz distribution and its applications. *Genus*, 48, 15–27.

Ricklefs, R.E. and Scheuerlein, A. (2001). Comparison of aging-related mortality among birds and mammals. *Experimental Gerontology*, 36, 845–857.

Sacher, G.A. (1966). The Gompertz transformation in the study of the injury–mortality relationship: application to late radiation effects and ageing. In: Lindop, P.J. and Sacher, G.A., eds. *Radiation and Ageing*. London: Taylor & Francis, pp. 411–441.

Sacher, G.A. and Trucco, E. (1962). The stochastic theory of mortality. *Annals of the New York Academy of Sciences*, 96, 985–1007.

Shryock, H.S. and Siegel, J.S. (1975). *The Methods and Materials of Demography*, vol. 1. Washington, DC: U.S. Government Printing Office.

Stearns, S.C., Ackermann, M. and Doebeli, M. (1998). The experimental evolution of aging in fruitflies. *Experimental Gerontology*, 33, 785–792.

Wachter, K.W. and Finch, C.E. (Eds.). (1997). *Between Zeus and the Salmon: The Biodemography of Longevity*. Washington, DC: National Academy Press.

Weibull, W. (1951). A statistical distribution function of wide applicability. *Journal of Applied Mechanics*, 18, 293–297.

Weismann, A. (1891). *Essays upon Heredity and Kindred Biological Problems*. Oxford: Clarendon Press.

Williams, G.C. (1957). Pleiotropy, natural selection, and the evolution of senescence. *Evolution*, 11, 298–311.

Wilmoth, J.R. (1997). In search of limits. In: Wachter, K.W. and Finch, C.E., eds. *Between Zeus and the Salmon: The Biodemography of Longevity*. Washington, DC: National Academy Press, pp. 38–64.

Wilmoth, J. (2001). How long can we live? *Science debate* 2001. Available at http://www.sciencemag.org/cgi/eletters/291/5508/1491.

Wilmoth, J., Deagan, L.J., Lundstrom, H., and Horiuchi, S. (2000). Increase of maximal lifespan in Sweden: 1861–1999. *Science*, 289, 2366–2368.

7

The Metabiology of Life Extension

Michael R. Rose

The Darkling Plain

Despite hysteria on both sides, extending human life now seems about as difficult as building an atomic bomb in 1935. But unlike the atomic physicists of that time, who were motivated by the threat of Hitler, biologists generally are not inclined to develop the tools appropriate to the problem of extending human life. A few biologists have set about developing the tools required for such life extension, and they may yet triumph over the hostility of the National Institutes of Health, the medical establishment generally, and many of their religiously or politically biased allies. On the other hand, this lonely band of biologists could succumb to the Alice-in-Wonderland illusions of the anti-aging movement, with its dubious nostrums and raging optimism. What would be surprising is the success of any effort to extend human life substantially on this darkling plain, where benighted armies clash over biological ideologies. Surprising, but perhaps not impossible.

Here I will argue that the fundamental science of extending life is well developed in its theoretical and experimental foundations. Like atomic physicists in the period from 1935 to 1945, who had the option to create atomic weapons, we *could* accomplish significant life extension. The basic science is there. Whether or not we *will* is not my concern.

Irrespective of human aspirations, the scientific perception of aging and death has grown considerably more complex over the past decade. Old assumptions about the nature and pattern of aging have been exploded, with consequences as yet dimly perceived. It is my purpose to sketch some of the consequences for possible future life extension in a preliminary manner. It will be the work of the next few decades to improve on these preliminary sketches.

I will not weep or gnash teeth over the decline of former beliefs about life extension. There was an abundance of confusion and cross-purposes before. Much of this confusion was generated by the unfounded, not to say bizarre, notion that the duration of life—a complex quantitative problem—could be understood or manipulated using simplistic verbal concepts like species survival, loss of *program*, and so on. Now that life span data have gone far beyond these quaint ideas, we have to accept the need for theory appropriate to the problem. And not the least of these needs is a theory that can satisfactorily address the technical issues of life extension.

Here I outline what I consider the deepest, or if you prefer highest, biological issues inherent in life extension. These issues are essentially mathematical, and the relevant data are massively quantitative. But I will only hint at the mathematical and experimental development required to understand life extension fully. My hope is that the main quantitative themes of the field can be apprehended with a few graphs that emphasize the heuristic import of otherwise technically demanding findings.

To outline my argument, I begin with the most elementary facts about life, death, aging, and biological immortality. From there, I point out that we have theoretical tools that can make sense of these elementary facts. With the elementary facts and a few theoretical devices, I address the biological prospects for life extension.

Biological Immortality

Some demographers of sensitive disposition dislike the term *immortal*, but biologists have used it for some time to describe organisms or cells that do not undergo detectable aging. Reproductive cells have gone from one generation to the next, dividing and fusing, dividing and fusing, for hundreds of millions of years, yet still some demographers find that they can't countenance the term *biologically immortal.* Since this term already exists and has been used to describe a particularly interesting biological situation, it seems awkward to do away with it.

A similar situation existed with respect to the term *adaptation* in evolutionary biology in the 1980s. Adaptation is, of course, one of the most important ideas in biology, with origins in the work of Aristotle, the founder of academic biology. But ideological controversies arising over the application of evolutionary biology to human affairs, particularly by Richard Dawkins (e.g., 1976) and E.O. Wilson (e.g. 1975), led some Marxist evolutionary biologists, like R.C. Lewontin, to attack the use of the adaptation concept (e.g., Gould and Lewontin, 1979). Many biologists were intimidated by the ferocity and eloquence of this attack and retreated from the idea of adaptation. By the mid 1990's, the situation had become ridiculous, and most evolutionary biologists were fed up with being harangued for using the everyday terms of their discipline (Rose and Lauder, 1996).

Biological immortality is also a term that we can't do without. It must, of course, be distinguished from absolute, or mythological, immortality. All living things can die, and no professional biologist would suppose otherwise. But there still seems to be a profound difference between aging organisms that undergo a pervasive process of deterioration leading to death, irrespective of good living conditions, and those that do not, or no longer, undergo such a process.

There are some, especially in the gerontological community, who cling to the notion that aging affects all living things. Perhaps the core of this misunderstanding is the assumption that only aging can kill organisms kept in the laboratory. This is obviously not the case. Deleterious inherited mutations can kill organisms at any age or time. In addition, it is virtually impossible to keep organisms in the laboratory free of all diseases. Recondite viruses and bacteria will kill some organisms in laboratory cultures. Showing the absence of aging does not mean demonstrating the complete absence of death.

Instead, aging hinges on increasing mortality rates or declining fertility with respect to chronological age. That is, aging is about changing survival and reproduction. Aging can be defined as a persistent decline in the chance of survival or the chance of reproduction, even under the best conditions (Rose, 1991).

Given this definition, we can say what biological immortality means. It means generally flat rates of mortality and reproduction as a function of age. The best data of this kind known to me were collected by Martinez (1998), who studied mortality rates in *Hydra*, the aquatic animal that looks like a tiny tree. Martinez demonstrated convincingly that these organisms show no systematic increase in mortality rates over very long periods. Bell (1984) collected similar data in a few other small aquatic animals. Samples of some species showed aging, while other species did not. Significantly, the species that did not show aging reproduced without sex.

Aging is not a biological universal, and cases of biological immortality occur. This fact inspires great theoretical optimism about the project of life extension. If some organisms have biological immortality, then merely prolonging life is a much less daunting project.

Aging Organisms

I will continue with the mortality rate perspective on aging. If some organisms do not show steady increases in mortality rates with age, then aging organisms would simply be those that do show such increases. For some time, it was thought that aging species had increasing mortality rates throughout adulthood, an assumption embodied in the Gompertz equation for age-specific mortality

$$u(x) = A \exp(\alpha x), \tag{1}$$

where x is age, A is independent of age, and αx is age-dependent. The αx term produces an exponentially increasing mortality rate as a function of age, where the exponent is α. This equation has been fit to mortality data from a wide range of species (see, Finch, 1990).

The scientific sleight of hand in applying the Gompertz equation was twofold. Firstly, it had no theoretical justification whatsoever. It was merely a brute fact from curve-fitting. Secondly, the fit of the equation manifestly breaks down at early and very late ages. The lack of fit to early mortality has generally been known for a long time but was not of concern because juveniles were not supposed to be aging. (This is an assumption that we will return to.) The lack of fit to very late mortality was noticed first in human data (e.g., Greenwood and Irwin, 1939; Comfort, 1964; Gavrilov and Gavrilova, 1991). But human survival data are hard to interpret scientifically, given the confusing effects of wars and improvements in medical practice.

Things changed when two laboratories estimated mortality rates at very late ages in insects (Carey et al., 1992; Curtsinger et al., 1992).

Their findings were devastating. Carey and Curtsinger inferred that mortality rates either plateau or drop in late life. Subsequent studies have found this result again and again (e.g., Fukui et al., 1993; Vaupel et al., 1998; Drapeau et al., 2000).

The facts of death are shown in Figure 7.1. In the juvenile period, mortality rates fall or hold steady. They do not in any case show sustained increases. In the next phase of life, the aging phase, mortality rates increase exponentially, which looks like a linear increase on a logarithmic scale, the one used in Figure 7.1. In the third phase of life, mortality rates are roughly constant, though they tend to maintain a very high level. Organisms that reach such elevated ages can be said to be biologically immortal, in that they no longer age.

Broadly speaking, the difference between organisms that show aging and those that do not hinges on the existence of a protracted period of acceleration in mortality rates. This period of acceleration is flanked by two *plateau* periods in which mortality rates do not exhibit any consistent trends with respect to age. Organisms that don't age just have a single plateau that defines their mortality rates. The explanation of these facts is our next item of business.

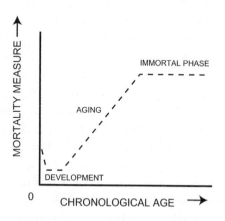

Figure 7.1. Mortality versus age. The mortality measure is a logarithmic function used to linearize mortality data that increases exponentially. At early ages, mortality is generally steady or declining. Throughout most of adulthood, logarithmic measures of mortality rates generally rise linearly, which supports the Gompertz model and similar models. Very late in life, mortality rates flatten with respect to age and sometimes even fall.

The Ultimate Cause of Mortality Patterns

There is an odd thing about causation in biology. When asked why a moth has two prominent yellow spots, one on each wing, an evolutionary biologist might answer "Because of selection for coloration that will scare birds away," while a developmental biologist will answer "Because of the production of a particular pigment during metamorphosis." Both will be right, and the evolutionary biologist will accept that, but the developmental biologist often won't.

Nothing is more puerile in aging research than the continuing search for a unifying general theory of aging among cell and molecular biologists. That theory has already been developed by evolutionary biologists. This theory construction took place in the period between 1940 and 1980, beginning with J.B.S. Haldane (1941) and P.B. Medawar (1946, 1952) and concluding with W.D. Hamilton (1966) and Brian Charlesworth (e.g., 1980). This theory is mathematically satisfying and coherent at the level of pure formalism. But that doesn't mean it's right.

It is more important that the evolutionary theory of aging has received a significant number of corroborations (reviewed in Rose, 1991) from comparisons of species and from experimental evolution. Though the evolutionary theory is not complete, for reasons that will be discussed here, it is the only credible contender for a general theory of aging. Put another way, just as Mendelian genetics is the best basis for the study of inheritance, even when it has to be amended, the evolutionary theory of aging has so far been the best basis for understanding aging and likely will continue to be.

At the center of the evolutionary theory of aging is the concept of the force of natural selection. To understand this force, let's start with natural selection. Natural selection, sometimes quickly but more often slowly, sifts genes in a way that usually increases the ability of organisms to survive and reproduce. This is fully analogous to the sorting action of the market, which usually rewards profitable firms over less profitable firms. Natural selection is evolution's steering mechanism, although it is important to bear in mind that it steers each population separately. Natural selection does not cosmically order all life on earth to one overarching plan.

Natural selection is an amazing thing, but it is not all-powerful. There are many circumstances where natural selection will be ineffectual. For example, if the environment changes rapidly, natural selection will not be able to keep up, resulting in species that are poorly suited to survive. The ecological changes that humans have produced in the past few centuries have produced a situation where large animals and plants, like whales and trees, have failed to adapt by natural selection. This has placed them in danger of extinction. When natural selection is too slow, survival and reproduction will be imperiled.

Older humans are somewhat like endangered whale species. Natural selection is weak where our health later in life is concerned. The source of this weakness can be understood in several ways. One way to think of it is to consider selection on a gene that kills everyone who has it. If that gene kills during childhood, it will be completely eliminated in a single generation. Natural selection is strong. But if it kills during old age, it will not be eliminated by natural selection, because the carriers of that gene have already finished reproducing. Their future survival doesn't matter for the transmission of their genes, good or bad. Natural selection is too feeble at advanced ages.

The evolutionary theory of aging explains the survival rates of Figure 7.1 as a result of this *weakness* of natural selection. When this weakness is low, as it is during childhood, mortality rates under ideal conditions are low. When it is high, mortality rates are high, even with the best of medical care. Hamilton (1966) first calculated the *force*, or strength, of natural selection. The concept of its weakness is a trivial inversion.

The weakness of natural selection is plotted in Figure 7.2. While this plot is crude, exact values for the force of natural selection can be calculated for any particular population, including human populations (e.g., Hamilton, 1966; Charlesworth, 1980). This figure shows how evolutionary biologists expect mortality rates under protected conditions to evolve to a first approximation. At early ages, natural selection is not weak, and mortality rates in laboratory or zoo populations are expected to be low—although not zero, because of other things that can cause death, such as genetic diseases (Tay-Sachs disease, cystic fibrosis, etc.). During the middle part of life, reproductive adulthood, natural selection becomes progressively weaker. This is expected to produce steadily increasing mortality rates, which we call *aging*, even under ideal conditions.

Finally, at the very end of life, the force of natural selection, and thus its weakness, reaches a plateau from which it does not budge.

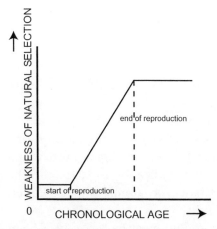

Figure 7.2. Because of the work of W.D. Hamilton, evolutionary theory expects that natural selection will not be weak before the start of reproduction in a population. After the start of reproduction, as shown, natural selection becomes steadily weaker. The shape of this curve is not necessarily linear, but it does rise steadily during the reproductive period of the population. Once reproduction has ceased, the weakness of natural selection reaches a stable maximum, from which it does not increase or decrease. Qualitatively, the curve plotted in this figure parallels that of Figure 7.1

After increasing steadily to its maximum, the weakness of natural selection doesn't increase further. This provides an explanation for the late-life mortality plateau of Figure 7.1, as has been shown in explicit simulations (Mueller and Rose, 1996), although the last word has still to be said about this part of the theory (cf. Charlesworth and Partridge, 1997; Pletcher and Curtsinger, 1998; Charlesworth, 2001). Evolutionary theory can explain the overall features of mortality rates, both with respect to aging and with respect to its cessation.

As a footnote to this theoretical discussion, evolutionary theory predicts that organisms that reproduce by splitting their bodies into two equal parts will not age. (This includes organisms as diverse as bacteria, sea anemones, juniper, and trembling aspen.) Natural selection favors the indefinite survival of such lineages, and the nonaging condition coincides closely with this vegetative reproduction (Rose, 1991). It does so because there is no adult phase of weakening natural selection. After the single reproductive act, two juveniles are recovered, with no adult to undergo aging. Natural selection stays in its first phase at all ages. These species always have biological immortality.

The Postponement of Aging

Given the seemingly arrogant claim of evolutionary biology to have figured out the basic theory for aging, it must be possible for evolutionary techniques to postpone aging fairly simply. Modern physics received its dramatic vindication in 1945, with the successful explosion of weapons based on atomic physics. Powerful theory should give powerful results.

And indeed, evolutionary biologists have been deliberately postponing aging since the 1970s (Rose, 1991). Almost all of these experiments have used the fruit fly *Drosophila*, but there have also been experiments with other insects (Tucic et al., 1996) and even mice (Nagai et al., 1990). These experiments have had one general feature in common: the increasing weakness of natural selection during adulthood is delayed over many generations by delaying the onset of successful reproduction. This effect of delayed reproduction on aging follows straightforwardly from the evolutionary theory, because delayed reproduction extends the first phase of natural selection, when it is strong. Once natural selection on adults has been strengthened, the experimenter metaphorically stands back and lets evolution increase the frequency of genes that postpone aging without controlling the specific genes involved. Evolution does the work.

A striking feature of these experiments is that there is apparently nothing that resists the postponement of aging in the experimental setting. In other words, the physiology of real animals does not forestall the extension of life. It may be difficult for quacks to extend life, but it is not difficult for evolution or for the biologists who control evolution.

Life extension could be as basic an application of biology in the twenty-first century as electricity was for the physics of the twentieth century. This does not mean that it was a trivial matter to make the twentieth century one that massively exploited electricity. It involved a huge amount of work, and electrical engineering continues to be one of the most important endeavors of our civilization. Life extension is a comparable task. The biological findings of today have as much potential for the extension of human life as research on electricity had for human technology.

The Metabiology of Life Extension

It is important to understand the fundamental possibilities before embarking on some wildly optimistic attempt to extend human life. That is, some overall scientific structure is needed for the task of extending human lives, like a relief map for a mountain-climbing venture. I will now offer some ideas concerning the fundamental biology of human life extension.

The first point is that conventional medicine has long been in the life extension business. Any number of modern medical procedures reduce mortality rates over more or less the whole spectrum of ages, from blood transfusion to repair of broken limbs. Such procedures have extended life, and the medical profession does not appear to be too chagrined about it. In terms of crude mortality-rate changes, this type of life extension is shown in Figure 7.3. Louis Pasteur, for example, had an impact on human survival of this kind. This type of mortality rate reduction no longer attracts the disapprobation of most theologians.

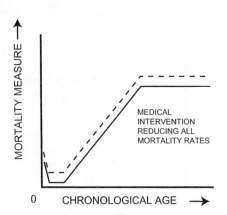

Figure 7.3. Mortality versus age plotted in the same way as in Figure 7.1. Normal mortality levels are plotted as a dashed line. Mortality levels after medical intervention are plotted as a solid line. Medical intervention can be thought of as life extension that is not age-dependent.

Other methods of changing mortality rates might be similarly considered in a practical vein. Since there is extensive evidence that associates earlier reproduction with increased mortality (Finch, 1990; Rose, 1991), a natural method of extending life would be to prolong the period of juvenility, perhaps by hormonal treatment. This is shown in Figure 7.4. This would allow extended periods of resistance to infection, cancer, and heart disease, as well as fostering the indefinite prolongation of education, which seems to be the goal of university educators everywhere. Perhaps the greatest problem facing this proposal is a lack of sizable graduate schools at which the endlessly juvenile might be warehoused. Since we academics have already adopted this lifestyle, we might be excused for any intemperate enthusiasm that we express for this approach to extending the human life span.

The type of proposal that seems to arouse the ire of some Christian theologians and a remarkably diverse range of political ideologues is the reduction in the rate of aging shown in Figure 7.5. It is, on the other hand, this type of proposal that sparks the enthusiasm of the anti-aging community. What both sides seem to neglect is the fact that this type of mortality rate intervention will have fairly minor effects on life expectancy. A large number of deaths will occur in a cohort of *slow agers* before there is much reduction in mortality rates at the later adult ages with this type of perturbation. Put another way,

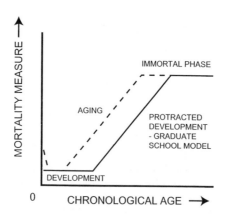

Figure 7.4. As in Figure 7.3, but with intervention extending the prereproductive period. This type of life extension gives more years, but no increase in the adult phase of life.

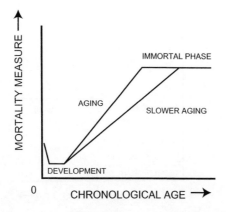

Figure 7.5. As in Figure 7.3, but with different patterns of aging labeled on the graph. With slower aging, the acceleration in mortality rates with adult age is reduced, leading to a shallower incline. Because the biggest changes in mortality rates occur at later ages, when many persons will have already died, this may be a less efficient way to extend life. Mortality rates rise to very high levels in any case.

anti-aging may not be a particularly good approach to the extension of life in terms of the number of years of additional life gained. On the other hand, face lifts are not particularly effective medical procedures for the recovery of youthful beauty, but their awkward evocation of such youth nonetheless attracts a significant clientele. Anti-aging may always have its devotees for this reason.

Recent research on the evolution of mortality, however, hints at the possibility of completely different approaches to the extension of the human life span. Since mortality rates normally plateau, and aging ceases, in cohorts preserved from exogenous death, what if that mortality plateau could be brought forward to earlier ages at earlier levels of physiological robustness? This possibility is diagrammed in Figure 7.6. It implies a kind of arrest in aging at some middle age, before the attainment of the very high mortality rates of individuals well past reproductive ages. Individuals who have been medically treated in this manner would no longer age. They would nonetheless suffer from an impairment in their ability to survive, depending on the age at which the arrest occurs. This idea was published some time ago, in the 1970 science fiction novel *One Million Tomorrows* by Bob Shaw. An interesting assumption in that novel is that the cessation of aging would require the termination of

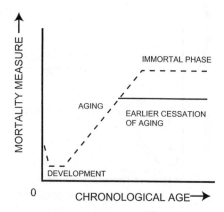

Figure 7.6. As in Figure 7.3, but in this case intervention takes the form of reducing the age at which the mortality rate stabilizes. This type of intervention reduces the period over which aging causes accelerating mortality.

reproductive function. Again, the data associating mortality with reproduction make this a tantalizing speculation. But we have no reason to accept such a connection between reproduction and immortality at this time.

Finally, Figure 7.7 proposes a type of mortality rate intervention that no one has discussed in print, to my knowledge: progressive con-

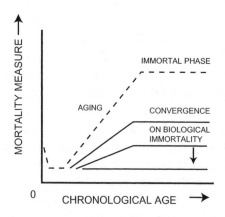

Figure 7.7. As in Figure 7.3, but in this case intervention both slows the rate of aging and terminates aging at an earlier age. If this intervention were progressively successful, the mortality pattern would converge on that of biologically immortal organisms.

vergence on biological immortality. It seems incredible to consider interventions that would both slow aging and reduce the age at which aging ceases. But data from my laboratory (Rose et al., 2002) indicate that we have been able to achieve the early stages of this transformation using evolutionary techniques applied to fruit flies. We have not fully eliminated aging, but we have both decelerated aging and reduced the level of mortality during the immortal phase of life, that is, when our flies are highly infirm but no longer aging. We already know that flies of this kind live a long time, and do so with remarkable retention of biological function.

What Can Be Done?

We have just considered a spectrum of scenarios for the extension of life. Most of these scenarios are attainable in laboratory animals by the combination of genetic, nutritional, and other interventions. Most of these interventions, unfortunately, are entirely impractical in humans. Massive genetic engineering of humans for an increased life span, a reasonable option in fruit flies, is a practically doubtful proposition in humans (Rose, 2000; Stock and Campbell, 2000). Nutritional restriction—that is, chronic dieting—reduces rodent mortality rates (e.g., Masoro, 1988), but it is unlikely to be adopted by the vast majority of people, who barely control their waistlines with the advent of middle age.

What is the practical situation with respect to postponing human aging using feasible methods? Like other parts of medicine, it seems to me that surgical and pharmaceutical interventions will be most important in any attempt to extend human life span. Of course, quack medications to postpone human aging have been around for millennia. The task before us is to consider whether modern biology and medicine can do better.

I think that the main barriers to past work on extending the life span were, on the one hand, magical thinking and, on the other, basic ignorance about the evolution of mortality rates. Magical thinking remains with us today, not just in the religiously inspired anti-aging interventions of traditional cultures, but also in credulous leaps from in vitro cell biology to the consumption of unproven nutritional supplements. Yes, substance X may prolong the growth of cells in culture, but that is no warrant to buy large quantities of a powder form of X and spread it on your salad. Despite the fact that the manufacture, distribution, and sale of such badly tested supplements is a billion-dollar industry, it has nothing to do with the future of life span extension—except perhaps as a monumental distraction from useful efforts to reduce mortality rates.

Biologists have more than their share of responsibility. It is our failure to solve the problems of life span extension that provided the opportunity for quackery, self-delusion, and magical thinking. At the core of the failure of biology to solve this problem was the focus on simple pathways of causation within cell and molecular biology. Such a focus works well for most features of functional biology because such things as eyes and kidneys are carefully built by natural selection. They are functional devices to be figured out by a kind of reverse-engineering detective work.

But the great increase in mortality rates brought about by aging is not a functional feature of organisms. It is instead a collapse of function brought on by the collapse in the strength of natural selection at later ages. As such, it has an evolutionary logic unlike that which cell and molecular biologists generally, and even most evolutionary biologists, are trained in.

Because later life is not a triumph of focused adaptation, its biology is a product of evolutionary accidents. Such accidents draw in many genes, because they are not focused by powerful selection. This makes the shaping of mortality in later life a function of *many* biochemical mechanisms, not a few. This does not preclude getting results from the manipulation of single pathways; such work has been a growth industry in aging genetics. But any assumption that such single pathways will control all aspects of aging is chimerical.

Fortunately, modern genomics has reached the point where it can study thousands of genes at one time. Even though we now know that aging is a many-headed monster (Rose and Long, 2002), we are also in a position to study just such biological problems with the new technologies that are available.

But the existence of this opportunity is very different from embracing it. Biologists like myself are always willing to perform another study in the endless quest for more information. And there are those who have an agenda that precludes effective life extension, people whose clamoring, imprecations, and grandstanding foster the temptation to focus on anchoretic research among biologists who would otherwise change the world.

References

Bell, G. (1984). Evolutionary and nonevolutionary theories of senescence. *American Naturalist*, 24, 600–603.

Carey, J.R., Liedo, P., Orozco, D., and Vaupel, J.W. (1992). Slowing of mortality rates at older ages in large medfly cohorts. *Science*, 258, 457–461.

Charlesworth, B. (1980). *Evolution in Age-Structured Populations*. London: Cambridge University Press.

Charlesworth, B. (2001). Patterns of age-specific means and genetic variances of mortality rates predicted by the mutation-accumulation theory of ageing. *Journal of Theoretical Biology*, 210, 47–65.

Charlesworth, B. and Partridge, L. (1997). Ageing: Leveling of the grim reaper. *Current Biology*, 77, R440–R442.

Comfort, A. (1964). *Ageing: The Biology of Senescence*. New York: Holt, Rinehart & Winston.

Curtsinger, J.W., Fukui, H.H., Townsend, D.R., and Vaupel, J.W. (1992). Demography of genotypes: Failure of the limited life-span paradigm in *Drosophila melanogaster*. *Science*, 258, 461–463.

Dawkins, R. (1976). *The Selfish Gene*. London: Oxford University Press.

Drapeau, M.D., Gass, E.K., Simison, M.D., Muller, L.D., and Rose, M.R. (2000). Testing the heterogeneity theory of late-life mortality plateaus by using cohorts of *Drosophila melanogaster*. *Experimental Gerontology*, 35, 71–84.

Finch, C.E. (1990). *Longevity, Senescence, and the Genome*. Chicago: University of Chicago Press.

Fukui, H.H., Xiu, L., and Curtsinger, J.W. (1993). Slowing of age-specific mortality rates in *Drosophila melanogaster*. *Experimental Gerontology*, 28, 585–599.

Gavrilov, L.A. and Gavrilova, N.S. (1991). *The Biology of Lifespan: A Quantitative Approach* London: Harwood.

Gould, S.J. and Lewontin, R.C. (1979). The spandrels of San Marco and the Panglossian paradigm. A critique of the adaptationist program. *Proceedings of the Royal Society of London B*, 205, 581–598.

Greenwood, M. and Irwin, J.O. (1939). Biostatistics of senility. *Human Biology*, 11, 1–23.

Haldane, J.B.S. (1941). *New Paths in Genetics*. London: Allen & Unwin.

Hamilton, W.D. (1966). The moulding of senescence by natural selection. *Journal of Theoretical Biology*, 12, 12–45.

Martinez, D.E. (1998). Mortality patterns suggest a lack of senescence in *Hydra Experimental Gerontology*, 33, 217–225.

Masoro, E.J. (1988). Food restriction in rodents: An evaluation of its role in the study of aging. *Journal of Gerontology*, 43, B59–B64.

Medawar, P.B. (1946). Old age and natural death. *Modern Quarterly*, 1, 30–56.

Medawar, P.B. (1952). *An Unsolved Problem of Biology*. London: H.K. Lewis.

Mueller, L.D., Nusbaum, T.J., and Rose, M.R. (1995). The Gompertz equation as a predictive tool in demography. *Experimental Gerontology*, 30, 553–569.

Mueller, L.D. and Rose, M.R. (1996). Evolutionary theory predicts late-life mortality plateaus. *Proceedings of the National Academy of Sciences USA*, 93, 15249–15253.

Nagai, J., Lin, C.Y., and Sasada, H. (1990). Selection for increased length of reproductive life in mice. *Theoretical and Applied Genetics* 79, 268–72.

Pletcher, S.D. and Curtsinger, J.W. (1998). Mortality plateaus and the evolution of senescence: Why are old-age mortality rates so low? *Evolution*, 52, 454–464.

Rose, M.R. (1991). *Evolutionary Biology of Aging*. Oxford: Oxford University Press.

Rose, M.R. (2000). Aging as a target for genetic engineering. In: Stock, G. and Campbell, J., eds. *Engineering the Human Germline: An Exploration of the Science and Ethics of altering the Genes We Pass to Our Children*. New York: Oxford University Press, pp. 49–56.

Rose, M.R., Drapeau, M.D., Yadzi, P.G., Shah, K.H., Moise, D.B., Thakar, R.R., Rauser, C.L., and Mueller, L.D., (2002). Evolution of late-life mortality in *Drosophila melanogaster. Evolution*, 56, 1982–1991.

Rose, M.R. and Lauder, G.V. (Eds.). (1996). *Adaptation*. San Diego, CA: Academic Press.

Rose, M.R. and Long, A.D. (2002). Ageing: The many-headed monster. *Current Biology* 12, R311–R312.

Shaw, B. (1970). *One Million Tomorrows*. New York: Ace Books.

Stock, G. and Campbell, J. (Eds.). (2000). *Engineering the Human Germline: An Exploration of the Science and Ethics of Altering the Genes We Pass to Our Children*. New York: Oxford University Press.

Tucic, N., Glicksman, I., Seslija, D., Milanovic, D., Mikuljanac, S., and Stojkovic, O. (1996). *Journal of Evolutionary Biology*, 9, 485–503.

Vaupel, J.W., Carey, J.R., Christensen, K., Johnson, T.E., Yashin, A.I., Holm, N.V., Iachine, I.A., Kannisto, V., Khazaeli, A.A., Liedo, P., Longo, V.D., Zeng, Y., Manton, K.G., and Curtsinger, J.W. (1998). Biodemographic trajectories of longevity. *Science*, 280, 855–860.

Wilson, E.O. (1975). *Sociobiology: The New Synthesis*. Cambridge, MA: Belknap Press.

8

Extending Human Longevity: A Biological Probability

Robert Arking

*I*f life is a good thing, then death calls too soon. Fables abound about the search for long life or immortality, and about the unforeseen effects such a gift might bestow. But that quest has now moved from myth to laboratory report, with the result that we as a society shall likely soon be faced with the prospect of being able to significantly extend our individual life spans. I am one of many engaged in this quest, and I think it is time to consider seriously what modern biogerontology is fashioning for us. Some have said that significant extension of the human life span is basically impossible, that it is unrealistic to think that we can conquer every one of the age-related diseases that break our bodies, and so a priori rule out the prospect. Others have seen life extension breakthroughs in every new vitamin, drug release, or discovery of the latest anti-aging gene, and perhaps their perennial optimism is the main component of their opinion. I believe these extreme positions to be both wrong and incapable of providing us with useful debating positions. In this chapter, I will lay out the scientific evidence that strongly suggests that longevity extension is presently a real if somewhat limited phenomenon in the laboratory but one that will move out into the larger society over the next generation.

How prescient should the reader consider this writer to be when discussing something that has not yet happened? The library is littered with failed prophecies. History may provide a guide. People have speculated on the possibility of human flight since time immemorial. The Montgolfiers' balloon ascents in 1793 nurtured these speculations, and the thought of human flight spread in the popular and technical press. More than a century passed before the Wright brothers made the first successful powered heavier-than-air flight in December 1903. But their success did not appear out of the blue. Theirs was the coolheaded and logical culmination of several decades of focused research on the problems of flight by men such as George Cayley, Otto Lilienthal, Octave Chanute, and Samuel Langley. By the end of the nineteenth century, serious students of aviation considered it to be physically possible for humans to fly in a powered aircraft. They did not believe they were chasing an illusion, and they succeeded in convincing hardheaded governments and wealthy patrons to sponsor the necessary experiments. By 1900, the solution was seen to involve developing the appropriate technology and engineering: what was the best way to control yaw, pitch, and roll while maximizing lift? Some, such as Langley, developed complicated and inefficient solutions. The Wright brothers, using their own funds, logically homed in on the problem and showed us how to fly. The study of biogerontology is today where aeronautical science was in 1900. Laboratory data have made some of us sure of attaining a goal that many skeptics once considered impossible, and although we know the general problems that need to be solved, we are still unsure of the exact methods by which these interventions in the aging process can best be achieved. The Wright brothers of biogerontology are likely out there working in a lab someplace, yet to make their accomplishment known.

The Problem

Let us first define some terms so that we know what we are talking about. We are most definitely *not* talking about immortality. There are both theoretical and practical reasons why immortality is not possible, and I bring it up only to rule it out of bounds. We are *not* talking about a simple extension of the human life cycle as we know it today. The elderly are healthier today than in the past (Manton and Gu, 2001), and the number of centenarians will increase in the near future for various demographic reasons (Vaupel, 1997). This is likely a good thing, but there seems to be little enthusiasm among laypeople for using science to allow them to become even older and more frail elders and even less scientific reason for thinking such an outcome is feasible or desirable.

What *is* both biologically feasible and socially desirable is the doubling of the human *health span*. We are generally at our healthiest during the period from 20 to 55 or so. Teenagers may be stronger and more resilient than their parents, but they suffer from raging hormones and unformed minds. And increasing numbers of us begin to suffer from the ravages of age-related diseases once we enter our late 50s or early 60s, although this transition varies greatly from individual to individual. So if we designate the 35-year period from age 20 to 55 as our health span, then our practical task is the doubling of our health span to a 70-year period covering the ages from 20 to 90. To slow the rate of aging so that we will be as physically and mentally alert at age 90 as we are today at age 55 strikes me and others as a desirable goal. The senescent or aging period would likely not be affected and would be about the same in both length and degree as that which we now experience from the ages of 55 to 85 years or so. This limited goal has the virtues of being consistent with both biological theory and data; we have already accomplished this task with laboratory animals. The attainment of this goal by multiple laboratories using different systems can be interpreted as a robust proof of the principle that longevity can be significantly increased via a doubling of the health span. As Yogi Berra might have said, "It's 1900 all over again."

good concept

It is a fact that there was an extraordinary increase in life span in the United States during the twentieth century. Why then hasn't the health span increased as well? And what does that failure have to say about the validity of this chapter? In the United States, white women in 1900 had an average life span of 48 years and a maximum life span of 103 years, while in 2000, white women had an average life span of 87 years and a maximum life span of 118 years. This 40-year difference in average life span did not come about because of scientific advances in anti-aging medicine. It began with the elimination by mid-century of the 24% prepuberty mortality characteristic of the 1900 cohort. These young girls, no longer killed by accidents or infectious diseases, now survived and died as old ladies of various age-related diseases. This decreased mortality was initially due to the widespread development of good public health measures (i.e., sanitary sewers and drinking water installations) during the 1920s, and only later to antibiotics and improved medical care. This illustrates an important point: our individual survival and longevity fundamentally depends on the health practices of the entire society. We do not survive by ourselves alone. During the second half of the twentieth century, we saw the same deferred mortality affecting middle-aged women as better medical treatment coupled with an increased awareness of what constituted a healthy lifestyle allowed them to survive the heart attacks and other ills that would otherwise have taken their lives. The elderly became more healthy as the century's decades rolled past, they are more physically and mentally independent than their parents were, and they are now surviving longer than ever. Since there are more of them, the probability of some proportion of them surviving for more than a century increases as well, and so the increase in maximum life span is mostly the result of their increased numbers. But none of these social and medical interventions had the slightest effect on the aging process. A healthy 65-year-old in 1900 would be physically indistinguishable from his or her counterpart in 2000. The fact that there are more of them today than yesterday stems solely from the fact that the past century's efforts were devoted to reducing early or premature mortality. If you do not die young, then you can live to be old. And you will still age in the same way as humans have throughout history. Other than the concept of prevention, nothing that was done in the past century could have had any effect on extending the human health span—nor did it. Altering the health span turns out to require substantial knowledge about the aging process.

The Aging Process

So, why do we age? Or as the Nobel laureate Francois Jacob wrote, "It is truly amazing that a complex organism, formed through an extraordinarily intricate process of morphogenesis, should be unable to perform the much simpler task of merely maintaining what already exists" (1982, p. 50). His implicit question comes in two parts. First is the longtime philosophical poser: why do we age? Second is the mechanistic consideration: how do we age? In the terminology of Ernest Mayr, one of the founders of modern biology, the first component addresses the nature of the ultimate process, while the second component addresses the details of the proximate mechanisms (1961). Thus, our answer to Jacob must involve a bipartite answer because our understanding of the mechanistic processes of aging depends crucially on our understanding the biological reason as to why we age.

"Nothing in biology makes sense except in the light of evolution." This famous statement by the well-known geneticist Theodosius Dobzhansky is again verified by the study of aging (Dobzhansky et al., 1977). The operation of natural selection means that some genetic variants of any population will be more successful (i.e., leave more copies of their genes in the next generation) than other variants, and these variants will be thereby favored. Most known populations are structured by age; that is, the population is composed of individuals of different age classes that each represents a different proportion of the population. The high mortality rates caused by predation, illness, and accidents that are common among wild populations of animals mean that only a few, if any, individuals survive long enough to show signs of aging and senescence. Thus, in any wild population, there are many more young breeding adults than old adults, and in each generation the genetic contributions to the next generation come predominantly from young adults. One consequence of this age structure is that deleterious genetic variants that act late in life (to produce cancers, for example) will not be selected against by natural selection; their carriers will likely either have died from environmental hazards before reaching old age or else will have survived but as postreproductive adults. In either event, they are not contributing genes to the next generation and so are invisible to the operation of natural selection. Another consequence is that favorable genetic variants with the potential, for example, to delay the onset of senescence and extend longevity will not be selected for because these variants are expressed only in those few surviving postreproductive individuals who are also invisible to the operation of natural selection (Rose, 1991).

From an evolutionary point of view, the name of the game is to play again (i.e., the whole point of being a reproductive adult is to pass copies of your genes to the next generation). This is a game that no one can win but anyone can lose simply by failing to transmit sufficient copies of one's genes to the next generation. For a wild population, there is no evolutionary value in any trait—including extended longevity—if that trait does not materially assist in playing the game. Evolutionary value exists in living long enough to reproduce, but there is usually no increased reproductive (i.e., Darwinian) fitness associated with living so long that one is postreproductive (Mayr, 1961).

But we live so long already; then why are we not capable of reproducing and living much longer that we do now? Why is our health span not longer? The answer involves energy. Organisms must channel and apportion their energies to the broad categories of reproductive activities versus the maintenance and repair of their bodies. Although the energy cost of making an egg or a sperm probably stays more or less constant over time and is likely the same for both young and old, this is not the only energy cost involved in reproduction. The energy costs of courtship, pregnancy, and child rearing are high and represent a significant investment of energy by the organism. In addition, as every weary parent knows, some energy must be devoted to the repair and maintenance of the body if the organism is to survive reproduction. It is reasonable to assume that even a well-fed organism has only a limited amount of energy available. Thus, the problem facing the organism is how best to allocate its finite amounts of metabolic energy to maximize both reproduction and repair.

Thomas Kirkwood (1987) did a theoretical analysis that showed that increasing the amount of energy expended on bodily repair results in increased survivorship but decreased fecundity, and vice versa. It is not possible to maximize both outcomes simultaneously. (Think of maximizing simultaneously both savings and spending within your family budget.) A choice must be made. Repair requires more energy than reproduction. Thus, allocating sufficient energy to maximize repair will reduce fecundity and thereby decrease the organism's Darwinian fitness. In most cases, decreased fecundity over a longer life span yields fewer copies of an individual's genes in the next generation than does higher fecundity over a shorter lifetime. On the other hand, increasing fecundity will decrease the energy available for repair and likely result in shortened longevity. Since maximizing Darwinian fitness is the operative principle of natural selection, wild populations normally maximize fitness and thereby inevitably set their repair processes at some level lower than that required for a very long period of bodily repair. Hence we age and die. It is easy to see why this theory was named the *disposable soma* theory. Let us not mystify it. This process is nothing more than the cost–benefit analysis most of us have made when faced with the decision of whether to continue to invest our hard-earned money in repairs of the old car or in the purchase of a new car. At some point, the cost of repairs exceeds the cost of purchase, and so the old car is junked and a new one obtained.

Given that we modern humans have a very low and culturally controlled reproduction, it is reasonable to question whether this disposable soma theory still applies to us. Yes it does, for we evolved under its aegis, and the control mechanisms of the body that set fitness and repair levels are not reversed by one century of nonheritable demographic change. The concept provides us with a plausible mechanism by which evolution can act, and which has shaped us into what we are today. And, of course, Shakespeare foresaw this relationship and gave it to us in Sonnet 12:

> When I do count the clock that tells the time,
> and see the brave day sunk in hideous night; . . .
> Then of thy beauty do I question make,
> That thou among the wastes of time must go, . . .
> And nothing 'gainst Time's scythe can make defence
> Save breed, to brave him when he takes thee hence.

And so we age, not because of some philosophically satisfying cosmic reason that requires our senescence and death, but simply because the body's energy allocations are such that our failure to repair ensures that there is no reason not to age. This biological conclusion may seem dark and despondent to some. Who, after all, wants to believe that his or her death serves no larger purpose at all? The major religions of the world are based on the opposite premise. I, however, find it liberating. Jacob compared embryonic development to adult aging and saw a paradox. What biogerontologists see today is the fact that there is no evidence for the existence of a genetically based aging program. We do not have an organismal death program built into our genes. *We are not required to age.* And if we age only because there is no biological reason for us not to age, then this clearly implies that we need not age (or at least not age so quickly) if we can supply our bodies with a relevant biological reason not to age. It is the business of we biogerontologists, then, to provide these reasons.

The Laboratory Interventions

So, then, how good are our reasons? One obvious limitation of the laboratory record is that there are no human data: one cannot experiment on humans for both ethical and practical reasons. There are four species of multicellular animals that constitute most of the recent research into longevity extension (Weindruch, 1995). Two of these *model systems*—the mouse and the rat—are mammals commonly used in biomedical research. The other two are invertebrates much beloved of geneticists—the fruit fly and the worm. (The latter is not the earthworm one sees coming up for air after a heavy rain has soaked the lawn; rather, it is a very small (956 cells altogether) nematode worm that eats bacteria and has been developed over the past quarter century to the point where it is an exquisite genetic tool.) The mouse, fruit fly, and worm are extraordinarily well known genetically and thus lend themselves to modern genetic investigations. The rat has been well studied physiologically and its genome is now being sequenced, which will add depth to the physiological knowledge. Some labs focus on the use of in vitro cell cultures to investigate the biology of the individual cells of the mammalian organism. Is it not reckless to extrapolate from such a limited basket of dissimilar laboratory animals to humans? If the proper study of mankind is man, then why are we studying flies and worms? Of course, part of the answer is that they are cheap to raise in the laboratory (money is important) and they do not live very long (time is important). But the most important reason is that the genes each of them carry are homologous to the genes we carry and often have similar, if not identical, functions. For example, some 62% of the genes that are known to cause human diseases are known to exist in flies and to give rise to similar disorders when mutated (Banfi et al., 1966). The same genes that control the segmentation and organization of the fly embryo control the segmentation of the human (consider your vertebrae and ribs as evidence of your segmented nature). The genes now known to play various roles in animal aging are known to be operative in humans and seem to play similar roles. By investigating these model organisms, we investigate ourselves by proxy. The tricky part is to be able to translate the findings appropriately from mice, flies, and worms into insights relvant to humans, who are more complex than any of the model systems.

Patterns of Aging

One important similarity is that all these organisms probably age in the same three ways (Arking et al., 2002). Compared to their normal-lived controls, experimental animals can live long by (*1*) increasing their early survival rate, (*2*) increasing their late survival rate, or (*3*) delaying the onset of senescence. The first two longevity patterns are conceptually interesting but are dead ends so far as our goal of doubling the human health span is concerned. Each of these patterns of longevity extension suffers from the fact that, while they decrease the mortality rate at either the beginning or end of life, they do not affect the basic aging rate. The organisms age normally, but they seem to be somewhat more resistant to the various stresses that kill off their normal comrades. Exercising humans have higher early and midlife survival and a lower level of morbidity; they age, however, in a normal fashion and show no real decrease in late-life mortality. Centenarians, on the other hand, seem to have a higher late life survival rate, but though they have lower rates of morbidity and mortality, no one would mistake a centenarian for a middle-aged person. They have aged in a normal fashion but are a bit healthier than their normal fellows. Their health span is not affected, only their late-life mortality. These two extended longevity patterns are not useful clues for us to use in the attainment of our goals.

The most interesting alteration involves the third type, the delay in the onset of senescence. There are many examples of this pattern in animals but none in humans. Yet this is the one we want. This is the pattern that doubles the health span of our laboratory model systems. In Figure 8.1, I have graphed the survival curves of normal- and long-lived fruit flies created in our laboratory by means of artificial selection for increased longevity (Dudas and Arking, 1995; Arking et al., 2000). It is clear that both the mean and maximum life span values of the long-lived experimental strains are shifted to the right relative to the normal-lived controls. If we assume that the flies' health span covers the period of time from birth until 10% of the initial population has died, then the low mortality and high survival characteristic of the first 30 days of the normal-lived animals' life span has been extended so that it now spans the first 60 days of the long-lived animals' life span. The health span has been doubled but the senescent period occupies the same length of time (~35 days) in both strains, and thus a smaller proportion of the maximum life span

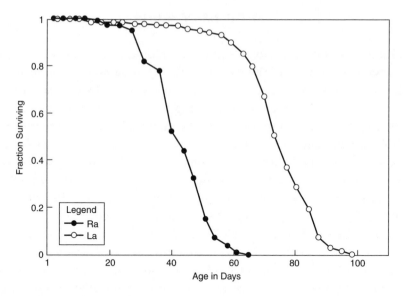

Figure 8.1. Survival curves of normal-lived control flies and of the long-lived experimental flies derived from them by selectively allowing only the longer-lived experimental animals of each generation to breed. Over the course of 21 generations, this artificial selection regime led to the creation of flies with significantly extended longevity. *Source:* redrawn after Arking et al., 2000.

in the long-lived flies. These data demonstrate that the health span and the senescent span are two separate phases of the life span, and that longevity extension via health span doubling is possible. Similar kinds of delayed-senescence, extended-longevity survival curves are seen in animals that have been put on a stringent diet, or have genetic changes that give them the ability to defend themselves better against the effects of oxidative stress, or have other sorts of genetic changes that shift their metabolism so that it focuses on repair rather than reproduction. The fact that each of the model organisms can express this delayed-senescence, extended-longevity pattern strongly suggests that the potential to double the health span is already built into each species, including mammals. Our task is not to introduce alien mechanisms into organisms but rather to discover how to activate the already existing longevity mechanisms effectively and safely. In this sense, what we are doing is natural.

What would be the outcome of such knowledge? If one projects a survival curve for contemporary U.S. women on the simplifying assumption that they would follow the same survival and mortality kinetics as do our delayed-onset-of-senescence fruit flies, then there would be no real decrease in survival (and therefore no increase in age-related mortality) until the age of about 102 years. The 82-year health span in this projected population is double that of the 41 years characteristic of contemporary normal-lived humans. If we can understand the mechanisms in the fly that delay the onset of senescence and then make them happen in humans, we will have achieved our goal. Doubling the health span in these laboratory organisms is perhaps akin to the Wright brothers' early experiments with unpowered flight in the gliders that preceded their historic achievement.

Is it realistic to believe that the extension of longevity in laboratory organisms foretells a comparable achievement in humans? All of the genes known to be involved in delaying the onset of senescence in our laboratory model systems are known to have homologues in humans. This implies that the relevant mechanisms are already in place. One concept that has been well established by the molecular and genomic revolutions in biology is that cellular processes are highly conserved across species and kingdoms. The obvious diversity of life on earth masks but does not obscure the fact that living forms share the same basic genomic, metabolic, and regulatory mechanisms. In light of this fact, it seems reasonable to conclude that the present failure to induce the delayed-senescence, extended-longevity pattern in humans represents a transient limitation of our knowledge rather than a permanent limitation imposed by human biology. So the question now becomes one of understanding the biological mechanisms that regulate this delayed-senescence, extended-longevity pattern and deciphering the cellular signals that control its expression by the organism.

Mechanisms of Aging

In the early days, biogerontology had little data and lots of theories. As the amount and quality of hard data have increased, the multiplicity of theories has been decreased to a small handful of robust biological mechanisms that each play some role in regulating the aging process. The two most important general mechanisms that are known to generate a delayed-senescence, extended-longevity pattern in one or more of our laboratory models are (1) resistance to oxidative stress and (2) metabolic changes. Let us briefly summarize the findings supporting each of these mechanisms.

Oxidative stress. We need oxygen. Without it, we cannot generate enough energy to live and we quickly die. But the oxygen that keeps us alive is a double-edged sword, for it can also break down within the cell to yield highly chemically reactive molecules of various kinds collectively termed *reactive oxygen species* (ROS) or, less accurately, *free radicals.* These reactive molecules combine chemically with any of the cell's components and transform them into oxygen-based damage products. This structural transformation of the molecules alters their function, usually for the worse. The damage process usually entails the generation and release of another ROS molecule, and so the destructive process continues to rampage throughout the cell until it is actively stopped by some *antioxidant* molecule. This destructive process is generally referred to as *oxidative stress.* In lay terms, one might envision the cell as undergoing something akin to a self-perpetuating rusting.

The oxygen we breathe in is transported to a subcellular organelle called the *mitochondrion,* located inside every cell. Here it is used in the final stages of converting the energy in our food to a form of chemical energy useful to the cell. Depending on their energy needs, cells might have from 10 to several hundred mitochondria per cell. Since most of the cell's oxygen is located in these mitochondria, this is where most of the cell's ROS are generated. And unfortunately, the nearest targets for these highly reactive ROS molecules are the lipid membranes and protein enzymes that compose the mitochondrion itself. These components can be repaired. But the mitochondrion is unique in that it is the only animal cell organelle to have its own genetic system. The 1 to 10 mitochondrial DNA molecules in every mitochondrion are very vulnerable to oxidative damage, and this damage cannot be repaired. Damaged mitochondria are less effective at producing useful energy, and they soon become almost nonfunctional. These damaged mitochondria are not repaired or recycled by the cell but instead simply accumulate. Eventually the resulting energy shortage inhibits the cells' normal functioning, and the tissues begin to show the functional loss characteristic of aging. It is likely this process that underlies the old observation that a good young athlete can beat a good old athlete any time. This particular process is known as the *Mitochondrial Free Radical Theory of Aging,* and it has been observed in both laboratory model systems and humans (Harman, 1994; de Grey, 1999).

Organisms contain a very elaborate system with which to defend themselves against the depredations of oxidative stress. This system seems to be reasonably effective at getting rid of most (but not all) of the ROS molecules that are generated in young animals and thereby keeping the level of oxidative stress to some low (but measurable) level. Eventually the failure to repair completely causes increasing inefficiencies in the body's antioxidative stress defense mechanisms. This then allows oxidative stress and cell damage to increase at a compound rate, and the age-related loss of function soon becomes apparent. This process has been speeded up in mutant flies (Phillips et al., 1989), worms (Honda and Matsuo, 1992), and mice (Melov et al., 2001) in which the antioxidative stress defense genes were made inactive. Such mutant organisms aged and died very quickly. The mice exhibited systemic failures similar to these observed in various age-related diseases. It occurred to many investigators that perhaps one could extend the organism's health span by increasing the level of its antioxidative stress defense mechanisms. Genetic engineering techniques were used independently by several laboratories to introduce extra copies of certain of these defense genes into otherwise normal flies (Orr and Sohal, 1994; Parkes et al., 1998; Sun and Tower, 1999). The flies now lived longer, displaying a delayed-senescence, extended-longevity pattern. Equally interesting was the observation derived from our selection experiments, in which a normal-lived population gave rise eventually to long-lived descendants by breeding only the longer lived flies of each generation. After some 22 generations, the descendants had a much higher level of antioxidative stress defenses, a lower level of oxidative damage, and lived long via a delayed onset of senescence (Dudas and Arking, 1995; Arking et al., 2000). When challenged, the flies really did turn on their antioxidative stress defenses and aged more slowly. The geneticists' logic was followed by the flies themselves. Other experiments showed that certain mutants in nematode worms also up-regulate (i.e., turn on to a higher degree) certain antioxidative stress defense genes—the same ones as are operative in the fly—and the resulting worms also live long via a delayed onset of senescence (Larsen, 1993; Taub et al., 1999). However, using genetic engineering techniques to insert extra copies of these same oxidative stress defense genes into mice has not yet resulted in creating an extended longevity pattern in those animals (Huang et al., 2000), although these genes can be turned on by caloric restriction (see below). There appears to be some qualitative difference between mice and the other laboratory models in this regard. I suspect that it has to do with the richer and more complex control and regulatory processes operative in mammals relative to the invertebrates; a more complex control system may well require a more sophisticated type of intervention.

The overall conclusion seems to be that appropriate enhancement of the antioxidative stress defense genes, and thus of their protein products, is capable of significantly delaying the onset of senescence in some model organisms and thereby leading to a significant extension of the organisms' health span.

Metabolic changes. The first intervention known to delay the onset of senescence in mammals and significantly increase the health span was reported in 1934 (McCay et al., 1934). Reducing the number of calories in the animal's diet by about 40% while keeping the different nutrients at normal levels results in extraordinarily healthy, long-lived mice and rats (and flies and worms as well) (Yu, 1994). These findings have been replicated hundreds of times and are probably the most robust experimental findings in the field. Similar experiments are underway in primates such as macaque monkeys, and while these long-term experiments are still in progress and thus incomplete, the available data suggest that a similar response may be happening in primates. No human experimental data exist, but it is a common finding that there are no obese centenarians.

Caloric restriction radically changes the animal's metabolism such that it becomes a physiologically different organism from its normally fed sib. Many, perhaps all, of these differences can be attributed to a shift in the animals' functions from growth and reproduction to repair. The calorie-restricted animals age more slowly and maintain their tissue integrity well into old age; the molecular signaling systems that underlie the cells' functioning are likewise maintained; the animals' progression of age-related diseases (including cancers) is greatly retarded; they have a greater degree of protection against exogenous carcinogens and a more effective immune system; and they show either a significant delay or a complete elimination of the onset of many normal age-related pathologies. Not only do such calorically restricted animals age much more slowly—their survival curves are similar to those of the long-lived flies shown in Figure 8.1—but they also stay physically healthier and mentally active much longer than their normally fed controls. On the other hand, calorically restricted animals grow more slowly than normal and are less fecund than normally fed animals; this presumably represents the trade-off in energy allocation brought about by this dietary regime.

Why not apply this simple and proven regimen to humans? Various attempts have amply demonstrated that the overwhelming majority of people in Western society will not willingly undergo a 40% reduction in caloric intake even when the trade-off might be extended longevity. Therefore, we need to understand the cellular processes underlying the body's response to caloric restriction if we wish to induce its expression by other means.

Insulin is a protein hormone that plays a vital role in regulating the cell's response to glucose. Insulin and the subcellular signaling system associated with it are not unique to humans but are widespread in animals, being found even in species where molecules different from but similar to insulin are used instead. This insulin or insulin-like signaling system (ISS) is thought to play a major role in the organism's response to caloric restriction. Decreasing the intake of calories has the effect of partially repressing the activity of the ISS. If one uses mutations to inactivate components of the ISS and thus bring about a genetically based repression of the ISS, one finds that the mutated flies and worms live long and express a delayed onset of senescence (Braeckman et al., 2001; Clancy et al., 2001; Tatar et al., 2001). The molecular basis for the apparent ability of the ISS to bring about a shift in the body's emphasis from growth to repair lies in the fact that the subcellular signaling system controlled by the insulin molecule eventually results in the activation or repression of two diametrically opposed sets of genes. One set includes the same antioxidative stress defense genes discussed above, and the other set includes genes that bring about the rapid bodily growth and high reproductive rate of the organism. When the ISS is activated by high amounts of insulin in the blood (the results of a high-caloric diet), the antioxidative stress defense genes are repressed and the progrowth genes are activated. The animal grows quickly, is highly fecund, and dies young. When the ISS is repressed because there are low amounts of insulin in the blood (the results of caloric restriction), the defense genes are activated and the growth genes are repressed. The animal grows slowly, is less fecund, and lives long. It seems that the ISS might be one of the body's molecular switches that bring about the change in energy allocations predicted by evolutionary theory.

These data suggest that altering metabolism from a progrowth to a prorepair stance by somehow repressing the insulin signaling system might be a worthwhile approach to delaying the onset of senescence.

The Pharmaceutical Interventions

Laboratory work has so far identified two potentially useful biological mechanisms that, when genetically manipulated, yield a delayed-senescence, extended-longevity pattern in our model organisms. Increased resistance to oxidative stress and/or altered metabolism both seem to be effective and robust longevity extension mechanisms. But the genetic manipulations we use in the lab are not likely to be well received a therapeutic tools. Genetic engineering of humans is currently risky, expensive, possibly ineffective, ethically challenging, and certainly political poison. Does this end the game? No. Once these two longevity extension mechanisms were identified, many scientists independently tried to develop pharmaceutical interventions by feeding various drugs suspected of regulating these two processes to their laboratory animals. Six of these experiments have shown various signs of success (Babar et al., 1999; Bickford et al., 2000; Melov et al., 2000; Kang et al., 2002; Larsen and Clarke, 2002; Roth et al., 2002). Although these independent experimenters used different intervention strategies and administered different molecules to their laboratory animals, they each recorded significant increases in the animals' health span and/or a significant extension of the animals' functional abilities. A recent experiment, by Kang et al. (2002), may serve as an example of this category of data. They fed a drug called *4-phenylbutyrate* to their fruit flies throughout all or part of their lives. This dietary pharmaceutical intervention resulted in a delayed onset of senescence in the treated flies, with survival curves similar to that shown in Figure 8.1. It turns out that this drug alters the manner in which the DNA normally wraps itself about certain chromosomal proteins, and this alteration significantly changes the pattern of gene expression in the animal. Some genes are repressed and others are enhanced. One of the genes most significantly enhanced is an antioxidative stress gene identical to that found to be highly effective in extending longevity in genetically engineered flies and worms. So it is possible, although not yet proven, that this drug may bring about its longevity extension effects by increasing the expression of these antioxidant genes and thus increasing the animal's resistance to oxidative stress. Another interesting observation from this experiment is that different strains of flies needed different drug doses in order to yield the same result. This implies the existence of genetically based individual differences in response to drug-based longevity interventions. No reports are yet available regarding the existence of various side effects or trade-offs. Since there is no free lunch, we should expect some other effects.

The pharmaceutical extension of longevity via a delayed onset of senescence has been proved in principle by these six experiments despite their individual limitations. It is now necessary to fully understand how these drugs exert their effects and to develop more effective drugs that will work on mammals as well. The basic research has defined at least two robust anti-aging mechanisms and has shown that pharmaceutical interventions are conceptually possible and technically feasible. Just like the Wright brothers in 1900, we know an awful lot about our subject but not quite enough to fly under our own power yet.

Do We Need a Complete Understanding of Aging Prior to Intervening in the Process?

There are other mechanisms that the laboratory data suggest might also be involved in regulating the rate of aging. Perhaps the most persuasive one is the cell senescence/telomere theory. Excepting stem cells, our body cells either divide very rarely (i.e., nerve cells, muscle cells) or they divide either continuously (i.e., blood cells, skin cells) or when stimulated (i.e., liver cells). Those cells that do divide seem to have some upper limit on the number of divisions they can undergo. There is some evidence that the telomerase enzyme may play some still not understood role in regulating this process. The failure to maintain cell numbers in our different tissues may underlie some aspects of our age-related loss of function. The operative part of the cell senescence theory may not be the actual number of divisions the cells undergo but the probability that nondividing senescent cells alter their pattern of gene expression from one that inhibits oxidative damage and permits division to one that permits oxidative damage and inhibits both cell repair and cell division. If so, then one could merge the cell senescence/telomerase theory, the oxidative damage theory, and the metabolic change theory into one general aging theory based on harmful changes in gene expression shifting the cell from a "youthful" preventive stance to an "older" damage-permitting stance (Fossel, 2000). Such a general theory of aging is itself highly speculative; the necessary data are only beginning to be collected, and so it presently exists only in our imaginations.

Yet the fact that we have accomplished successful interventions into the aging process in the absence of a complete understanding suggests that total comprehension is dispensable; it is desirable but not required. How can this be? The evolutionary considerations discussed above make it clear that organisms are usually geared toward reproduction as opposed to repair. What this means is that any population of animals will contain very few, if any, individuals that are optimally configured for repair. Most if not all individuals will have one or more physiological processes that are less than optimal. Tweaking any one of them—oxidative stress resistance, metabolic change, or some other—will have the effect of making that organism better in that one respect. Other physiological processes not directly affected by the intervention will either show no change or else a secondary and dependent change induced by the initial perturbation. The animal will have some measurable improvement in at least one of the several aging processes that operate in its body and will, as a result, age more slowly and live healthier and longer. This is, in effect, what we have done with the flies and worms. The very specific interventions used appear to have brought about a global effect on the organism. They live longer despite our ignorance of exactly what kind of control cascade brought this effect about. An interesting implication falls out of this observation. The more complex an organism is, the greater the number of different regulatory and control processes affecting aging mechanisms it will possess. More complex organisms should have more potential sites where intervention could take place (Johnson, 2002). In principle, mammalian aging should be able to be altered by more interventions than will work in flies and worms. The greater role that cell division, for example, plays in mammalian aging relative to the invertebrates, and the probable relationship between cell division and altered gene expression patterns, bolster this point. But having a greater number of potential drug targets is not an unmitigated blessing. The trade-off is that the mammalian interventions probably need to be very biologically specific in order to be effective. We have seen some interventions that work in flies and worms so far fail in mice, possibly because they were not specific enough to coax the mammalian regulatory systems into altering the organism's gene expression patterns. It is likely that deciphering these specificities will constitute much of the research necessary to the development of a successful mammalian pharmaceutical intervention.

Future Likelihoods

If the twentieth century was the century of physics, then the twenty-first century is likely to be the century of biology. What began a few decades ago with the efforts of a few biologists to better understand the biology of the aging process has now progressed to the point where the work is no longer some ivory tower curiosity but rather a young science with the unexpected prospect of eventually giving rise to a transforming world technology. Its findings to date are attracting wider attention both inside (Harris, 2000; Barinaga, 2001) and outside the field of science (viz., this volume). The doubling of the human health span will have wide and deep repercussions on society, and I leave it to others in this volume and elsewhere to discuss those implications. The successful pharmaceutical intervention that achieves this doubling in a mouse or monkey will be analogous to the Wright brothers' flight at Kitty Hawk in 1903: it will demonstrate that the mammalian and primate life spans can be significantly extended in a beneficial manner. But it will not be immediately useful. That flight by the Wright brothers did not, by itself, transform our society. The development of an airborne world crucially depended on the development by a variety of other individuals and companies of the physical and conceptual infrastructure necessary to the development of a future aviation industry. Only then did people fly. Perhaps the future development and spread of the health span–doubling interventions discussed here might follow the same path. (But perhaps not: if the interventions are not widely available, then violence may ensure; Kirkwood, 1999.) So then the key points to our possible future seem to be whether it will be possible to intervene successfully and double the health span of a laboratory mammal; whether such interventions will have a similar and benign effect in humans; and whether the necessary mobilizing of capital and talent to take full advantage of the current and future developments appears to be taking place.

Now that it has been empirically demonstrated that the health spans of invertebrates can be pharmaceutically extended, it seems biologically reasonable that the same outcome is likely with mammals. This may well take some time; after all, the extended life span of such an experimental mouse will be about 4 or 5 years. (But perhaps the experiments are already in progress.) And then there will be the need to replicate and confirm these findings. Perhaps one decade will be sufficient. Macaque monkeys live for 35 years, so an extended longevity experiment would take even longer. However, these times may be serious overestimates since it is possible to use biomarkers (i.e., physiological parameters indirectly marking the underlying rate of aging) to determine during their lifetime if the animals were in fact aging more slowly. Suites of biomarkers have been developed and validated for both humans and other mammals, although they are strain specific and not sufficiently predictive at an early age. Still, their judicious use might permit the rational design of overlapping experiments and thus speed up the testing process, although the gold standard of aging research will still be the life span and morbidity numbers. Perhaps another decade will suffice to produce good data in monkeys indicating whether the interventions are slowing down the rate of aging or not, though not a complete assessment of their lifetime effects on the animals. The details of human tests will depend critically on the state of the data and on the ethical and political constraints on such testing at that time; it is unrealistic to discuss that murky event now.

The mobilization of talent and capital is taking place even though it seems clear that there is no "magic pill" coming out of the laboratories in the near term (Holden, 2002). In addition to the National Institute on Aging (NIA) several private foundations and biotechnology companies such as Geron and American Cell Technologies are focused on developing the field of *therapeutic cloning*, in which stem cells with the ability to form any part of the body can be manipulated so as to grow into individual tissues or organs in vitro. Such "replacement parts" would then be transplanted into individual recipients. This is a logical strategy: if one cannot yet alter the underlying aging rate, then one can replace the specific organs that are showing signs of life-threatening age-related failure. One hopes that this approach will be successful, for it is likely to be the major new intervention available in the near term, and many of us may need this autotransplant protocol. But it is more useful to slow the aging rate, as has been argued above. The NIA and major foundations are sponsoring some of the work in this area. But more interesting are the multiple small startup biotechnology companies pursuing this goal, each in its own way (Holden, 2002). These may represent the coalescing of talent and capital into the infrastructure needed to translate the present and future laboratory data into a useful intervention. Not all will survive, but enough likely will to form the core companies that can develop and make practical the pharmaceutical interventions that will double our health span.

At the turn of the nineteenth and twentieth centuries, optimists predicted only good things to flow from the ability to fly. No one then foresaw all the constructive or destructive applications of airplanes. The gap between the predicted and actual effects of powered flight was huge. The same is likely to be the case with the predictions of the effect of extended longevity on our society. All our writing will not let us know the texture of that future society. We live in a risk-averse world, and many would not go forward without detailed knowledge of the consequences. We need to ask if we really wish the Wright brothers had failed (or worse, that their success was ignored and suppressed) and that we still lived in a flightless society.

Note Added in Proof

The health span of mice has been significantly extended in a manner similar to that of Figure 8.1 by Holzenberger et al. (2003) and by Bluher et al. (2003). The former investigators genetically decreased the effective concentration of the insulin-like growth factor-1 (IGF-1) while the latter group genetically inactivated the insulin receptor in the mice adipose tissue only. In both cases the health span was increased while the senescent span stayed more or less the same. Both treatments bring about their effects by manipulation of the ISP, a fact which illustrates the evolutionary conservation of this mechanism. The greater complexity of the mammal is indicated in the former case by the sex-specificity of the outcome, and in the latter case, by the longevity determinant role of adipose tissue. In addition, two FDA approved glucoregulatory drugs (metformin and phenformin) have been shown to act as candidate CR mimetic drugs (Spindler et al., 2003; Ingram, 2003). The genie is out of the pill bottle.

Acknowledgments

I thank Linda Avila, Robert Avila, Richard Arking, and Jonathan Arking for their constructive comments and criticism.

Suggestions for Further Reading

Arking, R. (1998). *Biology of Aging: Observations and Principles*, 2nd ed. Sunderland, MA: Sinauer Press.

Austad, S. (1997). *Why We Age: What Science Is Discovering about the Body's Journey through Life.* New York: Wiley.

Hayflick, L. (1994). *How and Why We Age.* New York: Ballantine Books.

Science magazine website on aging: www.sageke.sciencemag.org

References

Arking, R., Burde, V., Graves, K., Hari, R., Soliman, S., Saraigya, A., Sathrasala, K., Buck, S., Wehr, N., and Levine, R. (2000). Selection for longevity specifically alters antioxidant gene expression and oxidative damage patterns in *Drosophila. Experimental Gerontology*, 35(2), 167–185.

Arking, R., Novoseltsev, J., Hwangbo, D.-S., Novoseltsev, V., and Lane, M. (2002). Different age-specific demographic profiles are generated in the same normal-lived *Drosophila* strain by different longevity stimuli. *Journal of Gerontology: Biological Sciences*, 57A, B390–B399.

Babar, P., Adamson, C., Walker, G.A., Walker, D.W., and Lithgow, G.J. (1999). P13-kinase inhibition induces dauer formation, thermotolerance and longevity in *C. elegans. Neurobiology of Aging*, 20(5), 513–519.

Banfi, S., Borsani, G., Rossi, E., Bernard, L., Guffanti, A., Rubboli, F., Marchitiello, A., Giglio, S., Coluccia, E., Zollo, M., Zuffardi, O., and Ballabio, A. (1996). Identification and mapping of human cDNAs homologous to *Drosophila* mutant genes through EST database searching. *Nature Genetics*, 13(2), 167–174.

Barinaga, M. (2001). Life extension—our salvation or our ruin? Available at http://sakeke.sciencemag.org/cgi/content/full/sageke;2001/1/ns1

Bickford, P.C., Gould, T., Briederick, L., Chadman, K., Pollock, A., Young, D., Shukitt-Hale, B., and Joseph, J. (2000). Antioxidant-rich diets improve cerebellar physiology and motor learning in aged rats. *Brain Research*, 866(1–2), 211–217.

Bluher, M., Kahn, B.B., and Khan, C.R. (2003). Extended longevity in mice lacking the insulin receptor in adipose tissue. *Science* 299:572–574.

Braeckman, B.P., Houthoofd, K., and Vanfleteren, J.R. (2001). Insulin-like signaling, metabolism, stress resistance and aging in *Caenorhabditis elegans. Mechanisms of Ageing and Development*, 122(7), 673–693.

Clancy, D.J., Gems, D., Harshman, L.G., Oldham, S., Stocker, H., Hafen, E., Leevers, S.J., and Partridge, L. (2001). Extension of life-span by loss of CHICO, a *Drosophila* insulin receptor substrate protein. *Science*, 292(5514), 104–106.

de Grey, A.D.N.J. (1999). *The Mitochondrial Free Radical Theory of Aging.* Austin: R.G. Landes.

Dobzhansky, T., Ayala, F.J., Stebbins, G.L., and Valentine, J.W. (1977). *Evolution*. San Francisco: W.H. Freeman.

Dudas, S.P. and Arking, R. (1995). A coordinate upregulation of antioxidant gene activities is associated with the delayed onset of senescence in a long-lived strain of *Drosophila*. *Journal of Gerontology: Biological Sciences*, 50A, B117–B127.

Fossel, M. (2000). Cell senescence in human aging: A review of the theory. *In Vivo*, 14(1), 29–34.

Harman, D. (1994). Free-radical theory of aging. Increasing the functional life span. *Annals of the New York Academy of Sciences*, 717, 1–15.

Harris, J. (2000). Intimations of immortality. *Science*, 288(59),

Holden, C. (2002). The quest to reverse time's toll. *Science*, 295, 1032–1033.

Holzenberger, M., Dupont, J., Ducos, B., Leneuve, P., Geloen, A., Evans, P.C., Cervera, P., and LeBouc, Y. (2003). IGF-1 receptor regulates lifespan and resistance to oxidative stress in mice. *Nature* 421:182–187.

Honda, S. and Matsuo, M. (1992). Lifespan shortening of the nematode *Caenorhabditis elegans* under higher concentrations of oxygen. *Mechanisms of Ageing and Development*, 63(3), 235–246.

Huang, T.T., Carlson, E.J., Gillespie, A.M., Shi, Y., and Epstein, C.J. (2000). Ubiquitous overexpression of CuZn superoxide dismutase does not extend life span in mice. *Journal of Gerontology: Biological Sciences*, 55A, B5–B9.

Ingram, D.K. (2003). Development of caloric restriction mimetics as a pro-longevity strategy. *Biogerontology* 4 (suppl. 1):45 (abstr.).

Jacob, F. (1982). *The Possible and the Actual*. New York: Pantheon Books.

Johnson, T.E. (2002). Commentary on article by Geoge Martin. *Mechanisms of Ageing and Development*, 123, 77–78.

Kang, H.L., Benzer, S., and Min, K.T. (2002). Life extension in Drosophila by feeding a drug. *Proceedings of the National Academy of Sciences of the USA*, 99(2), 838–843.

Kirkwood, T. (1987). Immortality of the germ-line versus disposability of the soma. In: Woodhead, A.D., and Thompson, K.H., eds., *Evolution of Longevity in Animals: A Comprehensive Approach*. Basic Life Sciences, vol. 42. New York: Plenum Press, pp. 209–218.

Kirkwood, T. (1999). *Time of Our Lives: The Science of Human Aging*. Oxford and New York: Oxford University Press.

Larsen, P.L. (1993). Aging and resistance to oxidative damage in *Caenorhabditis elegans*. *Proceedings of the National Academy of Sciences of the USA*, 90, 8905–8909.

Larsen, P.L. and Clarke, C.F. (2002). Extension of life-span in *Caenorhabditis elegans* by a diet lacking coenzyme Q. *Science*, 295(5552), 120–123.

Manton, K.G. and Gu, X. (2001). Changes in the prevalence of chronic disability in the United States black and nonblack population above age 65 from 1982 to 1999. *Proceedings of the National Academy of Sciences of the USA*, 98(11), 6354–6359.

Mayr, E. (1961). Cause and effect in biology. *Science*, 134, 1501–1506.

McCay, C.M., Crowell, M.F., and Maynard, L.A. (1934). The effect of retarded growth upon the length of life span and upon the ultimate size. *Journal of Nutrition*, 10, 63–79.

Melov, S., Doctrow, S.R., Schneider, J.A., Haberson, J., Patel, M., Coskun, P.E., Huffman, K., Wallace, D.C., and Malfroy, B. (2001). Lifespan extension and rescue of spongiform encephalopathy in superoxide dismutase 2 nullizygous mice treated with superoxide dismutase-catalase mimetics. *Journal of Neuroscience*, 21(21), 8348–8353.

Melov, S., Ravenscroft, J., Malik, S., Gill, M.S., Walker, D.W., Clayton, P.E., Wallace, D.C., Malfroy, B., Doctrow, S.R., and Lithgow, G.J. (2000). Extension of lifespan with superoxide dismutase/catalase mimetics. *Science*, 289, 1567–1569.

Orr, W.C. and Sohal, R.S. (1994). Extension of life-span by overexpression of superoxide dismutase and catalase in *Drosophila melanogaster*. *Science*, 263(5150), 1128–1130.

Parkes, T.L., Elia, A.J., Dickinson, D., Hilliker, A.J., Phillips, J.P., and Boulianne, G.L. (1998). Extension of *Drosophila* lifespan by overexpression of human SOD1 in motorneurons. *Nature Genetics*, 19(2), 171–174.

Phillips, J.P., Campbell, S.D., Michaud, D., Charbonneau, M., and Hilliker, A.J. (1989). Null mutation of copper/zinc superoxide dismutase in *Drosophila* confers hypersensitivity to paraquat and reduced longevity. *Proceedings of the National Academy Sciences of the USA*, 86(8), 2761–2765.

Rose, M.R. (1991). *Evolutionary Biology of Aging*. New York: Oxford University Press.

Roth, G.S., Lane, M.A., Ingram, D.K., Mattison, J.A., Elahi, D., Tobin, J.D., Muller, D., and Metter, E.J. (2002). Biomarkers of caloric restriction may predict longevity in humans. *Science*, 297(5582), 811.

Spindler, S.R., Dhahbi, J.D., Mote, P.L., Kim, H.J., and Tsuchiya, T. (2003). Rapid identification of candidate CR mimetics using microarray. *Biogerontology* 4 (suppl. 1):89 (abstr.).

Sun, J. and Tower, J. (1999). FLP recombinase-mediated induction of Cu/Zn-superoxide dismutase transgene expression can extend the life span of adult *Drosophila melanogaster* flies. *Molecular and Cellular Biology*, 19(1), 216–228.

Tatar, M., Kopelman, A., Epstein, D., Tu, M.P., Yin, C.M., and Garofalo, R.S. (2001). A mutant *Drosophila* insulin receptor homolog that extends lifespan and impairs neuroendocrine function. *Science*, 295(5514), 107–110.

Taub, J., Lau, J.F., Ma, C., Hahn, J.H., Hoque, R., Rothblatt, J., and Chalfie, M. (1999). A cytosolic catalase is needed to extend adult lifespan in *C. elegans* daf-C and clk-1 mutants. *Nature*, 399(6732), 162–166.

Vaupel, J.W. (1997). The remarkable improvements in survival at older ages. *Philosophical Transactions of the Royal Society of London Series B, Biological Sciences*, 352(1363), 1799–1804.

Weindruch, R. (1995). Animal models. In: Masoro, E.J., ed. *Aging* (*Handbook of Physiology*, Section 11). New York: Oxford University Press, Chap. 3.

Yu, B.P. (1994). *Modulation of Aging Processes by Dietary Restriction*. Boca Raton, FL: CRC Press.

9

Eat Less, Eat Better, and Live Longer: Does It Work and Is It Worth It? The Role of Diet in Aging and Disease

Gemma Casadesus, George Perry, James A. Joseph, and Mark A. Smith

*U*nless a cure is found, the number of individuals afflicted by, and dying from, Alzheimer's (AD) and Parkinson's disease (PD) is projected to rise exponentially such that, by the middle of the twenty-first century, 30% of the aged population will be afflicted by motor and/or cognitive declines. Even though the mechanisms resulting in the onset of AD and PD are unknown, it is clear that oxidative stress, a cellular condition associated with free radical damage, is centrally involved such that oxidative stress is one of the earliest alterations of AD (Olanow, 1992; Smith et al., 1995, 1996, 2000; Jenner and Olanow, 1996; Finch and Cohen, 1997; Nunomura et al., 2001). Oxidative stress, albeit at lower levels than those seen in neurodegenerative disease, is also centrally involved in aging (Harman, 1992) and likely plays a critical role in the cognitive and functional declines apparent in many aged individuals.

Unfortunately, the aged brain, due to alterations in the neuronal plasma membrane, molecular structure, and physical properties (e.g., increased rigidity), is especially vulnerable to the damaging consequences of oxidative stress (Joseph and Roth, 1988b; Joseph et al., 1996a, 1998a, 2001; Perry et al., 2000, 2002). Certainly, endogenous antioxidant levels in brain regions such as the hippocampus, cortex, and striatum are reduced during aging, and plasma concentrations of antioxidant enzymes have been shown to be reduced in both normal old humans and subjects affected by neurodegenerative disease (Sofic et al., 1992; Zhang et al., 1993; Gsell et al., 1995). Therefore, the aged brain is not only subject to an increased concentration of free radicals but is also less well equipped than a younger brain to detoxify such excess free radicals. Therefore, it is not surprising that diseases of oxidative stress that affect cognitive and motor performance, such as AD and PD, both show age-related increases in prevalence.

Belying behavioral changes, functional declines occurring at the cellular level are also evident in the aged brain. For example, muscarinic receptor sensitivity significantly declines with age, and such declines can be mimicked by exposure to cellular oxidants (Joseph et al., 1996b, 1988a,b). Furthermore, cellular calcium buffering is functionally affected by the aging process in a vicious cycle, which induces further generation of oxidants via activation of xanthine oxidase, culminating in cell death (Cheng and Sun, 1994; Landfield and Eldridge, 1994; Joseph et al., 1999).

The pleotropic effects of oxidative stress include declines in the endogenous antioxidant system, abnormalities in protein function, oxidation of cell membrane lipids, and damage to DNA and RNA (Hazelton and Lang, 1985; Semsei et al., 1989; Smith et al., 1991; Joseph et al., 1996c; Tokumaru et al., 1996; Sayre et al., 1997). Conversely, the causes of oxidative stress are likely related to decreased antioxidant defenses such as an increased ratio of oxidized to total glutathione, with concurrent reduction in glutamine synthetase, bcl-2, membrane lipid peroxidation, lipofuscin accumulation, or redox metal imbalance (Olanow, 1992; Carney et al., 1994; Smith et al., 1997; Sadoul, 1998; Gilissen et al., 1999).

Given the role of oxidative stress in aging and disease, the issue is whether, by detoxifying free radicals, one can be afforded protection at the cellular level and whether this leads to restoration of function. The goal of this review is to critically discuss two alternative strategies that are proposed to offer protection against oxidative damage and specifically against the oxidative stress experienced by the brain during aging and disease. The first strategy, caloric restriction, has been postulated for many years to exert its positive benefits by enhancing endogenous protection against insults such as oxidative stress. The second strategy consists of increasing the dietary consumption of antioxidants through foods and antioxidant supplementation. The question is, which is more effective, less or better?

Less

The restriction of food and therefore of calories, either by alternate-day feeding or daily consumption of 40%–60% fewer calories, extends ends the life span in animals such as mice, rats, and primates (Blackwell et al., 1995; Sheldon et al., 1995; Keenan et al., 1996; Sohal and Weindruch, 1996; Duffy et al., 1997; Roth et al., 1999; Hubert et al., 2000). Indeed, dietary restriction more than doubles the 2-year survival rate of rats (Laroque et al., 1997). Similarly, even in models of accelerated aging, dietary restriction increases the median and maximal life span, decreases oxidative stress, and results in functional and cellular benefits (Kim and Choi, 2000).

Caloric restriction appears to decrease the sensitivity to oxidative stress by both lowering the metabolic rate, with consequent reductions in oxidant generation, and by eliciting a mild stress that primes the oxidant defense system. Combined, these adaptations increase the capacity of the body to face age-related oxidative insults (Mattson, 2000).

Mechanisms of Caloric Restriction

As indicated above, caloric restriction prolongs the life span by several different, but interrelated, mechanisms that attenuate oxidative stress by both increasing endogenous antioxidant systems to detoxify free radicals and reducing age-associated cellular sources of free radicals such as redox-active metals (Xia et al., 1995; Choi et al., 1998; Cook and Yu, 1998; Dubnov et al., 2000). Additionally, caloric restriction leads to the induction of endogenous protective cellular stress mechanisms that prime cells for further insults, much as a vaccine prevents disease by prealerting cellular defense mechanisms.

The role of molecular oxidative damage and caloric intake in the aging process has, and continues to be, one of the major foci of aging research. In particular, the mechanisms underlying age-associated increases in oxidative stress and the consequent macromolecular damage, as well as the mechanisms by which dietary restriction apparently attenuates such changes, have become hot topics. The fundamental observation is that dietary restriction reduces damage to cellular macromolecules such as proteins, lipids, and nucleic acids. For example, levels of 8OHdG, a product of DNA oxidation, are significantly reduced in calorically restricted animals compared to ad libitum–fed animals (Sohal et al., 1994). Caloric restriction leads to reductions in cellular oxidants such as hydrogen peroxide and increases the activity of endogenous antioxidant enzymes (Sohal et al., 1994; Xia et al., 1995). Moreover, caloric restriction acts to decrease sources of damage. For example, caloric restriction decreases iron accumulation and reduces ferritin levels (Choi et al., 1998; Cook and Yu, 1998). Iron deposits accumulate in aged brain and nerve tissue, and iron, together with hydrogen peroxide, can lead to excess production of free radicals and associated damage (Smith et al., 1997; Sayre et al., 2000).

Another mechanism by which caloric restriction may afford protection is by inducing a chronic low level of stress since caloric restriction has also been shown to mildly increase circulating corticosteroid levels (Mattson, 2000). Additionally, glucocorticoid receptor expression is significantly decreased in food-restricted subjects, perhaps due to glucocorticoid-mediated feedback suppression. Since glucocorticoid receptor inhibits the expression of several genes including those encoding heat shock protein-70, down-regulation of glucocorticoid receptor expression during periods of caloric restriction would lead to an increased level of these neuroprotective proteins (Guo et al., 2000).

A final mechanism thought to be important in modulating the protective effects of caloric restriction is stress-activated protein expression that, in turn, increases the levels of other neuroprotective agents such as neurotrophic factors. For example, brain-derived neurotrophic factor (BDNF) in calorically restricted animals is but one factor that is positively regulated by neuronal signals in the hippocampus (Patterson et al., 1992; Knipper et al., 1994; Korte et al., 1995; Lessmann, 1998; Duan et al., 2001). Such increases in neurotrophic factors lend protection against a variety of insults including those associated with aging, such as a reduction in seizure-induced damage to hippocampal neurons (Duan et al., 2001). Furthermore, increased BDNF levels are associated with increases in neurogenesis in the dentate gyrus of calorie-restricted animals (Lee et al., 2000). Since neurogenesis, in particular the survival rates of newly generated neurons, is not only decreased during the aging process but also closely associated with behavioral declines, the functional consequences of caloric restriction are of significant interest.

Behavioral Modulation by Caloric Restriction

Given the profound biochemical and cellular benefits of caloric restriction, it is not surprising that the benefits of caloric restriction translate into improved behavioral outcomes in aged animals. During aging, striatal function and behaviors such as psychomotor performance and rotational behavior display age sensitivity, and these effect can be significantly attenuated, if not completely abrogated, by caloric restriction (Ingram et al., 1987; Stewart et al., 1989; Joseph et al., 1996b, 1998a,b,c). However, the beneficial behavioral effects of caloric restriction appear to decrease when the regimen is implemented later in life, although some parameters still show improvement (Means et al., 1993; Bellush et al., 1996; Markowska, 1999).

Caloric Restriction Effects on Neurodegenerative Disease

Caloric restriction may be partially effective in retarding or reversing symptoms of neurodegenerative diseases such as AD and PD. Responsiveness to excitotoxic injury in transgenic mice that express mutant presenilin-1, which is associated with AD, is reduced by caloric restriction (Zhu et al., 1999). Protection against neurotoxic injury was also reported in animal models of PD (Duan and Mattson, 1999). Notably, a link between AD and caloric intake has been made by case control studies showing that patients who go on to develop AD eat up to 500 more calories per day than controls in the decade prior to disease (Smith et al., 1999). Supporting this, meta-analysis of world dietary habits shows that there is a strong correlation between the prevalence of AD and average caloric intake (Grant, 1999; Grant et al., 2002).

Summary

Overall, caloric restriction can successfully modulate a wide array of age-sensitive parameters. Variability across studies is substantial (especially in behavioral studies), and the onset and duration of caloric restriction are crucial. The most beneficial effects of caloric restriction are induced when the animals are placed under this regimen early in life. Therefore, while caloric restriction has utility in revealing mechanisms of aging, application of this diet may have extremely limited application to humans.

Better

Diets or supplements high in antioxidant activity offer an alternative to caloric restriction in fighting oxidative damage that is associated with aging. There have also been a number of studies examining the putative benefits of antioxidants in altering, reversing, or forestalling age-related and degenerative neuronal and behavioral trends (Joseph et al., 1998c, 1999; Launer and Kalmijn, 1998; Lynch, 1998; Pitchumoni and Doraiswamy, 1998; Smith et al., 1999; Youdim and Joseph, 2001).

All plants, including food plants (fruits and vegetables), synthesize a vast array of polyphenolic compounds, which are not involved in primary metabolism but instead serve a variety of protective functions to enhance the plant's survivability. Such *secondary compounds* are largely responsible for the beneficial effects of dietary fruits and vegetables. In this regard, a multitude of polyphenolic structures have been identified (Macheix and Fleuriet, 1990) in fruits, vegetables, nuts, seeds, grains, and herbs. These structures possess antioxidant, antiallergenic, anti-inflammatory, antiviral, and anticarcinogenic activities (Edenharder et al., 1993; Mayne, 1996; Fotsis et al., 1997; Middleton, 1998; Eastwood, 1999; Hollman and Katan, 1999). Flavonoid intake has a negative correlation with disease including a decreased incidence of stroke, coronary heart disease, and cancer (Willett, 1994; Keli et al., 1996; Knekt et al., 1996).

Antioxidant Supplementation Through Foods

An impressive body of literature suggests that the intake of fruits and vegetables may reverse or forestall age-related neuronal degeneration and behavioral deficits (Joseph et al., 1998c, 1999; Launer and Kalmijn, 1998; Lynch, 1998; Pitchmoni and Doraiswamy, 1998; Youdim and Joseph, 2001). Similarly, dietary intake of fruits and vegetables is associated with a reduced risk of developing AD (Smith et al., 1999).

Given the capacity of fruits and vegetables to reduce a vast array of age-related deficits, most of which result from oxidative stress, it is plausible that these beneficial effects are associated with the antioxidant levels of these foods. Recently, the antioxidant capacity of certain fruits and vegetables has been quantified using the Oxygen Radical Absorbance Capacity procedure (Cao et al., 1993, 1996; Wang et al., 1996). Various fruits and vegetables ranging from strawberries to spinach have been shown to have a high antioxidant capacity and are effective in improving both neuronal and behavioral changes related to aging and neurodegenerative disease.

Despite the paucity of studies investigating the capacity of fruits and vegetables to modulate aging and neurodegenerative disease, current data suggest that fruit and vegetable supplementation is as effective as vitamin E and *Ginkgo biloba* (see later). These effects may be mediated by antioxidant-flavonoid action. *Water-soluble protein*, an isolated radical scavenger from broad beans with high antioxidant and anti-inflammation capabilities, increases the endogenous activity of catalase as well as the glutathione concentration in both young and old cells (Okada and Okada, 2000). Similarly, and with regard to the brain, Manda, a product prepared by yeast fermentation of several fruits and black sugar, high in various flavonoids, suppresses the age-related increase in lipid peroxidation in the hippocampus and striatum but not in cerebral cortex (Kawai et al., 1998). Analysis of hippocampal-related function shows that the use of garlic extract can promote the survival of neurons derived from various regions of the neonatal brain (i.e., increased neurogenesis) and that the administration of aged garlic extract, at 2% (w/w) of the diet, increases the survival rate, decreases atrophy in the frontal brain areas, and enhances performance in both passive and active avoidance as well as cognitive performance in a unique strain of senescence accelerated mouse (Moriguchi et al., 1994, 1997a,b; Nishiyama et al., 1996; Zhang and Liu, 1996).

Long-term and short-term supplementation with various fruits and vegetables also modulates age-related neuronal and behavioral changes (Joseph et al., 1998a,b,c, 1999). For example, both short- (8 weeks) and long-term (6 months) dietary supplementation with spinach, strawberry, or blueberry extracts in the diet was effective in reversing age-related deficits of neuronal and behavioral function in aged rats. Specifically, aged rats showed improved performance when compared to nonsupplemented controls in tests of motor function such as rod walking and the accelerating rotarod, which rely on balance and coordination and are at least partially modulated by the cerebellum. These findings were associated with improvements in cerebellar function, as shown by improved cerebellar beta-adrenergic sensitivity (Bickford et al., 2000). In addition, antioxidant supplementation improved hippocampus-dependent working memory (short-term memory), as assessed in the Morris water maze in comparison to nonsupplemented animals (Joseph et al., 1999). These findings suggest that age-related deficits in motor and cognitive function can be reversed by nutritional intervention, possibly through the improvement of neuronal metabolic processes.

Vitamin E

Vitamin E, particularly α-tocopherol, is an antioxidant that provides protection to neurons (Erin et al., 1984; Joseph and Roth, 1988b; Behl, 1999). Mechanistically, vitamin E parallels many of the protective features of caloric restriction, including effects on oxidative stress (Behl et al., 1994) and calcium homeostasis (Huang et al., 2000), as well as stress-related signaling, transcriptional regulation, and apoptosis (Brigelius-Flohe et al., 2002).

Behavioral modulation by vitamin E. Vitamin E deficiency results primarily in neurological dysfunction in humans (Brigelius-Flohe et al., 2002), indicating a key role in neuronal function. Supporting this idea, vitamin E supplementation reverses age-related or oxidative stress–induced cognitive and motor deficits in various species, such as improvements in passive avoidance tasks and spatial memory (Ichitani et al., 1992; Joseph et al., 1998c).

Cognitive improvement is also evident in human studies. Daily oral supplementation with 300 mg of vitamin E (and 1000 mg vitamin C) for 12 months improves short-term memory, motor performance, and visuospatial skills (Sram et al., 1993; La Rue et al., 1997).

Vitamin E effects on neurodegenerative disease. α-Tochopherol, with or without selegiline, increased the level of independence and delayed deterioration of living performance but did not affect cognitive test scores in patients with AD (Sano et al., 1996, 1997). Factors such as the temporal initiation of treatment might be important in its efficacy (Sram et al., 1993).

In vitro studies show the capacity of vitamin E to modulate AD-related pathology. For example, vitamin E attenuates the oxidative toxicity mediated by amyloid-β (Aβ) (Behl et al., 1994). In vivo, vitamin E also blocks the effects of Aβ-induced neurotoxicity. For example, Y-maze and Morris water maze performance were significantly impaired in rats receiving continuous intraventricular injections of Aβ in comparison to control rats. These deficits were prevented by daily repetition of orally administered α-tocopherol 3 days before the start of Aβ infusion until the end of testing (Huang et al., 2000).

Vitamin E supplementation is also likely to play a role in improving the symptoms of PD. Recent studies demonstrated that injected vitamin E led to 74% and 68% reductions in contraversive and ipsiversive rotations, respectively. These behavioral changes were associated with an 18% reduction of tyrosine hydroxylase staining in ipsilateral substantia nigra pars compacta cells (Roghani and Behzadi, 2001). Clinical interventions have demonstrated that high doses of vitamin C (3000 mg/day) and vitamin E (3200 IU/day) administered to PD patients 1–8 years prior to levodopa treatment delay pharmacological treatment by 2–3 years (Fariello, 1990; Fahn, 1991). Other studies found that vitamin E treatment has no effect on motor or cognitive performance in patients with PD (Parkinson Study Group, 1989, 1993, 1996a,b, 1998).

Like caloric restriction, the effectiveness of vitamin E depends on the onset, dose, and duration. Furthermore, combinations of antioxidants may be more effective in forestalling the symptoms of neurodegenerative diseases. For example, AD and PD symptoms are more effectively reduced when caloric restriction and vitamin E are given in combination (Fariello, 1990; Fahn, 1991; Kontush et al., 2001).

Gingko Biloba

EGb761, a standardized extract of *Ginkgo biloba*, contains numerous flavonglycosides and proanthocyanidins. It acts as a potent free radical scavenger and inhibitor of NADPH-oxidase. In vivo studies, while sparse, have demonstrated that Ginkgo extract is effective in attenuating free radical damage produced by hypoxia (Oberpichler et al., 1988).

In vitro studies show that EGb761 provides potent neuroprotection against oxidative stress and attenuation of death-signaling pathways (Xin et al., 2000). In addition, EGb761 can modulate endogenous lipid peroxidation and the activity of the endogenous antioxidant enzymes, catalase and superoxide dismutase, in the hippocampus, striatum, and substantia nigra of rats. Pretreatment with EGb761 was also shown to be protective in neuronal cultures exposed to 1-Methyl-4-phenyl-1,2,3,6-Tetrahydropyridine, but not to 6-hydroxydopamine (Oyama et al., 1996).

Behavioral modulation by Ginkgo biloba. *Ginkgo biloba* has been shown to have beneficial effects on behavioral aging and perhaps on AD (reviewed in Christen, 2000; Defeudis and Drieu, 2000). In a similar fashion to supplementation with vitamin E, supplementation with *Ginkgo biloba* extract is also effective in reducing age-related deficits in behavior. For example, acquisition, performance, and retention in mice during an operant conditioning task are facilitated by oral supplementation with EGb761 (100 mg/kg/day) for 4 to 8 weeks (Winter, 1991). While chronic administration of EGb761 (50 mg/kg five times per week) from 7 months of age had no effect on continuous learning in the radial arm maze, it significantly decreased the number of errors made when compared to the performance of nonsupplemented counterparts. Additionally, the administration of EGb761 resulted in a dose-dependent decrease in total, retroactive, and proactive errors when delayed nonmatching to position performance was examined in aged rats. More importantly, rats supplemented with the extract lived significantly longer than the control rats, thus producing a caloric restriction–type effect (Winter, 1998).

Ginkgo biloba and neurodegenerative disease. Interest in examining the effects of *Ginkgo biloba* on neurodegenerative diseases such as AD has been promoted by its success in ameliorating neuronal and behavioral deficits in rats and humans. In vitro studies have demonstrated that *Ginkgo biloba* is effective in decreasing neurotoxicity associated with Aβ toxicity. For example, pretreatment of PC12 cells with EGb761 prevented, in a dose-dependent manner, the increases in free radical production, glucose uptake, apoptosis, and cell death induced by Aβ exposure. Additionally, EGb761 inhibits, in a dose-dependent manner, the formation of Aβ-derived diffusable neurotoxic soluble ligands, suggested to be involved in the pathogenesis of AD (Yao et al., 2001).

Primary cultured cells yield similar findings. In this regard, EGb761 protected hippocampal neurons against toxicity induced by

Aβ fragments and protected (for up to 8 hours) hippocampal cells from preexposure to Aβ 25-35 and Aβ 1-40 in a concentration-dependent manner (Bastianetto et al., 2000).

The association of AD with oxidative stress–related damage (Smith et al., 1996; Sayre et al., 1997, 2001) and the beneficial effects of EGb761 on cognitive behavior in animals have promoted various human trials to evaluate the efficacy of EGb761 for treating AD-type dementia. The effects of this extract on AD have been examined in patients with various degrees of AD symptomatology, and improvements have been noted in various cognitive and social functioning scales shown to be sensitive in AD. These studies demonstrated that EGb761 was both safe and capable of improving cognitive performance and social functioning in demented patients for 6 months to 1 year after treatment (Le Bars et al., 1997, 2000).

As Simple as Taking Antioxidants?

The majority of diet-related studies, especially in the field of aging, have focused on the effects of antioxidant supplementation. However, there are several reasons to think that antioxidants by themselves are insufficient to cause such robust effects on cognitive behavior (Joseph et al., 1998c, 1999). For example, while many fruits and vegetables, ranging from strawberries to spinach, have all been demonstrated to have a high antioxidant capacity (Cao et al., 1996; Wang et al., 1996), some are more effective than others—an effect seemingly unrelated to their antioxidant capacity. For example, cognitive performance, as evaluated using the Morris water maze, after long-term supplementation with strawberries, spinach, and vitamin E was significantly improved only by spinach and vitamin E. Moreover, while spinach reduced the latency and the distance swam to reach the platform, vitamin E reduced only the latter. More significant is the fact that all diets were balanced for their antioxidant capacity (Joseph et al., 1998c). These results illustrate that beneficial components (possibly phytochemicals) must play a role in the capacity of these diets to ameliorate cognitive output in aged rats. Conversely, strawberries, unlike spinach, were unable to modulate cognitive decline in aged rats, suggesting that the combined of antioxidant-independent properties of these diets may not have been the optimal one to modulate this type of output. Alternatively, the specific antioxidant phytochemicals may not all have equal access to the affected cells.

Studies of the effects of fruits and vegetables on neuronal parameters follow a similar pattern. For example, striatal slices harvested from blueberry-supplemented animal brain samples showed increased carbochol-stimulated guanosine triphosphatase (GTPase) activity and more efficient calcium buffering capacity. Nevertheless, while spinach supplementation did increase GTPase activity, it failed to improve calcium buffering (Joseph et al., 1999). Finally, strawberry supplementation was unable to modulate either of these parameters (Joseph et al., 1999). These findings again demonstrate that mechanisms or pathways independent of the intrinsic antioxidant activity present in these fruits and vegetables may be responsible. In *Ginkgo biloba*, the flavonoid fractions were better in attenuating lipid peroxidation, while the terpenoid constituents were more effective in reversing damage produced by $A\beta$ (Bastianetto et al., 2000; Zhou et al., 2000), whereas flavonoids, a "family" of active ingredients in fruits and vegetables, can modulate oxidative stress damage via a wide array of mechanisms (Ishige et al., 2001).

Phytochemicals contained in fruits and vegetables can display beneficial effects that are independent of their antioxidant activity. Therefore, the question becomes: by what mechanism are such phytochemicals working? For instance, phytochemicals can reduce inflammatory responses by antagonizing arachidonic acid transport or by suppressing the 5-lipoxygenase pathway, which can ultimately lead to improvements in cognitive behavior (Mirzoeva and Calder, 1996; Krischer et al., 1997; Frautschy et al., 2001). It is plausible that these independent properties may be acting in conjunction with the antioxidant properties of these fruits and vegetables to produce the differential effects seen in cognitive output. Alternatively, it is plausible that the various phytochemicals contained in these diets are taken up differently in the various brain regions. While this hypothesis has not yet been established, Martin and colleagues (1999) demonstrated that dietary vitamin E is not taken up equally in all brain regions. Thus, it is likely that phytochemicals may have an effect similar to that of vitamin E.

Compounds present in blueberries seem to play an especially beneficial role in preserving brain integrity in the aged animal, as demonstrated by the capacity of blueberries to reduce not only neuronal age-related deficits but also motor- and hippocampus-dependent cognitive deficits. Therefore, although it is important to determine how the interaction between these compounds can modulate cognition to produce future therapies, given that blueberries are already readily available to the general public, it is important to determine the mechanisms by which these fruits and vegetables, as a whole, cause these improvements.

The complex interaction of the substances in foods such as fruits and vegetables may be much more effective and much less expensive than the innumerable variety of anti-aging supplements found in today's market that are reported to contribute to successful aging. The question still arises, though, as to whether it might be more expedient to achieve successful aging through a diet containing an abundance of fruits and vegetables, especially those that are high in antioxidant activity, than via caloric restriction.

Conclusions

As chronicled above, caloric restriction, phytonutrients, and supplements can reduce age-related and experimentally induced oxidative stress damage and slow or even reverse the deleterious effects of aging. However, which is more effective, less or better?

While the mechanisms by which fruits and vegetables work have not been established, it is clear from epidemiological data that diets rich in antioxidants play a pivotal role in maintaining health (Ferro-Luzzi and Branca, 1995; Smith et al., 1999). In addition, the flavonoids in fruits and vegetables can modulate oxidative stress damage via a wide array of mechanisms and are involved in other physiological actions, such as the reduction of inflammatory responses (Mirzoeva and Calder, 1996; Krischer et al., 1997). While supplementation with one antioxidant (vitamin E) has not been shown to increase longevity, other studies suggest that vitamin E given in combination with other antioxidant agents may increase survival in rodents (Bezlepkin et al., 1996; Morley and Trainor, 2001). Furthermore, it may be possible to increase longevity with polyphenolics (i.e., EGb761) as well (Winter, 1998). Caloric restriction, on the other hand, has the capacity to mitigate age-related damage and to increase survival in both rodents and primates.

Given these observations, why is the proportion of people in the United States who are morbidly obese reaching epidemic levels? Sadly, and despite the fact that the popular media bombard the Western population with innumerable diets, the answer is lack of compliance. Based on this empirical evidence, the likelihood that people would willingly commit to a 20%–30% caloric intake drop is extremely small.

In addition to the compliance issue, the reduction of food intake in humans leads to decreased cognitive performance (Heatherton et al., 1993; Green et al., 1994). Thus, chronic dietary restriction may lead to depression, already a significant problem in the United States, and to lower cognitive performance, clearly not enhancing the quality of life. One explanation for the positive effects of caloric restriction on cognitive performance in laboratory animals (Beatty et al., 1987; Pitsikas et al., 1990) is the observation that the behavioral amelioration seen in diet-restricted animals is not due to the decrease in calories, but rather to a reduction in excess calories (Lopak and Eikelboom, 2000).

Various epidemiological reports have been cited as evidence for the beneficial effects of dietary restriction in humans (Harman, 1998). Researchers have suggested that the lower incidence of AD in less industrialized countries is due to lower caloric intake (Hendrie et al., 2001). However, it is also known that less industrialized countries rely predominantly on agricultural products (fruits and vegetables) and less on high-fat, processed foods than do inhabitants of highly industrialized countries (Caperle et al., 1996; Leotsinidis et al., 2000). Thus, it is difficult to consider these data as convincing evidence for the beneficial effects of caloric restriction in humans. An additional study cites lower caloric intake in China and Japan as an explanation for their lower incidence of AD (Grant, 1999; Grant et al., 2002); confounding this interpretation is that in addition to lower caloric intake, Asian diets are particularly high in phytoestrogens (soy products) (Nagata, 2000) and omega-3 fatty acids (fish) (Okita et al., 1995), both of which have been shown to be potent antioxidants (Grodstein et al., 2000; Umegaki et al., 2001) and beneficial in aging (Rodriguez-Palmero et al., 1997). Thus, it is difficult to determine whether the decreased incidence of AD in these countries is due to caloric restriction or higher intake of antioxidants. Similarly, one must be cautious about when to start the intervention. While significant effects are present when the supplementation regimens are begun during senescence (Joseph et al., 1999; Youdim and Joseph, 2001), the overwhelming majority of studies examining the effects of caloric restriction on aging parameters indicate that the benefits are lost if the regimen is begun during midlife or early senescence (Lipman et al., 1995, 1998).

Finally, there is the all-important quality-of-life issue. Food in our species is related not only to health, but also to culture and socioeconomical status. There are numerous individuals for whom the quality-of-life issue may be more important than successful aging. Thus, to reduce caloric intake by a significant percentage in order to extend life and increase protection against the deleterious effects of aging may be less desirable than suffering the consequences later. A diet high in fruits and vegetables and low in fat is by default a diet low in calories. People following an appropriate diet and exercise regimen are already practicing a form of caloric restriction. Therefore, it seems more appropriate to propose a diet rich in fruits and vegetables, which has the added benefits of antioxidant and anti-inflammatory effects that come from these nutrients.

In sum, a well-lived life can only be seen in terms of a lifetime of living and, in the view of the ancient Greeks, is characterized by moderation. Scientific support for this view is found in the health benefits of a balanced diet rich in fruits and vegetables, with the greatest health benefit, and the increase in longevity, coming from dietary restriction (Lin et al., 2002; Luchsinger et al., 2002). In this regimen, organisms consuming about 30% of calories below *ad libum* have approximately a 30%–50% increase in life span. Decreased free radicals, increased cellular stress, and altered hormonal balance are all thought to play a role but have yet to be confirmed by mechanistic studies. However, recent findings showing that the life span-extending effect of dietary restriction in yeast is related to whether glycolysis or the Krebs cycle dominates is important because it suggests that it is not the total caloric intake but the outcome of dominance of one pathway or another that is critical to life span control (Lin et al., 2002). Therefore, focusing solely on caloric restriction may miss the point in that the consequences of differing metabolism strategies may have critical outcomes. Seen in light of the admonition for moderation by the ancient Greeks, it appears that the good life is not marked by extremes of diet but rather by a balance in metabolism.

References

Bastianetto, S., Ramassamy, C., Dore, S., Christen, Y., Poirier, J., and Quirion, R. (2000). The Ginkgo biloba extract (EGb 761) protects hippocampal neurons against cell death induced by β-amyloid. *European Journal of Neuroscience*, 12, 1882–1890.

Beatty, W.W., Clouse, B.A., and Bierley, R.A. (1987). Effects of long-term restricted feeding on radial maze performance by aged rats. *Neurobiology and Aging*, 8, 325–327.

Behl, C. (1999). Vitamin E and other antioxidants in neuroprotection. *International Journal of Vitamin and Nutrition Research*, 69, 213–219.

Behl, C., Davis, J.B., Lesley, R., and Schubert, D. (1994). Hydrogen peroxide mediates amyloid beta protein toxicity. *Cell*, 77, 817–827.

Bellush, L.L., Wright, A.M., Walker, J.P., Kopchick, J., and Colvin, R.A. (1996). Caloric restriction and spatial learning in old mice. *Physiology and Behavior*, 60, 541–547.

Bezlepkin, V.G., Sirota, N.P., and Gaziev, A.I. (1996). The prolongation of survival in mice by dietary antioxidants depends on their age by the start of feeding this diet. *Mechanisms of Ageing and Development*, 92, 227–234.

Bickford, P.C., Gould, T., Briederick, L., Chadman, K., Pollock, A., Young, D., Shukitt-Hale, B., and Joseph, J. (2000). Antioxidant-rich diets improve cerebellar physiology and motor learning in aged rats. *Brain Research*, 866, 211–217.

Blackwell, B.N., Bucci, T.J., Hart, R.W., and Turturro, A. (1995). Longevity, body weight, and neoplasia in ad libitum–fed and diet-restricted C57BL6 mice fed NIH-31 open formula diet. *Toxicology and Pathology*, 23, 570–582.

Brigelius-Flohe, R., Kelly, F.J., Salonen, J.T., Neuzil, J., Zingg, J.M., and Azzi, A. (2002). The European perspective on vitamin E: Current knowledge and future research. *American Journal of Clinical Nutrition*, 76, 703–716.

Butterfield, D.A., Koppal, T., Subramaniam, R., and Yatin, S. (1999). Vitamin E as an antioxidant/free radical scavenger against amyloid beta-peptide-induced oxidative stress in neocortical synaptosomal membranes and hippocampal neurons in culture: Insights into Alzheimer's disease. *Reviews in the Neurosciences*, 10, 141–149.

Cao, G., Alessio, H.M., and Cutler, R.G. (1993). Oxygen-radical absorbance capacity assay for antioxidants. *Free Radical Biology and Medicine*, 14, 303–311.

Cao, G., Sofic, E., and Prior, R.L. (1996). Antioxidant capacity of tea and common vegetables. *Journal of Agriculture and Food Chemistry*, 44, 3426–3431.

Caperle, M., Maiani, G., Azzini, E., Conti, E.M., Raguzzini, A., Ramazzotti, V., and Crespi, M. (1996). Dietary profiles and anti-oxidants in a rural population of central Italy with a low frequency of cancer. *European Journal of Cancer Prevention*, 5, 197–206.

Carney, J.M., Smith, C.D., Carney, A.M., and Butterfield, D.A. (1994). Aging- and oxygen-induced modifications in brain biochemistry and behavior. *Annals of the New York Academy of Sciences*, 738, 44–53.

Cheng, Y. and Sun, A.Y. (1994). Oxidative mechanisms involved in kainate-induced cytotoxicity in cortical neurons. *Neurochemical Research*, 19, 1557–1564.

Choi, J.H., Kim, D.W., and Yu, B. (1998). Modulation of age-related alterations of iron, ferritin, and lipid peroxidation in rat brain synaptosomes. *Journal of Nutrition, Health and Aging*, 2, 133–137.

Christen, Y. (2000). Oxidative stress and Alzheimer disease. *American Journal of Clinical Nutrition*, 71, 621S–629S.

Cook, C.I. and Yu, B.P. (1998). Iron accumulation in aging: Modulation by dietary restriction. *Mechanisms of Ageing and Development,* 102, 1–13.

Defeudis, F.V. and Drieu, K. (2000). Ginkgo biloba extract (EGb 761) and CNS functions: Basic studies and clinical applications. *Current Drug Targets,* 1, 25–58.

Duan, W., Lee, J., Guo, Z., and Mattson, M.P. (2001). Dietary restriction stimulates BDNF production in the brain and thereby protects neurons against excitotoxic injury. *Journal of Molecular Neuroscience,* 16, 1–12.

Duan, W. and Mattson, M.P. (1999). Dietary restriction and 2-deoxyglucose administration improve behavioral outcome and reduce degeneration of dopaminergic neurons in models of Parkinson's disease. *Journal of Neuroscience Research,* 57, 195–206.

Dubnov, G., Kohen, R., and Berry, E.M. (2000). Diet restriction in mice causes differential tissue responses in total reducing power and antioxidant compounds. *European Journal of Nutrition,* 39, 18–30.

Duffy, P.H., Leakey, J.E.A., Pipkin, J.L., Turturro, A., and Hart, R.W. (1997). The physiologic, neurologic, and behavioral effects of caloric restriction related to aging, disease, and environmental factors. *Environmental Research,* 73, 242–248.

Eastwood, M.A. (1999). Interaction of dietary antioxidants in vivo: How fruit and vegetables prevent disease? *Quarterly Journal of Medicine,* 92, 527–530.

Edenharder, R., von Petersdorff, I., and Rauscher, R. (1993) Antimutagenic effects of flavonoids, chalcones and structurallly related compounds on the activity of 2-amino-3-methylimidazo[4,5-f]quinoline (IQ) and other heterocyclic amine mutagens from cooked foods. *Mutation Research,* 287, 261–274.

Erin, A., Spirin, M.M., Tabidze, L.V., and Kagan, V.E. (1984). Formation of alpha-tocopherol complexes with fatty acids. A hypothetical mechanism of stabilization of biomembranes by vitamin E. *Biochimica et Biophysica Acta,* 774, 96–102.

Fahn, S. (1991). An open trial of high-dosage antioxidants in early Parkinson's disease. *American Journal of Clinical Nutrition,* 53(Suppl. 1), 380S–382S.

Fariello, R.G. (1990). Biochemical profile of vulnerable neurons in neurodegenerative disorders. *International Journal of Tissue Reactions,* 12, 179–181.

Ferro-Luzzi, A. and Branca, F. (1995). Mediterranean diet, Italian-style: Prototype of a healthy diet. *American Journal of Clinical Nutrition,* 61(Suppl. 6), 1338S–1345S.

Finch, C.E. and Cohen, D.M. (1997). Aging, metabolism, and Alzheimer disease: Review and hypotheses. *Experimental Neurology,* 143, 82–102.

Fotsis, T., Pepper, M.S., Aktas, E., Breit, S., Rasku, S., Adlercreutz, H., Wahala, K., Montesano, R., and Schweigerer, L. (1997). Flavonoids, dietary-derived inhibitors of cell proliferation and in vitro angiogenesis. *Cancer Research,* 57, 2916–2921.

Frautschy, S.A., Hu, W., Kim, P., Miller, S.A., Chu, T., Harris-White, M.E., and Cole, G.M. (2001). Phenolic anti-inflammatory antioxidant reversal of

Aβ-induced cognitive deficits and neuropathology. *Neurobiology and Aging*, 22, 993–1005.

Gilissen, E.P., Jacobs, R.E., McGuinness, E.R., and Allman, J.M. (1999). Topographical localization of lipofuscin pigment in the brain of the aged fat-tailed dwarf lemur (*Cheirogaleus medius*) and grey lesser mouse lemur (*Microcebus murinus*): Comparison to iron localization. *American Journal of Primatology*, 49, 183–193.

Grant, W.B. (1999). Dietary links to Alzheimer's disease. *Journal of Alzheimer's Disease*, 1, 197–201.

Grant, W.B., Campbell, A., Itzhaki, R.F., and Savory, J. (2002). The significance of environmental factors in the etiology of Alzheimer's disease. *Journal of Alzheimer's Disease*, 4, 179–189.

Green, M.W., Rogers, P.J., Elliman, N.A., and Gatenby, S.J. (1994). Impairment of cognitive performance associated with dieting and high levels of dietary restraint. *Physiology and Behavior*, 55, 447–452.

Grodstein, F., Mayeux, R., and Stampfer, M.J. (2000). Tofu and cognitive function: Food for thought. *Journal of the American College of Nutrition*, 19, 207–209.

Gsell, W., Reichert, N., Youdim, M.B., and Riederer, P. (1995). Interaction of neuroprotective substances with human brain superoxide dismutase. An in vitro study. *Journal of Neural Transmission Supplement*, 45, 271–279.

Guo, Z., Ersoz, A., Butterfield, D.A., andMattson, M.P. (2000). Beneficial effects of dietary restriction on cerebral cortical synaptic terminals: Preservation of glucose and glutamate transport and mitochondrial function after exposure to amyloid beta-peptide, iron, and 3-nitropropionic acid. *Journal of Neurochemistry*, 75, 314–320.

Harman, D. (1992). Free radical theory of aging. *Mutation Research*, 275, 257–266.

Harman, D. (1998). Aging and oxidative stress. *Journal of the International Federation of Clinical Chemistry*, 10, 24–27.

Hazelton, G.A. and Lang, C.A. (1985). Glutathione peroxidase and reductase activities in the aging mouse. *Mechanisms of Ageing and Development*, 29, 71–81.

Heatherton, T.F., Polivy, J., Herman, C.P., and Baumeister, R.F. (1993). Self-awareness, task failure, and disinhibition: How attentional focus affects eating. *Journal of Personality*, 61, 49–61.

Hendrie, H.C., Ogunniyi, A., Hall, K.S., Baiyewu, O., Unverzagt, F.W., Gureje, O., Gao, S., Evans, R.M., Ogunseyinde, A.O., Adeyinka, A.O., Musick, B., and Hui, S.L. (2001). Incidence of dementia and Alzheimer disease in 2 communities: Yoruba residing in Ibadan, Nigeria, and African Americans residing in Indianapolis, Indiana. *Journal of the American Medical Association*, 285, 739–747.

Hollman, P.C. and Katan, M.B. (1999). Health effects and bioavailability of dietary flavonols. *Free Radical Research*, 31, S75–S80.

Huang, H.M., Ou, H.C., and Hsieh, S.J. (2000). Antioxidants prevent amy-loid peptide–induced apoptosis and alteration of calcium homeostasis in cultured cortical neurons. *Life Sciences*, 66, 1879–1892.

Hubert, M.F., Laroque, P., Gillet, J.P., and Keenan, K.P. (2000). The effects of diet, ad libitum feeding, and moderate and severe dietary restric-tion on body weight, survival, clinical pathology parameters, and cause of death in control Sprague-Dawley rats. *Toxicological Science*, 58, 195–207.

Ichitani, Y., Okaichi, H., Yoshikawa, T., and Ibata, Y. (1992). Learning behav-iour in chronic vitamin E–deficient and –supplemented rats: Radial arm maze learning and passive avoidance response. *Behavioral and Brain Research*, 51, 157–164.

Ingram, D.K., Weindruch, R., Spangler, E.L., Freeman, J.R., and Walford, R.L. (1987). Dietary restriction benefits learning and motor perfor-mance of aged mice. *Journal of Gerontology*, 42, 78–81.

Ishige, K., Schubert, D., and Sagara, Y. (2001). Flavonoids protect neuronal cells from oxidative stress by three distinct mechanisms. *Free Radical Biol-ogy and Medicine*, 30, 433–446.

Jenner, P. and Olanow, C.W. (1996). Oxidative stress and the pathogenesis of Parkinson's disease. *Neurology*, 47, S161–S170.

Joseph, J.A., Dalton, T.K., and Hunt, W.A. (1988a). Age-related decrements in the muscarinic enhancement of K^+-evoked release of endogenous striatal dopamine: An indicator of altered cholinergic-dopaminergic reciprocal inhibitory control in senescence. *Brain Research*, 454, 140–148.

Joseph, J.A., Dalton, T.K., Roth, G.S., and Hunt, W.A. (1988b). Alterations in muscarinic control of striatal dopamine autoreceptors in senescence: A deficit at the ligand–muscarinic receptor interface? *Brain Research*, 454, 149–155.

Joseph, J.A., Denisova, N., Fisher, D., Cantuti-Castelvetri, I., and Erat, S. (1998a). Membrane constituencies and receptor subtype contribute to age-related increases in vulnerability to oxidative stress. *Progress in Alzheimer and Parkinson Diseases*, 9, 53–58.

Joseph, J.A., Denisova, N., Villalobos-Molina, R., Erat, S., and Strain, J. (1996a). Oxidative stress and age-related neuronal deficits. *Molecular Chemistry and Neuropathology*, 28, 35–40.

Joseph, J.A., Erat, S., Denisova, N., and Villalobos-Molina, R. (1998b). Receptor- and age-selective effects of dopamine oxidation on receptor–G protein interactions in the striatum. *Free Radical Biology and Medicine*, 24, 827–834.

Joseph, J.A. and Roth, G.S. (1988a). Upregulation of striatal dopamine receptors and improvement of motor performance in senescence. *Annals of the New York Academy of Sciences*, 515, 355–362.

Joseph, J.A. and Roth, G.S. (1988b). Altered striatal dopaminergic and cholin-ergic reciprocal inhibitory control and motor behavioral decrements in senescence. *Annals of the New York Academy of Sciences*, 521, 110–122.

Joseph, J.A., Shukitt-Hale, B., Denisova, N.A., Bielinski, D., Martin, A., McEwen, J.J., and Bickford, P.C. (1999). Reversals of age-related declines in neuronal signal transduction, cognitive, and motor behavioral deficits with blueberry, spinach, or strawberry dietary supplementation. *Journal of Neuroscience*, 19, 8114–8121.

Joseph, J., Shukitt-Hale, B., Denisova, N.A., Martin, A., Perry, G., and Smith, M.A. (2001). Copernicus revisited: Amyloid beta in Alzheimer's disease. *Neurobiology of Aging*, 22, 131–146.

Joseph, J.A., Shukitt-Hale, B., Denisova, N.A., Prior, R.L., Cao, G., Martin, A., Taglialatela, G., and Bickford, P.C. (1998c). Long-term dietary strawberry, spinach, or vitamin E supplementation retards the onset of age-related neuronal signal-transduction and cognitive behavioral deficits. *Journal of Neuroscience*, 18, 8047–8055.

Joseph, J.A., Villalobos-Molina, R., Denisova, N., Erat, S., Cutler, R., and Strain, J. (1996b). Age differences in sensitivity to H_2O_2- or NO-induced reductions in K(+)-evoked dopamine release from superfused striatal slices: Reversals by PBN or Trolox. *Free Radical Biology and Medicine*, 20, 821–830.

Joseph, J.A., Villalobos-Molina, R., Denisova, N., Erat, S., Jimenez, N., and Strain, J. (1996c). Increased sensitivity to oxidative stress and the loss of muscarinic receptor responsiveness in senescence. *Annals of the New York Academy of Sciences*, 786, 112–119.

Kawai, M., Matsuura, S., Asanuma, M., and Ogawa, N. (1998). Manda, a fermented natural food, suppresses lipid peroxidation in the senescent rat brain. *Neurochemical Research*, 23, 455–461.

Keenan, K.P., Laroque, P., Soper, K.A., Morrissey, R.E., and Dixit, R. (1996). The effects of overfeeding and moderate dietary restriction on Sprague-Dawley rat survival, pathology, carcinogenicity, and the toxicity of pharmaceutical agents. *Experimental Toxicology and Pathology*, 48, 139–144.

Keli, S.O., Hertog, M.G., Feskens, E.J., and Kromhout, D. (1996). Dietary flavonoids, antioxidant vitamins, and incidence of stroke: The Zutphen study. *Archives of Internal Medicine*, 156, 637–642.

Kim, D.W. and Choi, J.H. (2000). Effects of age and dietary restriction on animal model SAMP8 mice with learning and memory impairments. *Journal of Nutrition, Health and Aging*, 4, 233–238.

Knekt, P., Jarvinen, R., Reunanen, A., and Maatela, J. (1996). Flavonoid intake and coronary mortality in Finland: A cohort study. *British Medical Journal*, 312, 478–481.

Knipper, M., Leung, L.S., Zhao, D., and Rylett, R.J. (1994). Short-term modulation of glutamatergic synapses in adult rat hippocampus by NGF. *NeuroReport*, 5, 2433–2436.

Kontush, A., Mann, U., Arlt, S., Ujeyl, A., Luhrs, C., Muller-Thomsen, T., and Beisiegel, U. (2001). Influence of vitamin E and C supplementation on lipoprotein oxidation in patients with Alzheimer's disease. *Free Radical Biology and Medicine*, 31, 345–354.

Korte, M., Carroll, P., Wolf, E., Brem, G., Thoenen, H., and Bonhoeffer, T. (1995). Hippocampal long-term potentiation is impaired in mice lacking brain-derived neurotrophic factor. *Proceedings of the National Academy of Sciences of the USA*, 92, 8856–8860.

Krischer, S.M., Eisenmann, M., Bock, A., and Mueller, M.J. (1997). Protein-facilitated export of arachidonic acid from pig neutrophils. *Journal of Biological Chemistry*, 272, 10601–10607.

La Rue, A., Koehler, K.M., Wayne, S.J., Chiulli, S.J., Haaland, K.Y., and Garry, P.J. (1997). Nutritional status and cognitive functioning in a normally aging sample: A 6-y reassessment. *American Journal of Clinical Nutrition*, 65, 20–29.

Landfield, P.W. and Eldridge, J.C. (1994). The glucocorticoid hypothesis of age-related hippocampal neurodegeneration: Role of dysregulated intraneuronal calcium. *Annals of the New York Academy of Sciences*, 746, 308–321.

Laroque, P., Keenan, K.P., Soper, K.A., Dorian, C., Gerin, G., Hoe, C.M., and Duprat, P. (1997). Effect of early body weight and moderate dietary restriction on the survival of the Sprague-Dawley rat. *Experimental Toxicology and Pathology*, 49, 459–465.

Launer, L.J. and Kalmijn, S. (1998). Anti-oxidants and cognitive function: A review of clinical and epidemiologic studies. *Journal of Neural Transmission Supplement*, 53, 1–8.

Le Bars, P.L., Katz, M.M., Berman, N., Itil, T.M., Freedman, A.M., and Schatzberg, A.F. (1997). A placebo-controlled, double-blind, randomized trial of an extract of Ginkgo biloba for dementia. *Journal of the American Medical Association*, 278, 1327–1332.

Le Bars, P.L., Kieser, M., and Itil, K.Z. (2000). A 26-week analysis of a double-blind, placebo-controlled trial of the ginkgo biloba extract EGb 761 in dementia. *Dementia and Geriatric Cognitive Disorders*, 11, 230–237.

Lee, J., Duan, W., Long, J.M., Ingram, D.K., and Mattson, M.P. (2000). Dietary restriction increases the number of newly generated neural cells, and induces BDNF expression, in the dentate gyrus of rats. *Journal of Molecular Neuroscience*, 15, 99–108.

Leotsinidis, M., Alexopoulos, A., Schinas, V., Kardara, M., and Kondakis, X. (2000). Plasma retinol and tocopherol levels in Greek elderly population from an urban and a rural area: Associations with the dietary habits. *European Journal of Epidemiology*, 16, 1009–1016.

Lessmann, V. (1998). Neurotrophin-dependent modulation of glutamatergic synaptic transmission in the mammalian CNS. *General Pharmacology*, 31, 667–674.

Lin, S.J., Kaeberlein, M., Andalis, A.A., Sturtz, L.A., Defossez, P.A., Culotta, V.C., Fink, G.R., and Guarente, L. (2002). Calorie restriction extends *Saccharomyces cerevisiae* lifespan by increasing respiration. *Nature*, 418, 344–348.

Lipman, R.D., Smith, D.E., Blumberg, J.B., and Bronson, R.T. (1998). Effects of caloric restriction or augmentation in adult rats: Longevity and lesion biomarkers of aging. *Aging (Milano)*, 10, 463–470.

Lipman, R.D., Smith, D.E., Bronson, R.T., and Blumberg, J. (1995). Is late-life caloric restriction beneficial? *Aging (Milano)*, 7, 136–139.

Lopak, V. and Eikelboom, R. (2000). Pair housing induced feeding suppression: Individual housing not novelty. *Physiology and Behavior*, 71, 329–333.

Luchsinger, J.A., Tang, M.-X., Shea, S., and Mayeux, R. (2002), Caloric intake and the risk of Alzheimer disease. *Archives of Neurology*, 59, 1258–1263.

Lynch, M.A. (1998). Age-related impairment in long-term potentiation in hippocampus: A role for the cytokine, interleukin-1 beta? *Progress in Neurobiology*, 56, 571–589.

Macheix, J.-J. and Fleuriet, A. (1990). *Fruit Phenolics*. Boca Raton, FL: CRC Press.

Markowska, A.L. (1999). Life-long diet restriction failed to retard cognitive aging in Fischer-344 rats. *Neurobiology of Aging*, 20, 177–189.

Martin, A., Janigian, D., Shukitt-Hale, B., Prior, R.L., and Joseph, J.A. (1999). Effect of vitamin E intake on levels of vitamins E and C in the central nervous system and peripheral tissues: Implications for health recommendations. *Brain Research*, 845, 50–59.

Mattson, M.P. (2000). Neuroprotective signaling and the aging brain: Take away my food and let me run. *Brain Research*, 886, 47–53.

Mayne, S.T. (1996). Beta-carotene, carotenoids, and disease prevention in humans. FASEB *Journal*, 10, 690–701.

Means, L.W., Higgins, J.L., and Fernandez, T.J. (1993). Mid-life onset of dietary restriction extends life and prolongs cognitive functioning. *Physiology and Behavior*, 54, 503–508.

Middleton, E., Jr. (1998). Effect of plant flavonoids on immune and inflammatory cell function. *Advances in Experimental Medicine and Biology*, 439, 175–182.

Mirzoeva, O.K. and Calder, P.C. (1996). The effect of propolis and its components on eicosanoid production during the inflammatory response. *Prostaglandins, Leukotrienes and Essential Fatty Acids*, 55, 441–449.

Moriguchi, T., Matsuura, H., Itakura, Y., Katsuki, H., Saito, H., and Nishiyama, N. (1997b). Allixin, a phytoalexin produced by garlic, and its analogues as novel exogenous substances with neurotrophic activity. *Life Sciences*, 61, 1413–1420.

Moriguchi, T., Saito, H., and Nishiyama, N. (1997a). Anti-ageing effect of aged garlic extract in the inbred brain atrophy mouse model. *Clinical and Experimental Pharmacology and Physiology*, 24, 235–242.

Moriguchi, T., Takashina, K., Chu, P.J., Saito, H., and Nishiyama, N. (1994). Prolongation of life span and improved learning in the senescence accelerated mouse produced by aged garlic extract. *Biology and Pharmacology Bulletin*, 17, 1589–1594.

Morley, A.A. and Trainor, K.J. (2001). Lack of an effect of vitamin E on lifespan of mice. *Biogerontology*, 2, 109–112.

Nagata, C. (2000). Ecological study of the association between soy product intake and mortality from cancer and heart disease in Japan. *International Journal of Epidemiology*, 29, 832–836.

Nishiyama, N., Chu, P.J., and Saito, H. (1996). An herbal prescription, S-113m, consisting of biota, ginseng and schizandra, improves learning performance in senescence accelerated mouse. *Biology and Pharmacology Bulletin*, 19, 388–393.

Nunomura, A., Perry, G., Aliev, G., Hirai, K., Takeda, A., Balraj, E.K., Jones, P.K., Ghanbari, H., Wataya, T., Shimohama, S., Chiba, S., Atwood, C.S., Petersen, R.B., and Smith, M.A. (2001). Oxidative damage is the earliest event in Alzheimer disease. *Journal of Neuropathology and Experimental Neurology*, 60, 759–767.

Oberpichler, H., Beck, T., Abdel-Rahman, M.M., Bielenberg, G.W., and Krieglstein, J. (1988). Effects of Ginkgo biloba constituents related to protection against brain damage caused by hypoxia. *Pharmacolical Research Communications*, 20, 349–368.

Okada, Y. and Okada, M. (2000). Effect of a radical scavenger "water soluble protein" from broad beans (*Vicia faba*) on antioxidative enzyme activity in cellular aging. *Journal of Nutritional Science and Vitaminology (Tokyo)*, 46, 1–6.

Okita, M., Yoshida, S., Yamamoto, J., Suzuki, K., Kaneyuki, T., Kubota, M., and Sasagawa, T. (1995). n-3 and n-6 fatty acid intake and serum phospholipid fatty acid composition in middle-aged women living in rural and urban areas in Okayama Prefecture. *Journal of Nutritional Science and Vitaminology (Tokyo)*, 41, 313–323.

Olanow, C.W. (1992). An introduction to the free radical hypothesis in Parkinson's disease. *Annals of Neurology*, 32, S2–S9.

Oyama, Y., Chikahisa, L., Uhea, T., Kanemaru, K., and Noda, K. (1996). Ginkgo biloba extract protects brain neurons against oxidative stress induced by hydrogen peroxide. *Brain Research*, 712, 349–352.

Parkinson Study Group. (1989). Datatop: A multicenter controlled clinical trial in early Parkinson's disease. *Archives of Neurology*, 46, 1052–1060.

Parkinson Study Group. (1993). Effects of tocopherol and deprenyl on the progression of disability in early Parkinson's disease. *New England Journal of Medicine*, 328, 176–183.

Parkinson Study Group. (1996a). Impact of deprenyl and tocopherol treatment on Parkinson's disease in datatop subjects not requiring levodopa. *Annals of Neurology*, 39, 29–36.

Parkinson Study Group. (1996b). Impact of deprenyl and tocopherol treatment on Parkinson's disease in datatop patients requiring levodopa. *Annals of Neurology*, 39, 37–45.

Parkinson Study Group. (1998). Mortality in datatop: A multicenter trial in early Parkinson's disease. *Annals of Neurology*, 43, 318–325.

Patterson, S.L., Grover, L.M., Schwartzkroin, P.A., and Bothwell, M. (1992). Neurotrophin expression in rat hippocampal slices: A stimulus paradigm inducing LTP in CA1 evokes increases in BDNF and NT-3 mRNAs. *Neuron,* 9, 1081–1088.

Perry, G., Nunomura, A., Hirai, K., Zhu, X., Pérez, M., Avila, J., Castellani, R.J., Atwood, C.S., Aliev, G., Sayre, L.M., Takeda, A., and Smith, M.A. (2002). Is oxidative damage the fundamental pathogenic mechanism of Alzheimer's and other neurodegenerative diseases? *Free Radical Biology and Medicine,* 33, 1475–1479.

Perry, G., Raina, A.K., Nunomura, A., Wataya, T., Sayre, L.M., and Smith, M.A. (2000). How important is oxidative damage? Lessons from Alzheimer's disease. *Free Radical Biology and Medicine,* 28, 831–834.

Pitchumoni, S.S. and Doraiswamy, P.M. (1998). Current status of antioxidant therapy for Alzheimer's disease. *Journal of the American Geriatric Society,* 46, 1566–1572.

Pitsikas, N., Carli, M., Fidecka, S., and Algeri, S. (1990). Effect of life-long hypocaloric diet on age-related changes in motor and cognitive behavior in a rat population. *Neurobiology of Aging,* 11, 417–423.

Rodriguez-Palmero, M., Lopez-Sabater, M.C., Castellote-Bargallo, A.I., de la Torre-Boronat, M.C., and Rivero-Urgell, M. (1997). Administration of low doses of fish oil derived N-3 fatty acids to elderly subjects. *European Journal of Clinical Nutrition,* 51, 554–560.

Roghani, M. and Behzadi, G. (2001). Neuroprotective effect of vitamin E on the early model of Parkinson's disease in rat: Behavioral and histochemical evidence. *Brain Research,* 892, 211–217.

Roth, G.S., Ingram, D.K., and Lane, M.A. (1999). Calorie restriction in primates: Will it work and how will we know? *Journal of the American Geriatric Society,* 47, 896–903.

Sadoul, R. (1998). Bcl-2 family members in the development and degenerative pathologies of the nervous system. *Cell Death Differentiation,* 5, 805–815.

Sano, M., Ernesto, C., Klauber, M.R., Schafer, K., Woodbury, P., Thomas, R., Grundman, M., Growdon, J., and Thal, L.J. (1996). Rationale and design of a multicenter study of selegiline and alpha- tocopherol in the treatment of Alzheimer disease using novel clinical outcomes. Alzheimer's Disease Cooperative Study. *Alzheimer Disease Associated Disorders,* 10, 132–140.

Sano, M., Ernesto, C., Thomas, R.G., Klauber, M.R., Schafer, K., Grundman, M., Woodbury, P., Growdon, J., Cotman, C.W., Pfeiffer, E., Schneider, L.S., and Thal, L.J. (1997). A controlled trial of selegiline, alpha-tocopherol, or both as treatment for Alzheimer's disease. The Alzheimer's Disease Cooperative Study. *New England Journal of Medicine,* 336, 1216–1222.

Sayre, L.M., Perry, G., Harris, P.L.R., Liu, Y., Schubert, K.A., and Smith, M.A. (2000). In situ oxidative catalysis by neurofibrillary tangles and senile plaques in Alzheimer's disease: A central role for bound transition metals. *Journal of Neurochemistry*, 74, 270–279.

Sayre, L.M., Smith, M.A., and Perry, G. (2001). Chemistry and biochemistry of oxidative stress in neurodegenerative disease. *Current Medical Chemistry*, 8, 721–738.

Sayre, L.M., Zelasko, D.A., Harris, P.L.R., Perry, G., Salomon, R.G., and Smith, M.A. (1997). 4-Hydroxynonenal-derived advanced lipid peroxidation end products are increased in Alzheimer's disease. *Journal of Neurochemistry*, 68, 2092–2097.

Semsei, I., Rao, G., and Richardson, A. (1989). Changes in the expression of superoxide dismutase and catalase as a function of age and dietary restriction. *Biochemical and Biophysical Research Community*, 164, 620–625.

Sheldon, W.G., Warbritton, A.R., Bucci, T.J., and Turturro, A. (1995). Glaucoma in food-restricted and ad libitum–fed DBA/NNia mice. *Laboratory Animal Science*, 45, 508–518.

Smith, C.D., Carney, J.M., Starke-Reed, P.E., Oliver, C.N., Stadtman, E.R., Floyd, R.A., and Markesbery, W.R. (1991). Excess brain protein oxidation and enzyme dysfunction in normal aging and in Alzheimer disease. *Proceedings of the National Academy of Sciences of the USA*, 88, 10540–10543.

Smith, M.A., Harris, P.L.R., Sayre, L.M., and Perry, G. (1997). Iron accumulation in Alzheimer disease is a source of redox-generated free radicals. *Proceedings of the National Academy of Sciences of the USA*, 94, 9866–9868.

Smith, M.A., Joseph, J.A., and Perry, G. (2000). Arson: Tracking the culprit in Alzheimer's disease. *Annals of the New York Academy of Sciences*, 924, 35–38.

Smith, M.A., Perry, G., Richey, P.L., Sayre, L.M., Anderson, V.E., Beal, M.F., and Kowall, N. (1996). Oxidative damage in Alzheimer's. *Nature*, 382, 120–121.

Smith, M.A., Petot, G.J., and Perry, G. (1999). Diet and oxidative stress: A novel synthesis of epidemiological data on Alzheimer's disease. *Journal of Alzheimer's Disease*, 1, 203–206.

Smith, M.A., Sayre, L.M., Monnier, V.M., and Perry, G. (1995). Radical Ageing in Alzheimer's disease. *Trends in Neuroscience*, 18, 172–176.

Sofic, E., Lange, K.W., Jellinger, K., and Riederer, P. (1992). Reduced and oxidized glutathione in the substantia nigra of patients with Parkinson's disease. *Neuroscience Letters*, 142, 128–130.

Sohal, R.S., Ku, H.H., Agarwal, S., Forster, M.J., and Lal, H. (1994). Oxidative damage, mitochondrial oxidant generation and antioxidant defenses during aging and in response to food restriction in the mouse. *Mechanisms of Ageing and Development*, 74, 121–133.

Sohal, R.S. and Weindruch, R. (1996). Oxidative stress, caloric restriction, and aging. *Science*, 273, 59–63.

Sram, R.J., Binkova, B., Topinka, J., Kotesovec, F., Fojtikova, I., Hanel, I., Klaschka, J., Kocisova, J., Prosek, M., and Machalek, J. (1993). Effect of antioxidant supplementation in an elderly population. *Basic Life Sciences*, 61, 459–477.

Stewart, J., Mitchell, J., and Kalant, N. (1989). The effects of life-long food restriction on spatial memory in young and aged Fischer 344 rats measured in the eight-arm radial and the Morris water mazes. *Neurobiology of Aging*, 10, 669–675.

Tokumaru, S., Iguchi, H., and Kojo, S. (1996). Change of the lipid hydroperoxide level in mouse organs on ageing. *Mechanisms of Aging and Development*, 86, 67–74.

Umegaki, K., Hashimoto, M., Yamasaki, H., Fujii, Y., Yoshimura, M., Sugisawa, A., and Shinozuka, K. (2001). Docosahexaenoic acid supplementation–increased oxidative damage in bone marrow DNA in aged rats and its relation to antioxidant vitamins. *Free Radical Research*, 34, 427–435.

Wang, H., Cao, G., and Prior, R.L. (1996). Total antioxidant capacity of fruits. *Journal of Agricultural and Food Chemistry*, 44, 701–705.

Willett, W.C. (1994). Diet and health: What should we eat? *Science*, 264, 532–537.

Winter, E. (1991). Effects of an extract of Ginkgo biloba on learning and memory in mice. *Pharmacology, Biochemistry, and Behavior*, 38, 109–114.

Winter, J.C. (1998). The effects of an extract of Ginkgo biloba, EGb 761, on cognitive behavior and longevity in the rat. *Physiology and Behavior*, 63, 425–433.

Xia, E., Rao, G., Van Remmen, H., Heydari, A.R., and Richardson, A. (1995). Activities of antioxidant enzymes in various tissues of male Fischer 344 rats are altered by food restriction. *Journal of Nutrition*, 125, 195–201.

Xin, W., Wei, T., Chen, C., Ni, Y., Zhao, B., and Hou, J. (2000). Mechanisms of apoptosis in rat cerebellar granule cells induced by hydroxyl radicals and the effects of EGb761 and its constituents. *Toxicology*, 148, 103–110.

Yao, Z., Drieu, K., and Papadopoulos, V. (2001). The Ginkgo biloba extract EGb 761 rescues the PC12 neuronal cells from beta-amyloid-induced cell death by inhibiting the formation of beta-amyloid-derived diffusible neurotoxic ligands. *Brain Research*, 889, 181–190.

Youdim, K.A., and Joseph, J.A. (2001). A possible emerging role of phytochemicals in improving age-related neurological dysfunctions: A multiplicity of effects. *Free Radical Biology and Medicine*, 30, 583–594.

Zhang, J.R., Andrus, P.K., and Hall, E.D. (1993). Age-related regional changes in hydroxyl radical stress and antioxidants in gerbil brain. *Journal of Neurochemistry*, 61, 1640–1647.

Zhang, Y.G. and Liu, T. P. (1996). Influences of ginsenosides Rb1 and Rg1 on reversible focal brain ischemia in rats. *Zhongguo Yao Li Xue Bao*, 17, 44–48.

Zhou, L.J., Song, W., Zhu, X.Z., Chen, Z.L., Yin, M.L., and Cheng, X.F. (2000). Protective effects of bilobalide on amyloid beta-peptide 25-35-induced PC12 cell cytotoxicity. *Acta Pharmacologica Sin.*, 21, 75–79.

Zhu, H., Guo, Q., and Mattson, M.P. (1999). Dietary restriction protects hippocampal neurons against the death-promoting action of a presenilin-1 mutation. *Brain Research*, 842, 224–249.

10

Extending Life: Scientific Prospects and Political Obstacles

Richard A. Miller

*I*n the past two decades, biogerontologists have established that the pace of aging can be decelerated routinely in mammals by dietary or genetic means. These discoveries, still largely unappreciated by the lay and scientific public alike, overturn the common assumption that human aging is likely to be unalterable and raise the question of whether we can make use of our growing knowledge about aging to produce 90-year-old adults who are as healthy and active as today's 50-year-olds. This chapter deals with three related issues: first, why discussions of anti-aging medicines are no longer silly; next, why the development of anti-aging strategies is making so little headway; and lastly, whether further work in this area would be a good thing to do.

By *aging* I mean a process that converts healthy young adults into less healthy older ones with progressively increasing risks of illness and death. This definition, which looks fairly innocuous, is careful enough to be controversial, because there are many interesting areas of investigation—studies of childhood development, of specific late-life diseases, of death or proliferative ennui of cells in culture, of leaf abscission, of time-dependent changes in the chemical composition of wines, cheeses, and bones—that are sometimes proposed, in various combinations, as worthy of gerontological attention and extramural funding. Each of these areas may deserve study, and some of them may eventually provide insights into real aging, but to avoid confusion I will be talking only about the kind of aging that works on whole young bodies and turns them into old ones.

The idea that anti-aging interventions might someday be developed makes the assumption, remarkably controversial when carefully scrutinized, that there *is* an aging process, as contrasted to a set of aging processes that just happen to occur in rough synchrony within any one species and at different rates among different species. The majority of deep thinkers (Partridge and Harvey, 1993; Masoro, 1995; Holliday, 1999) in the gerontological community have convinced themselves that there is no aging process, no central clock that times the whole shooting match. The conviction of these *Multiplicitists* rests on profound awe at the complexity of aging, with its effects on proliferating cells, nonproliferating cells, extracellular matrices, cell-to-cell communication, gene expression patterns, cell structures, and the like. It is obvious that each of these age-related forms of disarray can be influenced by many genes, many more or less predictable progressive adaptations to environmental insults, and many forms of stochastic misadventure; ergo, the sum of these processes—which we call aging—must be more complicated still. From this perspective, a quest for anti-aging medicines resembles the alchemists' search for the sorcerer's stone, that is, serving as clear evidence that the alchemists' basic working worldview is inadequate.

The Case for an Aging Process

There is now, however, incontrovertible evidence, from many fronts, that aging in mammals can be decelerated, and that it is not too hard to do this. In ways to be presented in more detail below, caloric restriction (CR) surely slows aging down (Weindruch and Sohal, 1997), and methionine restriction may also do so (Orentreich et al., 1993). There are at least three spontaneous mouse mutants (dw, df, and lit) and two induced ones (GHR/BP and p66^{shc} knockouts) that reproducibly increase their life span by as much or more than CR, and do so through metabolic alterations that overlap with CR only partially (Brown-Borg et al., 1996; Migliaccio et al., 1999; Miller, 1999; Coschigano et al., 2000). Artificial selection for altered body size creates long-lived dogs (Li et al., 1996; Miller, 1999) and mice (Miller et al., 2000) (and possibly horses), does so over and over again, and does so in a few dozen to a few hundred generations. Natural selection for adaptation to environmental niches with low intrinsic hazards routinely produces new species (and in some cases subspecies or races) with extended longevity [Austad and Fischer, 1991; Austad, 1993], including, for example, at least three species of rodents (porcupines, naked mole rats, and capybaras) with longevity records 3- to 10-fold above those of common household and laboratory rodents. Indeed, nature can churn out long-lived variants from short-lived predecessors quickly and reliably, making bats, tortoises, flying squirrels, elephants, parrots and many other birds, tuna and rockfish, longevitous opossums, and people; the trick seems to be easy and (in the opossum, at least) takes an evolutionary eyeblink (Austad, 1993). Aging in mice, dogs, horses, and people is easily recognized: a creature with cataracts, weak muscles, poor immunity, incipient deafness, drastically reduced cardiopulmonary reserves, and several early malignancies is clearly old, but we cannot know whether it is 2, 12, 25, or 75 years old until we know to what species it belongs. It seems distinctly odd to maintain that each of these processes, and many more besides, are timed by independent clocks that just happen to count out 2 years in a mouse and 75 in a human, and it is equally odd to view as pure coincidence the ability of multiple single-gene mutations and at least one dietary modulation to slow all these down in synchrony. My own reading of the evidence is that the aging process is probably timed by a single clock (or perhaps a very small number of clocks), and we will call this view the *Unitarian thesis.*

Aging Is Both Unitarian and Multiplex

Is aging one process or many? When both answers to a question are clearly correct, the question is poorly phrased. An economy, for example, is clearly multiplex, with many interlocking, partially independent, parallel processes, and just as clearly subject to acceleration or deceleration through fairly simple means—an interest rate change, a war, massive deficit spending—that influence the much larger set of downstream processes. The time spent by gerontologists debating whether aging is a single process or many would be better devoted to trying to figure out the mechanistic links between the master clock whose existence is strongly suggested by the Unitarian argument and the many cell-specific, organ-specific, and organismwide processes that march in crude synchrony at species-specific rates.

Why Do We Age At All?

A remarkably large proportion of first-year medical students are confident of the same wrong answer to this question: the assertion that evolution promotes genes that cause aging in order to clear away old individuals and provide room for establishment of their progeny. This belief rests on a misunderstanding of how evolution works: (hypothetical) genes that accelerate aging would have little chance of becoming common in a population because their owners would, as they become enfeebled and then died, leave fewer offspring than would their colleagues that did not have the fast-aging gene. Evolutionary biologists have indeed developed a clear, consistent, and fairly well-tested understanding of why aging is so common (nearly universal) among plants and animals (Medawar, 1952; Williams, 1957). The key realization is that genes that have ill effects only at later ages—ages "late" with respect to the attainment of breeding age—are not exposed very strongly to the pressures of natural selection. Consider, for example, a hypothetical species (the grommit) whose environment is full of hazards; in their environmental niche even the healthiest young adults have a 50:50 chance each year of starving, being eaten, or succumbing to infection. A genetic mutant that greatly increased the likelihood of dementia, osteoporosis, or cataracts in 1-year-old grommits is likely to be weeded out by natural selection, because there are many 1-year-old grommits whose chances of reproducing would be diminished by any of these (and many similar) tribulations. But a mutation that caused ill effects in 10-year-old grommits has very little impact on reproductive success, because with 50% annual mortality there are very few grommits that live to 10 years of age. And indeed, a mutation that increased, even slightly, the reflex speed, or muscle strength, or immune response in 1-year-old grommits would be highly favored, even if as a side effect it caused serious illnesses in 10-year-olds. The consequence is clear: mutations with late-acting deleterious effects tend to accumulate in the genome of every species. If fully evolved grommits are then lucky enough to be transplanted to a zoo or laboratory in which the food supply is constant and predators, both infectious and carnivorous, have been banished, they find themselves suddenly confronted, at age 10 or so, with the fruits of this genetic burden: the losses in skin, bone, muscle, brain, immune, endocrine, and digestive functions that we so readily recognize as aging in our pets and in ourselves.

This argument shows why we age, but why then do we not age more slowly? Nature can make 20-year-old turtles, horses, and tunas; why does it shy away from evolving mice that age at the same slow rate? The catch is that genes that could slow down aging incur reproductive costs. It would not be worthwhile to print the *Michigan Daily* on stone tablets, because today's issue is likely to have little value in the next millennium; nor are titanium doors worth the price in an automobile likely to break down within a few dozen years. High-hazard niches, in which a mouse, however resistant to cancers and cataracts and osteopenia, is likely to be eaten within a year or so do not support selection of genes that postpone these age effects for decades, because mice that devote their energies to eating and breeding will do better than those that spend valuable capital on eye repair and anticancer surveillance.

Nature invests in longevity often, but it does so only in safe neighborhoods. Not all rodenty creatures burn their candles at both ends. Rodents that learn to fly or glide become, respectively, bats and flying squirrels, nearly every species of which is remarkably longevitous compared to nonflying animals of the same size (Austad and Fischer, 1991). Rodents that evolve protective spines become porcupines, among which most species are quite long-lived (Carey and Judge, 2000); the current world record for longevity in a porcupine is held by a Sumatran crested porcupine that made it to 27¼ years. Rodents that learn to live underground in thermocontrolled bunkers also do well; the naked mole rat, a 25 gram denizen of Ethiopia, Kenya, and Somalia, has lived at least 20 years in captivity, with rumors of 30-year-old specimens mooted wherever naked mole rat experts congregate. Nature discovered the backbone once, the flower once, hair once, and the hand once, but figures out longevity over and over, always when a species stumbles into a suitably safe niche where flying, body armor, large size, predator-free islands, or (for humans and naked mole rats) environmental control systems mitigate risk and provide a potential payoff for deceleration of senescence. This seems to be an easy trick to learn, and it would be of great practical and theoretical interest to find out whether the trick is performed in the same way—that is, using genetic alterations of the same set of biochemical pathways—in each phylogenetically distinct instance.

Anti-Geric Intervention: Slowing Aging in Laboratory Animals

Nature can slow down aging, and so, it turns out, can we. There are so far two approaches that work for sure: diminished total caloric intake and changes in genes that regulate the rate of early-life growth.

It has been known since the work of McCay (McCay et al., 1935) in 1935, replicated and expanded by Masoro and his colleagues (Maeda et al., 1985; Yu et al., 1985), that rats and mice given about 40% less food than they would eat on their own show life span extension of about 40% compared to fully fed controls. This basic observation has been repeated in about 100 experiments done in dozens of independent laboratories (Weindruch and Walford, 1988). The CR protocol differs from starvation in that CR rodents receive fully adequate amounts of proteins, vitamins, and minerals, fatty acids, and other nutrients; their diets are adjusted to provide adequate nutrition but with drastically fewer calories. Their life span is extended because the CR diet postpones whatever diseases are the key causes of death in each species and stock tested. Importantly, the CR diet does not merely postpone diseases and death; is seems to decelerate aging per se and in so doing retards age-related changes in (nearly) every system and cell type examined. Thus, for example, CR slows down the effects of aging on cells that divide frequently (such as bone marrow and gut-lining cells), cells that divide only rarely (such as bone cells), and cells that do not divide at all (such as neurons). It retards age changes in extracellular materials (such as collagen and the crystallin proteins of the eye lens), in intracellular processes (such as age-sensitive patterns of gene expression), and in systems that mediate intercellular communications (such as endocrine feedback loops). Thus CR seems to slow aging—and, indeed, the CR-mediated deceleration of aging is a key element in the argument that aging is indeed sensibly considered a unitary process with a varying rate. It will be highly informative to learn more about the ways in

which an apparently simple intervention leads to a delay or deceleration of age-related changes in so wide a range of apparently disparate
cell types and inter- and intracellular processes.

Caloric restriction works in rodents, and has been shown to
extend longevity in a wide range of other animal types, most of them
invertebrates. At least three research groups are now in the middle of
studies designed to determine if CR will retard aging in a nonhuman
primate, the rhesus monkey, and the data, though incomplete, so far
look fairly promising. The largest CR effects are seen in experimental protocols in which the dietary restriction is begun early in life,
for example in adolescents or young adults, but partial effects have
also been demonstrated in rodents first exposed to CR about 40%
through the average life span.

How does CR work? Of the dozen or so plausible ideas, only a few
have to date been disproven. McCay's original notion was that CR
extended the life span by preventing growth to full body size, but this
is wrong: CR produces dramatic life span extension even if begun at
an age when the animal is already a full-sized adult. Calorie-restricted
rodents are typically very lean, suggesting that the lack of adipose tissue is a key element in their extended youthfulness, but imposition of
CR on a mouse with a genetic mutation that leads to extreme obesity
produces a very-long-lived, fat mouse. The idea that CR slows aging by
diminishing the rate at which food is converted to energy (and thus
the rate at which metabolism produces toxic, oxidizing by-products)
was disproven by studies showing that the small body size of CR
rodents balances their lower food intake, so that the amount of fuel
(or oxygen) used per gram of body mass is not lower in CR than in
control rodents (McCarter et al., 1985). Several other theories,
though, are still fully plausible, including notions that the long,
healthy lives of CR rodents are due to their low glucose levels, high
insulin sensitivity, mildly elevated glucocorticoid levels, or changes in
gene expression that represent adaptive responses to metabolic hard-
ship. Determining the mechanism by which CR slows aging, and discovery of a technique for inducing these changes without CR per se,
would constitute a major landmark in medical research.

In the context of public health and preventive medicine, it is
critical to note that CR does not merely postpone death, that is, does
not merely create a prolonged interval of late-life disability. Calorie-
restricted rodents remain healthy and active at ages at which control
littermates have long since all died. Studies of exercise capacity, for

example, show that while ordinary rats, given access to a running wheel, typically put in about 1000 m/day for their first few months of adult life, running drops off quickly and rarely exceeds 200 m/day after the age of 8 months. Calorie-restricted rodents, in contrast, typically run 4000–5000 m/day at least until 2 years of age (the median life span for controls) and are still devotedly running 1000 m/day at 3 years of age. Autopsy studies of CR animals at the end of their life span typically show very low levels of arthritic, neoplastic, and degenerative change, and in functional tests of immunity, memory, muscle strength, and the like, they typically resemble much younger animals of the control group.

For about 50 years the CR protocol was the only established method for producing very old, very healthy rodents. This situation changed in 1996 with the discovery that the Ames dwarf mutant mouse, known since 1961 as an example of small stature due to deficits of pituitary hormones, lived about 50% (and females up to 70%) longer than nonmutant control mice (Brown-Borg et al., 1996). Small stature in these mice results from deficits in the production of growth hormone, thyroid hormones, and prolactin. Since that time two laboratories, including my own (Miller, 1999), have documented a similar degree of life span extension in the closely related Snell dwarf mouse, and a third group (Coschigano et al., 2000) has shown exceptional longevity in an engineered mutant that can make growth hormone but cannot respond to it. A fourth mutation with defective activation of the growth hormone pathway, the *little* mutant lit/lit, also shows extended longevity (about 20%–25% over controls) when raised on a diet relatively low in fat (Flurkey et al., 2001). Snell and Ames dwarf mice, unlike the other two mutants, also are deficient in production of thyroid hormones and prolactin, one or both of which may contribute to the especially dramatic longevity effect in these two models. Characterization of the pathophysiology of these long-lived mutant mice is much less advanced than studies of the CR effect, but it is already apparent that Snell dwarf mice, at least, are not only long-lived but also relatively slow to develop age-related changes in the immune and connective tissues (Flurkey et al., 2001). It thus seems likely that thorough characterization will show that these mutants are authentic examples of decelerated or postponed aging. These observations are not in conflict with the claims that administration of growth hormone to elderly people may help alleviate some of the ill effects of aging, such as loss of muscle mass (Rudman et al., 1990), because it is quite plausible that the effects of growth hormone early in life may be different from those it exerts at advanced ages.

The association between alterations in body size and longevity seen in these mutant mice seems likely to prove reproducible in other rodents and other species of mammals. The most dramatic example comes from a comparison of body weight and longevity among breeds of purebred dogs. Using statistics compiled by Norman Wolf from an archive of veterinary records (Li et al., 1996), I have shown by linear regression that the relationship between breed weight and mean breed longevity is very strong, with a squared correlation coefficient of 0.56 among the 16 breeds for which records were available (Miller, 1999). Thus, centuries of breeding to produce dogs whose size suited them for distinct tasks—small dogs as pets and rodent hunters, larger dogs for guard and military duty—has not only generated the intended wide variations in growth rate and ultimate size, but has also created unintended differences in life span. The high correlation coefficient supports the very provocative conclusion that 56% of the variation among extant breeds in longevity is due to the effects of genes whose main selective purpose is to regulate size and growth rate. The physiological basis for differences in size between related large and small breeds has been investigated in two cases only, but in both instances was shown to represent genetic differences in the response to growth hormone—smaller dogs producing less growth hormone and (as a consequence?) living longer. There is also some evidence, so far anecdotal, for exceptional longevity among miniature breeds of horses.

Dogs are dogs and mice are mice, but what about humans? The relationship between size and longevity genes in humans is difficult to tease apart, because socioeconomic advantages can contribute both to large body size and to good health outcomes. Nevertheless there is some evidence that after control for the potentially confounding effects of nonbiological influences, people of relatively short stature may be relatively long-lived, or at least relatively resistant to certain major classes of disease (Samaras and Storms, 1992; Davey et al., 2000). There are also some humans, on the European island of Krk, who exhibit short stature because of a mutation in the same gene responsible for the Ames dwarf mutation in mice. The limited evidence (Krzisnik et al., 1999) suggests that this particular variety of growth hormone deficiency in humans may, like the dwarf mutations in mice, be associated with exceptional longevity.

Thus, three lines of evidence—one genetic, one based on dietary restriction, and one phylogenetic—lead to an important conclusion: although the signs of aging are to a first approximation similar in all species of mammals, the pace at which these changes develop can be coordinately regulated, and in some cases by as simple a change as modification of a single base of DNA sequence or restriction of food availability. Fifty years ago, an assertion that the rate of aging might be deliberately modified would have represented a hunch or a statement of faith, without empirical foundation. Today it is clear that the rate of aging can differ among members of the same species, and differ radically between species as closely related as monkeys and humans. This set of new findings prompts an important question: what implications for public health would follow from the development of a simple intervention, such as a pill, that would lead to a dramatic decline in the rate of aging? What obstacles need to be overcome to attain this result? And would such a discovery be a good thing or, like television, gunpowder, and the internal combustion engine, a mixed blessing?

What Would an Anti-Aging Pill Do?

So: what if we figured out enough about CR or age-retarding mutations to be able to design strategies that could routinely produce centenarians whose physical and mental health (and life expectancy) resembled that of today's typical retiree—a pill, free of side effects, that could slow down aging to the extent that is now reproducibly attained in CR laboratory rodents? One can, without undue speculation, produce a plausible estimate about what such a pill would do to actuarial tables and life insurance rates. Typically, CR produces in rodents an increase in mean and maximal longevity of about 30%–40%. Similarly, the dwarf mutations of mice lead to an increase in both mean and maximal life span of about 25%–70%, and the longest-lived small dog breeds typically exceed the longevity of average-sized dogs by a similar amount. Restriction of the amino acid methionine, which like CR also produces growth retardation and life span extension (Orentreich et al., 1993; Richie et al., 1994), produces about a 30%–42% longevity booster, and a mutation that alters cellular resistance to irradiation seems to extend longevity in mice by 28% (Migliaccio et al., 1999). Thus, one can with some confidence expect that an effective anti-aging intervention might produce an increase in mean and maximal human life span of about 40%—a mean age at death of about 112 years for Caucasian American or Japanese women, with an occasional winner topping out at about 140 years. Claims in the popular press, even when made by accredited gerontologists, suggesting the possibility of 200- to 600-year-old people are not supported by any credible evidence.

Effective anti-aging interventions—those that mimic the known results of CR or the genes that produce fox terriers and miniature schnauzers—would be expected to produce 112-year-old people with the same highly variable set of abilities and disabilities seen in today's 78-year-olds. We can infer that CR, or something like it that worked in people, would not produce 112-year-olds that resemble today's supercentenarians in their precarious states of mental and physical health, because 3¼-year-old CR mice, our current best guides to what we'd expect to see in a 112-year-old CR-facsimile person, are still fairly vigorous and admirably free of degenerative changes. Interventions that slow down aging—at least the ones we know about so far—do not prolong the period of late-life suffering, but instead delay its appearance by increasing the length of healthy adult life.

Demographic considerations show that aging research has potentially the biggest bang for the buck, and has the prospect to improve public health to a far greater extent than research that works on only one disease at a time. Calculations based on estimations of life tables based in turn on the hypothetical elimination of specific causes of late-life illness illustrate this point very clearly. Figure 10.1, based upon calculations of S. Jay Olshansky (Olshansky et al., 1990), shows some illustrations of this idea. In 1985, for example, the typical 50-year-old American woman could look forward to another 32 years of life, with a mean age at death of about 82 years. The elimination of all forms of cancer—that is, the hypothetical adjustment of cancer mortality risks to zero at all ages above 50—would increase this woman's life expectancy by only 2.7 years, with death expected, on average, at about age 85. In fact, complete elimination of all deaths due to cancer, heart diseases, stroke, and diabetes would produce a mean life span of about 96 years, or a change in mean age of death of only 17% (i.e., from 82 to 96 years). The reason that the disease-at-a-time approach is so unproductive is indicated in Figure 10.2: most causes of death show an exponential, rather than a linear, increase in incidence across the last third of the life span, and thus elimination

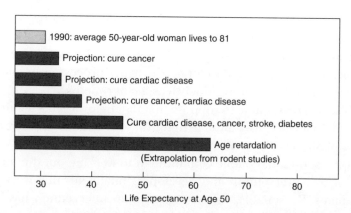

Figure 10.1. Remaining life expectancy of a 50-year-old Caucasian woman in the United States in 1985, at the then-current mortality risk schedule (top bar) or as projected under the assumption that adult mortality risks for specific diseases (cancer, cardiac disease, etc., as indicated) were reduced to zero from 1985 on. The bottom bar shows projected life expectancy if human adult mortality risks could be reduced to the same extent that caloric restriction reduces them in mice. *Source*: data from Olshansky et al., 1990.

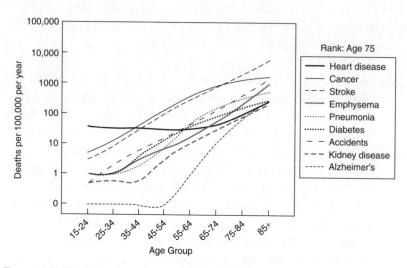

Figure 10.2. Number of deaths per 100,000 individuals at risk, by age decade, for the nine leading causes of death at age 75. *Source*: data from *Vital Statistics of the United States* (1997). Hyattsville, MD: National Center for Health Statsitics.

of any one of the major lethal illnesses buys only a short respite from the implacable march of the next illness in line. Figure 10.1 also shows an estimate of the longevity that one would expect if it should ever become possible to decelerate the aging process in humans to the extent that has been routinely feasible in rodents.

It seems reasonable to suppose that the discovery of a technique that can, in a laboratory animal, diminish to near zero the incidence of neoplasia, cardiovascular illnesses, and diabetic changes would prompt a substantial public commitment to working out the mechanism of the intervention and developing analogues that work well in humans. Reasonable, but wrong: such an intervention has been clearly established for decades, and yet its investigation receives such a small proportion of governmental research funding that it cannot be seen on a pie chart.

Obstacles to Applied Gerontology

Why is research on aging and longevity—despite its immense potential to prevent late-life illness and prolong active adult life—relegated to an obscure and dusty corner of the research establishment? I have eight reasons to suggest:

1. Most gerontologists who are widely known to the public are unscrupulous purveyors of useless nostrums. Fears of aging, illness, and death make most of us easy prey to confidence hucksters armed with bottles of potions and attractively polished testimonials. Amazon.com lists 57 titles on melatonin and another 20 on dehydroepiandrosterone (DHEA), most at sales rankings well above that for the *Journal of Gerontology: Biological Sciences*; at present, books about *HGH—The Amazing Medically Proven Plan to Reverse Aging* are gaining rapidly on last year's champions, *The Melatonin Miracle* and *The Superhormone* (aka DHEA). Scientists and their patrons—even those who have legitimate research interests in interventional gerontology— do not wish to be seen hanging out with snake oil vendors. Perhaps for these reasons, discussions of research into life span extension are carefully skirted in political discourse at the National Institutes of Health and among similar custodians of public funding. One can get away, sometimes, with cautious

circumlocutions ("we do research on the causes of late-life illnesses"), but to be safe, it is clearly better to focus on how to
"add life to years" and how "to learn the secrets contributing to
a healthy old age." A president who announces a war on cancer
wins political points; a president who publicly commits the
resources of the government to research on life span extension
would be deemed certifiable.

2. Senators' and voters' parents died of specific diseases. Cancer,
kidney diseases, acquired immune deficiency syndrome, lung
diseases, and Alzheimer's disease, all have enviable lobbies raising significant amounts of private funds for research and, more
importantly, convincing legislators to devote public funds
to disease-specific research programs. Lobbyists for basic aging
research, though doing the Lord's work, are thinner on the
ground. The problem is to a major extent one of public education: cancer and Alzheimer's disease are viewed officially as diseases and are thus in the realm of the theoretically curable,
like polio, but aging is proverbially inevitable, its opponents as
deluded as Canute. Those of us who have become convinced
that aging, whether it's considered a disease or not, is the root
of (nearly) all late-life illnesses, a fulcrum from which to shift
the timing of all the real diseases on the list, have not yet convinced those who have the power to do much about aging.

3. Aging experiments in mammals take more than 4 years to finish.
Young scientists need to write a lot of papers to get a postdoctoral fellowship, to get a job, and to get tenure. No responsible
mentor will advise a smart and ambitious protégé to go into
biogerontology research (except possibly in malleable but ques-
tionably relevant model organisms that have the grace to die in a
few weeks).

4. Worse yet, aging experiments in mammals usually do not
require fancy equipment or cutting-edge methodology. Smart
beginners can sometimes be seduced by the opportunity to learn
the hottest new methods and use expensive new equipment, but
alas, many gerontological questions of interest require only the
ability to distinguish live from dead mice. Learning to make this
distinction is not adequate preparation for getting an academic
or industrial position, and students know this.

5. Pharmaceutical firms can and do make excellent profits selling
anti-aging medicines that do not work. United States law permits

over-the-counter sales of medicines without proven efficacy as long as the sales pitch does not explicitly state that the substances are to be used to treat disease. Pharmaceutical firms are, to some extent, in business to make money, and if it's legal and more or less harmless to pour tap water into bottles labeled "Authentic Ann Arbor Springs Health Water," they see little reason to spend valuable marketing money on proving that the stuff slows down aging.

6. A pharmaceutical firm cannot test, let alone sell, actual anti-aging medicines in the expected lifetime of the firm's CEO. The good-guy CEO of PharmaInc, who wants to develop an agent that slows down aging, has a problem: it will be extremely difficult, and very time-consuming, to develop convincing evidence that a candidate drug slows down aging in people. Although there are interventions that slow down aging in rodents, there's no evidence that these would work if applied beyond approximately the middle of the life span. Caloric restriction has its largest effect if begun at juvenile or adolescent stages; it has a reproducible but smaller effect when applied at about midlife but no detectable effect if applied at later ages. But even if a potential anti-geric compound appears in animal models to postpone or decelerate aging when administered to middle-aged volunteers, documentation that it has an effect on longevity or late-life illnesses in humans is at minimum a 20-year exercise, and an expensive one with no certainty of success.

7. We don't know how to measure aging. Research on medicines to help hypertensives depended heavily on invention of a device to measure blood pressure. Research on antipyretics requires a thermometer, and research on antiobesity agents requires a scale. Aging is harder to measure than blood pressure, temperature, and weight, indeed so hard to measure that many authorities (the Multiplicitists limned above) are convinced that aging does not exist and cannot be measured per se. Informally, many researchers, like most members of the lay public, can use either visual clues or functional testing procedures (such as uphill races to avoid the maws of charging beasts) to sort acquaintances into age classes with a good deal of accuracy, but rigorous attempts to develop test batteries that do better than chronological age at identifying those middle-aged persons who resem-

ble younger ones in multiple dimensions have had little success so far. Traits that (*a*) can be measured innocuously in middle age, (*b*) predict the remaining life span and/or time before occurrence of some adverse late-life event of interest, and (*c*) predict the outcome of other age-sensitive tests in widely diverse experimental arenas (e.g., an immune test that predicts cataracts and muscle weakness and pulmonary compliance as well as life span) will deserve classification as biomarkers of aging and would be highly valuable as surrogate variables in tests for anti-geric interventions. No such biomarkers exist yet. Getting public or private money for such testing is very very difficult, and there is no organized program to develop such a biomarker battery. The absence of a well-validated method to measure biological age is a major impediment to the testing of agents thought likely to slow aging.

8. To be honest, we don't know what biochemical pathways control the rate of aging. There are still some scientific obstacles to be overcome, an area beyond the scope of this chapter, but see (Miller, 1997).

A Ninth Obstacle to Longevity Manipulation

There is a ninth obstacle preventing the discovery of effective anti-geric interventions, which deserves a separate heading and special consideration: gerontologiphobia. There is an irrational public predisposition to regard research on specific late-life diseases as marvelous but to regard research on aging, and thus on all late-life diseases together, as a public menace bound to produce a world filled with nonproductive, chronically disabled, unhappy senior citizens consuming more resources than they produce. No one who speaks in public about longevity research goes very far before encountering the widespread belief that research on life span extension is unethical, because it will create a world in which there are too many old people and not enough room for young folks. Pointing out that such an argument would inveigh, with equally fallacious force, against research on heart attacks, diabetes, and cancer (whose goals, like those of gerontology, are to allow people to live longer and healthier lives) does little good in practice to dispel this fixed belief. It also does little good to point out that a similar argument could have been made 200 years ago against penicillin, plumbing systems, and surgical anesthesia, each of which helps to produce people who remain healthy and productive to the age of 40 and sometimes even beyond.

A recent set of news articles about progress in extending the life span of worms elicited, on the *New York Times'* op-ed page, a letter from Thomas Lynch, a professional undertaker-poet, calling for a halt to aging research as a danger to the public (Lynch, 1999). This opinion stated, in part:

> The news, lately reported, that the life span of humans might be doubled in the next century is cause for sober and deliberate contemplation. . . . People are living longer but suffering diminishing returns on their death-care portfolios. Given adequate financing, given lucky breaks, how far could we go? . . . Let me hazard that "too far" is one possible answer. We are a species, and especially a country, for whom, like drunks with drink or politicians with other people's money, enough is never going to be enough. It was true of the arms race, deficit spending and TV violence, the impeachment hearings and high-tech stocks—our appetites are insatiable, our habits tend toward gluttony. . . . To the medicos, maybe "thanks but no thanks" is the thing we should say—as if we had learned to spread the wealth or leave it to our children, or failing that, to leave well enough alone.

While it is in a certain respect cheering to note that biogerontology has progressed to the point where the leading figures in the mortuary business have begun to feel alarmed, this cheer is muted by the realization that so many members of the educated public, while frequently interested in promoting their own longevity, view improving the longevity of their fellows as vaguely distasteful and somehow unwise.

So, in this context, it should be pointed out that the current alarming population crisis and depletion of nonrenewable resources has come about without the slightest aid from biogerontologists, who have not yet discovered anything that actually improves public health or prevents disease. It follows inexorably that placing obstacles in the path of aging research will not provide the key to resolving the population crunch. Proposals that do address the root causes of the problem—solutions based on access to birth control information and hardware, strong incentives for resource conservation, and changes in social attitudes about optimal family size, about the scheduling of reproductive efforts, and about the proper role of the human female—typically elicit strong opposition from powerful religious, economic, and political factions. The currently fashionable concern about the hypothetical ill effects of hypothetical future advances in biogerontology seems, from this perspective, a diversionary tactic, a sally to draw attention away from the authentic malefactors whose political connections are better than those of us lowly biogerontologists. Perhaps there are some who, after sober and deliberate contemplation, feel that our Malthusian ills are best addressed by strategies that constrain the productive life span of healthy adults rather than by controlling the supply of new people. Were I a member of such a group, I'd suggest that it devote its energies to removing seat belts from automobiles, insulin and antibiotics from the pharmacies, and anti-smoking campaigns from the schools, because compared to these interventions, picking on biogerontologists has at this point a pretty low yield. The gerontologiphobic position (*Lynchism*) seems to me indefensible, but it is common enough to present a formidable obstacle to progress in aging research.

Summary

If we—the good guys who favor preventive medicine and medical research—accept the idea that it would be worthwhile to prevent late-life illness and thus increase the period of healthy active life, then we ought to note that researchers are very far from developing any method that can, even in laboratory rodents, prevent cancer, osteoporosis, immunosenescence, heart or kidney disease or cataracts, or indeed, any other of the troublesome concomitants of old age. We can, however, routinely retard *all* of these tribulations at the same time, at least in laboratory mammals, by well-validated methods. We do not know how these interventions work, and are not likely to figure this out without substantial investment of money and brainpower. Those of us who are still enjoying life in our 40s and 50s, and even beyond, and still making contributions to the public weal, should be grateful to our predecessors who invented plumbing, X-rays, disinfectants, antibiotics, and insulin. We biogerontologists wish to do our share to earn the gratitude of the coming generations, and we now have some good reason for optimism. But the obstacles blocking the development of the hypothetical discipline of applied gerontology are at this point about 85% political and 15% scientific, and they will not be overcome by biologists alone.

Acknowledgments

This chapter appeared previously under the same title in *The Milbank Quarterly*, 80(1) (2002), 155–174.

References

Austad, S.N. (1993). Retarded senescence in an insular population of Virginia opossums (*Didelphis virginiana*). *Journal of Zoology*, 229, 695–708.

Austad, S.N. and Fischer, K.E. (1991). Mammalian aging, metabolism, and ecology: Evidence from the bats and marsupials. *Journal of Gerontology: Biological Sciences*, 46, B47–B53.

Brown-Borg, H.M., Borg, K.E., Meliska, C.J., and Bartke, A. (1996). Dwarf mice and the ageing process. *Nature*, 384, 33.

Carey, J.R. and Judge, D.S. (2000). *Longevity Records: Life Spans of Mammals, Birds, Amphibians, Reptiles, and Fish.* Odense, Denmark: Odense University Press.

Coschigano, K.T., Clemmons, D., Bellush, L.L., and Kopchick, J.J. (2000). Assessment of growth parameters and life span of GHR/BP gene-disrupted mice. *Endocrinology*, 141, 2608–2613.

Davey, S.G., Hart, C., Upton, M., Hole, D., Gillis, C., Watt, G., and Hawthorne, V. (2000). Height and risk of death among men and women: Aetiological implications of associations with cardiorespiratory disease and cancer mortality. *Journal of Epidemiology and Community Health*, 54, 97–103.

Flurkey, K., Papaconstantinou, J., Miller, R.A., and Harrison, D.E. (2001). Life span extension and delayed immune and collagen aging in mutant mice with defects in growth hormone production. *Proceedings of the National Academy of Sciences of the USA*, 98, 6736–6741.

Holliday, R. (1999). *Understanding Ageing.* Cambridge: Cambridge University Press.

Krzisnik, C., Kolacio, Z., Battelino, T., Brown, M., Parks, J.S., and Laron, Z. (1999). The "Little People" of the island of Krk—revisited. Etiology of hypopituitarism revealed. *Journal of Endocrine Genetics*, 1, 9–19.

Li, Y., Deeb, B., Pendergrass, W., and Wolf, N. (1996). Cellular proliferative capacity and life span in small and large dogs. *Journal of Gerontology: Biological Sciences*, 51a, B404–B408.

Lynch T. (1999). Why buy more time? *New York Times*, March 14, op ed page.

Maeda, H., Gleiser, C.A., Masoro, E.J., Murata, I., McMahan, C.A., and Yu, B.P. (1985). Nutritional influences on aging of Fischer 344 rats: II. Pathology. *Journal of Gerontology*, 40, 671–688.

Masoro, E.J. (1995). Aging: Current concepts. In: Masoro E.J., ed. *Handbook of Physiology, Section 11, Aging.* New York: Oxford University Press. pp. 3–21.

McCarter, R., Masoro, E.J., and Yu, B.P. (1985). Does food restriction retard aging by reducing the metabolic rate? *American Journal of Physiology*, 248, E488–E490.

McCay, C.M., Crowell, M.F., and Maynard, L.A. (1935). The effect of retarded growth upon the life span and upon ultimate body size. *Journal of Nutrition*, 10, 63–79.

Medawar, P.T. (1952). *An Unsolved Problem of Biology.* London: H.K. Lewis.

Migliaccio, E., Giorgio, M., Mele, S., Pelicci, G., Reboldi, P., Pandolfi, P.P., Lanfrancone, L., and Pelicci, P.G. (1999). The p66shc adaptor protein controls oxidative stress response and life span in mammals. *Nature*, 402, 309–313.

Miller, R.A. (1997). When will the biology of aging become useful? Future landmarks in biomedical gerontology. *Journal of the American Geriatrics Society*, 45, 1258–1267.

Miller, R.A. (1999). Kleemeier Award Lecture: Are there genes for aging? *Journal of Gerontology: Biological Sciences*, 54A, B297–B307.

Miller, R.A., Chrisp, C., and Atchley, W.R. (2000). Differential longevity in mouse stocks selected for early life growth trajectory. *Journal of Gerontology: Biological Sciences*, 55A, B455–B461.

Olshansky, S.J., Carnes, B.A., and Cassel, C. (1990). In search of Methuselah: Estimating the upper limits to human longevity. *Science*, 250, 634–640.

Orentreich, N., Matias, J.R., DeFelice, A., and Zimmerman, J.A. (1993). Low methionine ingestion by rats extends life span. *Journal of Nutrition*, 123, 269–274.

Partridge, L. and Harvey, P.H. (1993). Methusalah among nematodes. *Nature*, 366, 404–405.

Richie, J.P., Jr., Leutzinger, Y., Parthasarathy, S., Malloy, V., Orentreich, N., and Zimmerman, J.A. (1994). Methionine restriction increases blood glutathione and longevity in F344 rats. *FASEB Journal*, 8, 1302–1307.

Rudman, D., Feller, A.G., Nagraj, H.S., Gergans, G.A., Lalitha, P.Y., Goldberg, A.F., Schlenker, R.A., Cohn, L., Rudman, I.W., and Mattson, D.E. (1990). Effects of human growth hormone in men over 60 years old. *New England Journal of Medicine*, 323, 1–6.

Samaras, T.T. and Storms, L.H. (1992). Impact of height and weight on life span. *Bulletin of the World Health Organization*, 70, 259–267.

Weindruch, R. and Sohal, R.S. (1997). Seminars in medicine of the Beth Israel Deaconess Medical Center. Caloric intake and aging. *New England Journal of Medicine*, 337, 986–994.

Weindruch, R. and Walford, R.L. (1988). *The Retardation of Aging and Disease by Dietary Restriction.* Springfield, IL: Charles C Thomas.

Williams, G.C. (1957). Pleiotropy, natural selection, and the evolution of senescence. *Evolution,* 11, 398–411.

Yu, B.P., Masoro, E.J., and McMahan, C.A. (1985). Nutritional influences on aging of Fischer 344 rats: I. Physical, metabolic, and longevity characteristics. *Journal of Gerontology,* 40, 657–670.

11

An Engineer's Approach to Developing Real Anti-Aging Medicine

Aubrey D.N.J. de Grey

A nti-aging medicine does not yet exist in the sense in which the term *medicine* is generally used. Effective medicine nearly or completely eliminates the risk of death from its target cause; antibiotics, for example, cut American deaths from bacterial infections by a factor of 20 in the past century. All that we have to combat aging, at this point, is interventions that modestly (if at all) delay the onset and progression of age-related frailty. In the past few years, however, it has become possible to enumerate a comprehensive panel of technically feasible interventions that, jointly, would probably constitute real anti-aging medicine: that is, would probably reduce the risk of death from currently prevalent age-related causes to a level similar to our present risk of death from bacterial infections. The time frame for developing these interventions in laboratory mice has recently been authoritatively estimated to be around a decade from now. We don't know how long it would take thereafter to translate them to humans, but it might be only a couple of decades. As the population aged while in possession of these medicines, new aspects of aging would doubtless emerge that would need progressively more sophisticated medicine, but these might not be beyond us once aging's aura of immutability had at last been swept aside. Here I describe the main components of this panel of interventions and the reasons why an increasing number of biogerontologists feel that they will be so much more effective than anything we have today.

The Appropriate Mindset: Hints from Some of Our Longer-Lived Creations

Houses are one of civilisation's success stories. We are very expert at building houses that, with moderate maintenance, will remain intact and habitable essentially forever—certainly much longer than we can yet keep our own bodies intact and habitable. How do we do it?

They don't remain intact forever with *no* maintenance, of course. The weather constantly takes its toll. A frequent, and perhaps the most overt, way in which a totally unmaintained house eventually succumbs is via storm damage to its roof, which allows water to get into areas of the house that are not designed to tolerate it.

What does this earth-shattering insight have to do with aging? you're doubtless asking. Quite a lot, because it provides a remarkably accurate analogy—the best I know, and I've heard plenty—to explain why we don't have genuinely effective anti-aging medicine yet, why we will not develop it with our prevailing way of thinking about it, and also, very explicitly, how we must begin to think about it if we *are* to develop it. See Figure 11.1; the imagery may be a trifle Delphic at first sight, but in a couple of paragraphs it'll be clear.

Gerontologists pride themselves on their interest in the causes, rather than the symptoms, of age-related physiological decline. They stress the exponential rise with age in people's susceptibility to all manner of ailments, which means that an improvement in medicine to treat one or another of those ailments does nothing to lessen its severity, but only postpones it to a slightly (often *very* slightly) later age. They fully acknowledge the importance of geriatric medicine, as the only option for those who are already suffering from age-related disability, but they argue that only by tackling the underlying causative process—aging itself—can a really big difference be made in the length of the average person's healthy life. The geriatrician is thus caricatured as the householder who fails to replace dislodged roof tiles after a storm, but instead engages in increasingly frenzied and

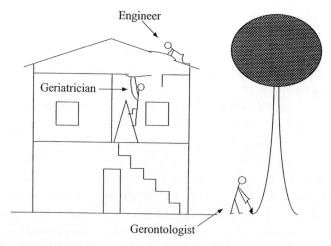

Figure 11.1. The difference between gerontologists, geriatricians, and engineers placed in a more familiar context.

futile running repairs of the fallen ceilings, collapsed staircases, and so on that result (at most a few years later) from the ingress of rain.

The above logic is completely correct. Unfortunately, gerontologists tend to take it too far. The ultimate, absolutely originating cause of aging is well known to us all: it is being alive in the first place. Maintaining all our bodily functions in a state compatible with life is an extraordinarily complex feat, achieved by the concerted action of tens of thousands of different proteins that are synthesized—under their own collective control, no less—in just the right places, times, and quantities to keep disintegration at bay. It's no surprise that this network of interactions has unintended side effects, which accumulate during life and finally overwhelm the processes that spawned them. Gerontologists' avowed intent, as basic scientists, is to improve our *understanding* of the mechanisms of that accumulation of damage. (Note that I use the term *damage* rather broadly here and throughout this chapter. I don't mean to restrict it, as is often done in gerontology, to random chemical damage, such as by free radicals, but instead to include more *programmed* deleterious changes such as shrinkage of the thymus.) When, if at all, they turn their attention to the more prosaic matter of actually *doing* something about aging, their preferred solution is to disrupt those molecular and cellular processes—to "clean up" the business of being alive so that its side effects are fewer and/or further between. The enormous attention paid to antioxidants, of which more later, is the most prominent example of this methodology.

Why is this wrong—even silly? Figure 11.1, in which the gerontologist plants trees as a windbreak, embodies three reasons. Firstly, a house surrounded by tall trees is somewhat less likely to lose tiles in strong winds, but damage will occur at some slower rate anyway; thus, focusing exclusively on a preemptive approach to house preservation is inappropriate. Secondly, those same trees may actually *increase* the risk of roof damage, since a storm that might otherwise have removed a couple of tiles might now remove a limb of a tree and propel it through the roof. And thirdly, the function of the house as a nice place to inhabit is diminished by all those trees blocking the view. So it is for antioxidants and other purely preventive measures: they do a very partial job, they have unquantifiable risks of long-term side effects, and they're no fun to have to take all the time anyway.

Of course, one has no right to call an approach silly unless one can do better, and that is where the house analogy comes into its own. There's no shame in basic scientists' not being terribly interested in goal-directed concepts such as anti-aging medicine: it's not what they're trained to do. To find a technical solution to a specific problem, you ask someone who has the appropriate training: an engineer. And, of course, if you ask any engineer (even a completely amateur engineer, in this case) what should be done to maintain a house in the face of periodic loss of roof tiles, the reply will always be "Replace the tiles when they come off." The tiles are the fulcrum of the process by which weather wrecks the house: not too early in that process, not too late, but just at the point where a modicum of timely, judicious action can preempt all that otherwise follows. In aging, as we will see, just the same applies. Rather than trying to stop damage (at the molecular and cellular levels) from happening in the first place, the effective approach to stopping it from snowballing out of control is to let it happen unhindered but periodically to repair it.

Clearly, one must actually devise ways to perform this repair: it may simply be technically infeasible, as for the householder with the right intentions but no scaffolding with which to gain access to the hole. Just a few years ago, in my view, some of the major aspects of aging were well beyond repair by any foreseeable biotechnology. That is not, however, my view now. In what follows, I shall survey the major categories of molecular and cellular damage that jointly comprise mammalian aging and, for each one, outline an approach to repairing this damage that is now probably within our technological reach to develop within a decade in mice, and perhaps capable of application to humans reasonably soon thereafter.

Aging as the Engineer Sees It

Gerontologists have been arguing about the definition of aging for as long as they have been studying it. The reason this debate has gone on so long—and has generated so much more heat than light—is not that aging is hard to define but that no definition suits all purposes. One that works well from a gerontologist's perspective is the following, due to Ed Masoro:

> Deteriorative changes with time during postmaturational life that underlie an increasing vulnerability to challenges, thereby decreasing the ability of the organism to survive
>
> (Masoro, 1995, p. 3)

This is gloriously general, applying just as well to fruit flies as to people. It's also extremely precise. It isn't, however, remotely useful for the design of anti-aging medicine. Here's another one:

> A collection of early-onset, slowly progressive, mutually synergistic degenerative processes, whose later stages are fatal but tend to be given "disease" status only if they fairly often kill or severely debilitate people before they reach their society's life expectancy
>
> (de Grey et al., 2002, p. 669)

This is clearly much less general, being focused only on humans, but it has the advantage of provoking a careful analysis of whether the things we call *diseases* are the only things that medicine is (or should be) intended to cure. Again, however, it doesn't give the slightest hint as to how to develop anti-aging medicine. Here's my best shot at a definition of aging that does what the engineer needs: A collection of cumulative changes to the molecular and cellular structure of the adult organism, which result from essential metabolic processes but which, once they progress far enough, increasingly disrupt metabolism, resulting in pathology and death.

What I've tried to do here is encapsulate the position of cumulative changes at the fulcrum of the process by which being alive leads to being dead. Without these cumulative changes, 40-year-olds would have the same physical composition as 20-year-olds, which means — societal considerations and the like aside—that they would have the same future life expectancy. The fact that 40-year-olds actually live, on average, nearly 20 years less than 20-year-olds is due 100% to the fact that their bodies have accumulated subtle (and, thereafter, increasingly unsubtle) changes.

So, what are these changes? They (the ones that we have any reason to think are deleterious, anyway) are hearteningly few in number.

Cell loss (without replacement)
Oncogenic nuclear mutations and epimutations
Cell senescence
Mitochondrial mutations
Lysosomal aggregates
Extracellular aggregates
Extracellular protein-protein cross-linking
Immune system decline
Endocrine changes

Check it yourself. What are we made of? Cells and stuff between cells. What are cells made of? Quite a variety of types of molecule—sugars, fats, proteins, nucleic acids and more—but almost all of them are ephemeral, constantly being imported and exported, synthesised and destroyed, and such things cannot accumulate damage. The only parts of cells that are long-lived enough to accumulate damage are our DNA (most of it in the nucleus, some in the mitochondria) and a residue of junk, varying in composition from one cell type to another, which many long-lived cells accumulate in special structures called lysosomes. (Actually, all our mitochondrial DNA and some cells' nuclear DNA is rather short-lived too, but it's functionally long-lived. Because new DNA is synthesised only by copying old DNA, damage to it can still accumulate, even though it's not all inflicted on physically the same molecule.) DNA suffers three major types of damage: mutations (changes to the sequence), epimutations (persistent changes to the decorations that control gene expression) and senescence-inducing changes. All three happen to nuclear DNA; only mutations happen to mitochondrial DNA. Outside the cell, the situation is even simpler. Nothing in our blood exists for very long at all. The proteins that form blood vessels, and indeed maintain the three-dimensional structure of all our tissues, are rather different; many of them are very long-lived, and they accumulate the damage referred to above as *cross-linking*. Also, especially in the brain and the artery wall, junk accumulates between cells.

The immune system relies heavily on the coexistence of a wide spectrum of different cell types, distinguishable by the presence or absence of certain proteins on the cell surface; also, within each such cell type, there needs to be a lot of genetic variation in special *hyper-variable* regions of the DNA that are deliberately scrambled in order to make the immune system so discriminating (capable of homing in on anything foreign while not destroying the body itself). This *poly-clonality* diminishes with age, and there are also changes in the relative and absolute abundance of the various cell types. Both of those changes seem to lead to a progressively impaired immune system. However, since all this complexity is laid down by a genetic system that is still there in the old individual, it might just recover on its own if its environment is restored to a youthful state. A finding hinting at this (Aspinall and Andrew, 2000) is that restoring youthful levels of certain growth factors stimulates regrowth of the thymus, an organ that produces many of the cell types mentioned above and loses as many as 90% of its cells during the first half of life.

The endocrine system is in the same boat—but luckily it is also a relatively straightforward system to repair directly if such repair turns out to be needed. Most glands secrete progressively less of the hormones that they make; this is generally not because they shrink in size (like the thymus), but because their constituent cells become less active. That could be because of the extracellular environment or it could be because of lysosomal junk. It's hard to see what else could drive it, so I'm optimistic that the endocrine system will fall off the list of things we need to fix. But also, since (by definition) these glands make substances that circulate in the blood, it doesn't matter which cells make them. We can therefore engineer other cells to do the same job, and we already know how to do this (MacColl et al., 1999).

Is that really all? I think so, if we restrict ourselves to things that matter in a (currently!) normal lifetime. The reason nuclear mutations (and epimutations) are qualified by the adjective *oncogenic* (cancer-promoting) in the above list is that mutations that do not promote cancer seem to be far too rare to be a problem in a lifetime as short as a century or two. Undegraded aggregates may form in parts of the cell other than lysosomes, but there is so far no strong evidence that they accumulate with age except in certain rare diseases. Extracellular structural proteins accumulate other types of damage in addition to cross-linking, but cross-linking is the only type that we have reason to suspect is bad for us. One part of the body that nonbiologists often think of as very long-lived, because it is so long-lived after death, is bone; in fact, though, our bone is being constantly destroyed and regenerated by specialized cells (osteoclasts destroying it and osteoblasts rebuilding it). Bone does deteriorate with age, but this is now well understood to be a direct result of an insufficiency of osteoblasts—in other words, it comes under "cell loss without replacement." Cartilage, the material that connects our bones to each other and to muscle, also deteriorates with aging, and again this seems to be largely because the cells necessary for its maintenance (chondrocytes) are depleted.

Some Popular Strategies That Don't Target the Fulcrum of Aging

By now you probably understand why antioxidants don't interest me very much. They can potentially slow down the rate of formation of many—perhaps all—of the types of damage listed in the two previous sections, but they don't get rid of that damage once it's done. Also, it is now clear that the reactive chemicals that antioxidants try to get rid of before they cause those types of damage are actually not as purely evil as was originally thought. Life has been generating, and thus tolerating, these chemicals for billions of years, and—as is the way of evolution—it has made the best of a bad job. Hydrogen peroxide, for example, is now known to be an important signaling molecule (Rhee, 1999); it's likely that its progenitor, superoxide, has similar roles. Thus, depleting these toxic chemicals may have nasty side effects, ones that we don't yet understand.

Another idea that has made a lot of headlines over the past decade or two is relengthening of telomeres as a reversal of cell senescence (Fossel, 2000). In some ways this is a splendid attack on the fulcrum of aging, because cell senescence is on my list of components of that fulcrum (though the evidence that it does us any harm in a normal lifetime is still highly equivocal). But in the past decade, it became clear that cell senescence can be caused not only by telomere shortening, but also by chromosome breakage. (This is no great surprise in hindsight, because the result of breaking a chromosome is a couple of new ends of DNA molecules, and those ends are not capped by the distinctive telomeric sequences: in other words, they look just like proper chromosome ends whose telomeres have shortened away to nothing.) Once a cell enters the senescent state, which entails a slew of changes of gene expression, it never spontaneously leaves it; thus, if senescent cells are bad for us, then we must find a way to unsenesce them. Or must we? A formally available alternative is to eliminate such cells and replace them by the division of others. (More on this in the next section.) But also, telomere relengthening won't work on cells that have gone senescent via chromosome breakage, because even if the new ends were given their own telomeres, one part-chromosome would have no centromere and so would be lost the next time the cell divides. Instead of this, the cell would have to be induced to put the chromosome back together again—something that it can usually do anyway, which it evidently had reason not to do in these cases. So the question of whether chromosome breakage or telomere shortening predominates in the genesis of senescent cells in vivo is rather pivotal. At this point we can't say for sure, but we do know that telomere length has no effect on mouse life span until telomeres get very short indeed, so we can say that if cell senescence matters at all in mouse aging, then it matters via the chromosome breakage route rather than the telomere shortening route. It's always possible that humans could be different, but I wouldn't bet on it.

A different tack, equally misguided in my view, is caloric restriction (CR). It's been known for over 60 years that if you feed a mouse or a rat a diet that contains a normal quantity of vitamins and other nutrients but a lot less than the normal number of calories, it tends to live considerably longer than if it can eat all it wants. This is the most thoroughly researched phenomenon in the whole of gerontology, and justifiably so, because until quite recently it has been the only reproducible way to increase the maximum life span of a normal mammal (i.e., one otherwise unhandicapped by environmental or genetic deficits). Moreover, the newly discovered ways to extend the mammalian life span seem mainly to involve crude genetic inductions of some of the mechanisms whereby CR does it, so in some senses CR is still the only method. But as a life-extending intervention for humans, it has three huge problems (even excluding people's fondness for food, which might potentially be gotten around by drugs). One is that we're so long-lived already that the same thing may not work for us. The second is that it may actually not work for "real" rodents either: recently, Steven Austad showed that mice recently derived from wild populations already live (when fed ad libitum) as long as CR-fed lab mice and that CR does not extend their life span at all (Harper et al., in press) In other words, the many decades that lab mice and their ancestors have spent in a captive environment may have simply resulted in their acquisition of mutations that make them intolerant of high-calorie diets. And finally, even CR of lab mice produces big life span increases only if it is begun when the mice are still growing: adult-onset CR gives at most a one-third increase (Weindruch and Walford, 1982), and CR onset in middle age or later (which is the only age at which people will realistically start taking a drug) gives no increase at all. Because of this, the search (Mattson et al., 2001) for drugs that induce the metabolic responses to CR seen in mice (and also in CR primates, though their life span is still unknown) is, in my view, rather pointless.

Feasible Strategies That Do Target the Fulcrum of Aging

Enough negativity: what *do* I recommend?

Cell loss without replacement is at the top of the list I gave earlier, and that's where it belongs. It certainly underlies neurodegeneration, osteoporosis, osteoarthritis, and sarcopenia; it's probably a major cause of immune senescence (specifically, loss of cells in the thymus); and it may well play a role in endocrine senescence too. Thus, cell therapy (the replenishment of cell types that are depleted with age) is as important a component of anti-aging medicine as any. I'm sure that all readers will be aware of the large body of work that is presently focused on cell therapy, so I won't detail it here; Anversa and Nadal-Ginard (2002), Armstrong and Svendsen (2000), Aspinall and Andrew (2000), Goldspink (1999), and Weissman et al. (2001) are authoritative contemporaneous reviews.

Why isn't cell therapy enough on its own? Two reasons. First, some damage is done to the stuff between cells rather than to cells themselves; second, some types of damage to cells don't cause them to die, but instead to become sick (and possibly toxic to other cells).

Look at extracellular damage first: it includes two items on my list, *cross-links* and *aggregates*. This may seem to be a rather arbitrary distinction, but in fact it's reasonable, because cross-linking describes what happens to molecules with structural roles, whereas aggregation describes what happens to nonstructural stuff that shouldn't be long-lived at all but occasionally forms clumps that are apparently hard for the body to get rid of. Techniques have emerged in the past few years that show huge promise in tackling both types of damage. Firstly, cross-linking of structural proteins seems to be dramatically reversed by a chemical called ALT-711 or, more technically, phenacyldimethylthiazolium chloride, which restores the arteries, cartilage, and skin of experimental animals to youthful elasticity and is currently in clinical trials (Vasan et al., 2001). Secondly, ways have been found (Brazil et al., 2000) to stimulate the immune system to take notice of extracellular aggregates, resulting in their engulfment by cells of the immune system (including, in the brain, the microglia).

That brings us neatly to intracellular lysosomal aggregates, because that's what extracellular aggregates become when they're engulfed. It is actually rather curious that cells should fill up with junk—whether junk taken up from outside, as just described, or junk of their own making. It's no surprise that there are some things that a cell simply lacks the machinery to break down, but there are other ways in which the observed result, lysosomal aggregates, might in theory be avoided. One is excretion. The junk accumulates exceedingly slowly, so surely it would be possible to spit it out (exocytose it, to use the biological term) in tiny chunks and have the bloodstream take it to the kidneys and out in the urine. Well, apparently not. We don't know the details, but for whatever reason, cells just don't tend to do this. With the exception of the liver, which does indeed spit stuff out in very much this way, cells seem to prefer to sequester their junk, not to discard it. Even though we don't understand this, we can be fairly confident that it would be a bad idea to try to change this policy; it has evolved, after all, in concert with a very long life span. One guess as to the reason is that the liver has unique options for garbage disposal: it can eject stuff directly into the gut via the bile duct, so that the kidneys never encounter it. The kidney has a very tricky filtration job to do as it is, and the burden of these specks of indigestible material might severely impair that process, which would certainly be very bad for us very quickly.

A second option is for the cell to divide, thereby diluting the junk. In fact, most gerontologists believe that cell division is a fabulously effective rejuvenation strategy, just so long as it's universal. There is only one multicellular animal that has been compellingly shown not to age at all, and it—*Hydra*—possesses no nondividing cells among its 20-odd cell types. Not a single cell in a *Hydra* is more than a few weeks old, but the organism can apparently live forever, certainly for several years (Martinez, 1998). So, in other words, we age because we have sacrificed the eternal rejuvenation of ubiquitous cell division in favor of the functional sophistication that necessitates having a lot of very long-lived cells. Sure enough, cells in the mammalian body that do divide do not accumulate much junk. But ones that don't divide do accumulate it and can't dilute it away.

A third ostensible option is cell death (with replacement, of course). This would work—except for the unpleasant business of disposing of the corpse. The indigestible junk in such a cell does not suddenly become digestible when the cell dies. Thus, nothing would actually be achieved by this.

The appropriate way to go, then, is completely different: as with the stuff outside cells, to break the junk down in situ so that the cells don't fill up after all. This can be done most feasibly, in my view, by gene therapy (or initially, in mice, by the well-established technique of germline transformation) to give cells extra enzymes that can degrade lysosomal material that our own enzymes cannot. Such enzymes seem to be easy to find in nature: the natural place to seek them is in soil microorganisms (bacteria and fungi, especially), since their possession of such enzymes is strongly suggested by the fact that these indigestible (by us) substances do not accumulate in the soil in which animals are forever dying and decaying. Preliminary work in my department in Cambridge has confirmed this optimism (de Grey, 2002).

Finally, we come to DNA. Mitochondrial DNA is extremely simple—it encodes only 13 proteins, about 0.02% of our total proteome. Unfortunately, those proteins are really, really necessary. Work has been going on for over 15 years to solve the problem of mitochondrial DNA damage in a totally comprehensive way—by making that DNA superfluous. Basically, all we need to do is make some fairly obvious changes to the DNA sequences encoding these proteins and then put that DNA into the *nucleus* of cells (de Grey, 2000). (As with lysosomal enhancement, this would be done first by germline transformation in mice and later by gene therapy in people.) The machinery to make this work all exists already in our cells, because the 1000 or so other proteins that make up mitochondria are already encoded by nuclear genes. And sure enough, in the past year or two, a couple of groups have got ten one gene working in exactly this way (de Grey, 2001). I have a small wager with the eminent biochemist Bruce Ames that all 13 will be working in cell culture by October 2005; I think I'll collect.

So, what about nuclear DNA? As I mentioned, it suffers not only mutations but also two other types of damage, epimutations and senescence-inducing changes. I'll address senescence-inducing changes first.

We don't know whether cell senescence really matters in aging, but the same is true of some of the other items on my list, such as mitochondrial DNA damage: it's enough at this point to know that it *might* matter. So, what to do about it? As noted earlier, it may result predominantly from telomere shortening or from chromosome breakage—possibly one in some cell types and the other in others—but to my mind, the balance of evidence is presently in favor of chromosome breakage being the prime culprit. We should not, therefore, put all our eggs in the telomere reconstitution basket. A promising alternative option, presently being aggressively pursued by Judith Campisi's group, is killing of senescent cells (Campisi, 2000); this would be equally effective on all senescent cells, irrespective of how they got that way. Unlike cells full of junk, a senescent cell can be cleanly and completely disposed of once it dies; the main problem, therefore, is identifying such cells and killing them without too much collateral damage (killing of nonsenescent cells). Progress in this direction has already been encouraging. A further problem must be considered, however: once gone, such cells must be replaced, and this necessarily entails division of some other cell—which, in consequence, is potentially pushed that bit closer to telomere-based senescence itself. There is thus a threshold where a selective killing approach would create as many senescent cells as it destroyed. I believe that concern about this possibility is unfounded, however, because the proportion of cells in the body (of any cell type not associated with overt disease, except possibly articular chondrocytes [Martin and Buckwalter, 2001]) that show any sign of being anywhere near senescence is so small that this threshold could not be reached until we are many centuries old.

Epimutations are irreversible alterations, either to the DNA or to the special proteins (histones) that it is wrapped around, which alter not its sequence but instead its ability to be appropriately decoded (Santini et al., 2001). They may not be quite so irreversible as sequence changes, but again, it is prudent to hedge our bets and fix them rather than bet our lives on their unimportance. There are several molecular types of epimutation. For present purposes, however, it is not necessary to go into details, because the harm that epimutations do and the approaches that I advocate for averting such harm are exactly the same as for bona fide mutations that change the sequence. Hence, in what follows, mutations and epimutations are not distinguished.

I mentioned earlier that, very probably, the only health problem posed by mutations (or epimutations) is cancer. A tumor starts from just one cell, so in order to avoid cancer for as long as we do, we have had to evolve DNA maintenance and protection systems so good that no cell acquires the necessary mutations. Other mutations affect one cell and do not cause that cell to proliferate, so they're astronomically less harmful. But the same DNA protection machinery protects against those nononcogenic mutations too, so they are comparably rare (Dolle et al., 2000). That's why I feel we can safely ignore all nuclear mutations and epimutations other than those leading to cancer.

My view, however—and that of many of my colleagues—is that cancer is the single hardest aspect of aging to tackle. This is because cancerous cells have to be removed completely. Get rid of 90% of your lysosomal junk, and you might be able to wait 60 years before the total amount of that junk reattains the pretreatment level. Get rid of 99% of a cancer and wait 1 year, if that, and the cancer will be just as serious as before. Worse than that, chances are that it'll be harder to treat the second time, because the reason you only got rid of 99% and not 100% was that the residual 1% had acquired (epi)mutations that made it resistant to your anticancer regimen. By the time of the second treatment, the whole cancer has this resistance trait, whereas for the lysosomal junk, only about the same proportion of the new junk will be resistant as was resistant the first time.

So, what to do? Until recently, in contrast to most of the other aspects of aging I've discussed, I've gone along with the biomedical consensus: we must pursue the messy but effective *cocktail* approach. That is, throw in every type of treatment we know and rely on one or another of them to catch pretty much every cancer cell. You've heard of all the prominent anticancer approaches: old ones like radiation therapy and chemotherapy, new ones like angiogenesis inhibitors (Kerbel, 2000) and immune stimulation (Pawelece et al., 2000), and future but foreseeable ones like telomerase inhibition (White et al., 2001). My present fear, however, is that this may not suffice—that the genomic instability that gives cancer its bite will outwit all these measures and we'll find our progress against cancer lagging behind progress against other aspects of aging. I therefore advocate exploration of a very ambitious, but potentially far more comprehensive and long-term, approach to combating cancer: total elimination of vital genes for telomerase and our other telomere maintenance mechanism, alternative lengthening of telomeres (ALT), from all our mitotic cells (de Grey et al., in preparation). This improves vastly on drug-mediated telomerase inhibition because the cancer cell cannot mutate to resist the drug; it would have to create a whole enzyme, telomerase, out of thin air. The idea, of course, sounds crazy at first hearing, because many of our tissues rely utterly on telomere maintenance in stem cells, but it may well be possible, because the technology already exists to repopulate the stem cells of the blood and (in mice) the gut, and the skin shouldn't be too tricky either. The telomere reserve of neonatal stem cells suffices for about a decade, judging from the age of onset of dyskeratosis congenita, a group of diseases associated with inadequate telomere maintenance, so in theory a decadal repopulation of all our stem cell populations with new ones whose telomeres had been restored ex vivo, but that had no telomere elongation genes of their own, should maintain the relevant tissues indefinitely while preventing any cancer from reaching a life-threatening stage. Cells already in the body would need either to be ablated when they became cancerous (but without killing the engineered cells) or to have their telomerase and ALT genes mutated in situ; both approaches are, again, already close to feasible in mice.

These strategies for engineered negligible senescence are listed in Table 11.1.

Implications for Humanity Tomorrow and Thus for Gerontology Today

If you're reading about the above technologies and the motivations for them for the first time, and you're thinking that they're all so logical as to be rather obvious, I have to agree. But remember, they're not so obvious unless one adopts an engineer's goal-directed approach to the problem. Hitherto, the only people with enough knowledge of

Table 11.1 Strategies for Engineered Negligible Senescence: Interventions to Reverse Aging in Rodents and Subsequently in Humans

Reversal of Possibly Life-Limiting Change	*Feasible Strategy That May Achieve It*
Digestion of lysosomal aggregates	Bacterial/fungal hydrolases (de Grey, 2002)
Apoptosis of senescent cells	Senescence marker-targeted toxins (Campisi, 2000; de Grey et al., 2002a)
Killing of age-related tumors	Telomerase/ALT deletion (de Grey et al., 2002a, in preparation)
Nuclear rescue of mtDNA mutations	Allotopic mt-coded proteins (de Grey, 2000, 2001)
Immune system restoration	IL-7-mediated thymopoiesis (Aspinall and Andrew, 2000)
Cleavage of AGE cross-links	Phenacyldimethylthiazolium chloride (Vasan, et al., 2001)
Clearance of extracellular aggregates	Immune-mediated phagocytosis (Brazil et al., 2000)
Cell replacement	Stem cell therapy (Armstrong and Svendsen, 2000; Weissman, et al., 2001; Anversa and Nadal-Ginard, 2002)
Hormone restoration	Genetically engineered muscle (MacColl et al., 1999)

Note: For details, see text and de Grey et al. (2002a,b).
AGE: Advanced Glycation Endproducts; ALT: Alternative Lengthening of Telomeres; IL-7: interlukin-7; CM+DNA: Mitochondrial DNA.

what the problem really is have been basic scientists, with curiosity-driven mindsets that are simply not geared to thinking in the way described here.

Several of the technologies that I have discussed here were unimagined, or at least unforeseeable, 10 years ago. By 1999 or so, however, nearly every one of them was the subject of a reasonable body of literature. In October 2000 I brought together a group of far-sighted and expert biogerontologists for a day's roundtable discussion of all these problems and technologies. The discussion continued by e-mail thereafter and culminated in a manuscript setting out our cautious, but at that time unprecedentedly optimistic, view of what might be possible in anti-aging research within the next decade and anti-aging medicine a modest interval thereafter. It was published, despite the vigorous complaint that it would "engender quite unwarranted optimism," in April 2002 (de Grey et al., 2002b); a follow-up article, involving three more experts and addressing sociological as well as biological issues, came out shortly afterward (de Grey et al., 2002b). I have campaigned energetically for the adoption by my colleagues of a more intervention-friendly public face, but this still remains the approach of a depressingly small minority of them. (I must, however, draw attention to a conspicuous recent exception [Miller, 2002]. Rich Miller and I disagree sharply about what approach is likely to succeed in greatly extending the maximum human life span in this century, and also about the scale of that progress—he foresees life expectancies of about 110 years, whereas I expect them to reach the thousands, though by then they will be unmeasurable [de Grey, in preparation]—but he is forthright in the view that the scientific obstacles to doing so are much less severe than the political ones.)

Many chapters in this volume consider the desirability of a greatly extended healthy life span, so I will say very little. As we concluded the follow-up article just mentioned (de Grey et al., 2002b), this inertia is in grave danger of making the evolutionary gerontologist Michael Rose correct in his 1996 prediction that we will some day more than double the human life span, but that when we do so, we will be ashamed that we took so long about it. We risk looking foolish, it is true, if our optimistic predictions are not borne out by the rate of progress in developing genuinely effective anti-aging medicine. Further, any biogerontologist who voices optimism about the future invariably risks misrepresentation by those who would have the public believe that anti-aging medicine already exists, and is often severely criticised by colleagues for doing so (Binstock, 2003; de Grey, 2003; Le Bourg, 2003). However, we risk being responsible for the deaths of (count them) over 100,000 people every day that this technology is not developed if we delay that progress by failing to speak and act to bring it about. To coin a phrase: I don't know much about ethics, but I know which risk I prefer to take.

References

Anversa, P. and Nadal-Ginard, B. (2002). Myocyte renewal and vertricular remodeling. *Nature*, 415, 240–243.

Armstrong, R.J. and Svendsen, C.N. (2000). Neural stem cells: From cell biology to cell replacement. *Cell Transplant*, 9, 139–152.

Aspinall, R. and Andrew, D. (2000). Thymic atrophy in the mouse is a soluble problem of the thymic environment. *Vaccine,* 18, 1629–1637.

Binstock, R.H. (2003). The war on "anti-aging medicine." *Gerontologist,* 43, 4–14.

Brazil, M.I., Chung, H., and Maxfield, F.R. (2000). Effects of incorporation of immunoglobulin G and complement component C1q on uptake and degradation of Alzheimer's disease amyloid fibrils by microglia. *Journal of Biological Chemistry,* 275, 16941–16947.

Campisi, J. (2000). Cancer, aging and cellular senescence. *In Vivo,* 14, 183–188.

de Grey, A.D.N.J. (2000). Mitochondrial gene therapy: An arena for the biomedical use of inteins. *Trends in Biotechnology,* 18, 394–399.

de Grey, A.D.N.J. (2001). Response to "approaches and limitations to gene therapy for mitochondrial diseases." *Antioxidant Redox Signal,* 3, 451–460, 1153–1154.

de Grey, A.D.N.J. (2002). The biomedical potential of transgenically enhanced lysosomal catabolism. *Trends in Biotechnology,* 20, 452–455.

de Grey, A.D.J.N. (2003). Fear of misrepresentation cannot justify silence about foreseeable life-extension biotechnology. *Bioessays,* 25, 94–95.

de Grey, A.D.J.N. (manuscript in preparation). Dating a singularity: An extrapolation of anti-aging biomdical progress that incorporates societal responses to ongoing progress.

de Grey, A.D.N.J., Ames, B.N., Andersen, J.K., Bartke, A., Campisi, J., Heward, C.B., McCarter, R.J.M., and Stock, G. (2002a). Time to talk SENS: Critiquing the immutability of human aging. Annals of the New York Academy of Sciences, 959(1), 452–462.

de Grey, A.D.N.J., Baynes, J.W., Berd, D., Heward, C.B., Pawelec, G., and Stock, G. (2002b). Is human aging still mysterious enough to be left only to scientists? *Bioessays,* 24(7), 667–676.

de Grey, A.D.N.J., Dokal, I., Fairbairn, L.J., Graham, G., Jahoda, C.A., Porter, A., and Artandi S.E.(manuscript in preparation). Total removal of in vivo telomere elongation capacity: An ambitious but possibly ultimate cure for all human cancers.

Dolle, M.E., Snyder, W.K., Gossen, J.A., Lohman, P.H., and Vijg, J. (2000). Distinct spectra of somatic mutations accumulated with age in mouse heart and small intestine. *Proceedings of the National Academy Sciences of the USA,* 97, 8403–8408.

Fossel, M. (2000). Human aging and progeria. *Journal of Pediatric Endocrinology and Metabolism,* 13 (Suppl. 6), 1477–1481.

Goldspink, G. (1999). Changes in muscle mass and phenotype and the expression of autocrine and systemic growth factors by muscle in response to stretch and overload. *Journal of Anatomy,* 194, 323–334.

Harper, J.M., Leathers, C., and Austad, S.N. (in preparation). A complex response to caloric restriction in wild-derived mice.

Kerbel, R.S. (2000). Tumor angiogenesis: Past, present and the near future. *Carcinogenesis*, 21(3), 505–515.

Le Bourg, E. (2003). A public debate about the feasibility of reversing human aging could be detrimental. *Bioessays*, 25, 93–94.

MacColl, G.S., Goldspink, G., and Bouloux, P.M. (1999). Using skeletal muscle as an artificial endocrine tissue. *Journal of Endocrinology*, 162 (1) 1–9.

Martin, J.A. and Buckwalter, J.A. (2001). Telomere erosion and senescence in human articular cartilage chondrocytes. *Journal of Gerontology: Biological Sciences*, 56a B172–B179.

Martinez, D.E. (1998). Mortality patterns suggest lack of senescence in hydra. *Experimental Gerontology*, 33(3), 217–225.

Masoro, E.J. (1995). Aging: Current concepts. In: Masoro, E.J., ed. *Handbook of Physiology, Section 11: Aging*. New York: Oxford University Press, pp. 3–21.

Mattson, M.P., Duan, W., Lee, J., Guo, Z., Roth, G.S., Ingram, D.K., and Lane, M.A. (2001). Progress in the development of caloric restriction mimetic dietary supplements. *Journal of Anti-Aging Medicine*, 4, 225–232.

Miller, R.A. (2002). Extending life: Scientific prospects and political obstacles. *The Milbank Quarterly*, 80(1), 155–174.

Pawelec, G., Heinzel, S., Kiessling, R., Muller, L., Ouyang, Q., and Zeuthen, J. (2000). Escape mechanisms in tumor immunity: A year 2000 update. *Critical Review of Oncogenes*, 11(2), 97–133.

Rhee, S.G. (1999). Redox signaling: Hydrogen peroxide as intracellular messenger. *Experimental and Molecular Medicine*, 31(2), 53–59.

Santini, V., Kantarjian, H.M., and Issa, J.P. (2001). Changes in DNA methylation in neoplasia: Pathophysiology and therapeutic implications. *Annals of Internal Medicine*, 134(7), 573–586.

Vasan, S., Foiles, P.G., and Founds, H.W. (2001). Therapeutic potential of AGE inhibitors and breakers of AGE protein cross-links. *Expert Opinions of Investigative Drugs*, 10(11), 1977–1987.

Weindruch, R. and Walford, R.L. (1982). Dietary restriction in mice beginning at 1 year of age: Effect on life-span and spontaneous cancer incidence. *Science*, 215(4538), 1415–1418.

Weissman, I.L., Anderson, D.J., and Gage, F. (2001). Stem and progenitor cells: Origins, phenotypes, lineage commitments, and transdifferentiations. *Annual Review of Cell Development and Biology*, 17, 387–403.

White, L.K., Wright, W.E., and Shay, J.W. (2001). Telomerase inhibitors. *Trends in Biotechnology*, 19, 114–120.

III

ETHICAL AND SOCIAL PERSPECTIVES ON RADICAL LIFE EXTENSION

12

An Unnatural Process: Why It Is Not Inherently Wrong to Seek a Cure for Aging

Arthur L. Caplan

Not everyone thinks it is a good idea to live longer lives. Some writers, perhaps, most notably Daniel Callahan, the cofounder of the Hastings Center, argue that the quest to extend life is not a self-evident good (Callahan, 1995; Barlow, 2002). A longer life, Callahan contends, is not necessarily a better life. Other writers, such as the philosopher/physician Leon Kass (2002), the political theorist Francis Fukuyama (Fukuyama, 2002), and the theologian Gilbert Meilander (2002) argue that the extension of life should not be pursued because lengthening life is not consistent with human nature. It is "unnatural" to extend human lives beyond the proverbial three score and ten that the demographers assure us is what the average citizen of an economically developed nation can expect.

Still, scientists are eagerly pursuing research in many species that might lead to life extension in human beings (Herndon et al., 2002). French scientists have produced mice that live 26% longer through genetic engineering (Fukuyama, 2002; Kristol and Cohen, 2002). Other scientists have produced longer-lived mice, rats, and primates by placing them early in life on low-calorie diets. Still others believe that by genetically engineering the telomeres of our chromosomes or replacing human growth hormone in our bodies, the changes associated with aging can be slowed or reversed and our lives extended by 30, 40, or even 50 years. We do not know enough about aging to know if any of these interventions can deliver a longer life. But research may provide answers to the question of what does and does not work. Are the scientists, physicians, and others working on techniques that might lead to significantly longer life spans for human beings engaged, as Callahan, Kass, Fukuyama, and others suggest, in unethical activities?

Callahan and those who worry about the personal, social, and economic consequences of life extension must show that our culture or other cultures are not clever enough or flexible enough to figure out how to cope with more life. In part, the resolution of the debate about the consequences of life extension rests on empirical facts.

Have we adjusted to changes in the life span in the past in our species such that longer lives are viewed as better lives? The answer to that question if one compares life for, say, the ancient Hittites, Hebrews, Greeks, and Romans and life for Americans or Italians or Japanese today would seem to be yes.

Few could seriously maintain that an average life span of 35 years would be preferable to the 75 enjoyed today even if many do spend their final years weak, demented, or debilitated. And it would be hard to argue that despite the problems of overpopulation and ageism, the quality of life for the average person has slipped so much during those years added from those lived by the ancients that we live more poorly or less happily today. Few, in other words, would trade their longer life span for the much shorter lives lived by their ancestors thousands of years ago.

Callahan is right to wonder about the consequences of both a longer life and the costs to society of pursuing a longer life. But the empirical evidence does not seem to bear out his case that trying to live longer must of necessity either bankrupt society or lead to lives of pain and misery. We need policies that ensure that a fair proportion of resources are devoted to the young, that seniority on the job does not become stasis in the workplace, and that we do not use medical technology overaggressively once life has become a burden or simply too painful to endure.

Those such as Kass, Fukuyama, and Meilander pose a more powerful critique of the war on aging. For theirs is an in-principle objection, not one linked to the possible negative consequences of life extension. They maintain that it is unnatural to live much longer than we now do. Of course, to make this argument hold, they must show why the extension of life is unnatural. Or to put the point another way, they must be able to show that aging and senescence are both natural processes and, as such, intrinsically good things. They need to show that the life span we now have is part of our human nature. Can that case be made? I do not think so.

Normality, Naturalness, and Disease

It may seem somewhat odd to question the naturalness of a process as familiar and universal as aging. After all, if aging is not a natural process, what is? While the prospect of aging may be greeted with mixed feelings, there would seem to be little reason to doubt the fact that aging is understood to be a normal and inevitable feature of human existence. The belief that aging is a normal and natural part of human existence is reflected in the practice of medicine. For example, no mention is made in most textbooks of medicine and pathology of aging as abnormal, unnatural, or indicative of disease. It is true that such texts often contain a chapter or two on the related subject of diseases commonly associated with aging or found in the elderly. But it is the diseases of the elderly, such as pneumonia, cancer, or atherosclerosis, rather than the aging process itself, that serve as the focus of description and analysis.

What is so different about the physiological changes and deteriorations concurrent with the aging process that these events are considered to be unremarkable, natural processes, while other, very similar, debilitative changes are deemed diseases constituting health crises of the first order when they occur in younger people?

Surely it cannot simply be the life-threatening aspects of diseases, such as cancer or atherosclerosis, that distinguish these processes from aging. For while it may be true that hardly anyone manages to avoid contracting a terminal disease at some point in life, aging itself produces the same ultimate consequence as these diseases—death. Our bodies break down, and death inevitably is the consequence.

Nor can it be the familiarity and universality of aging that inures medical science to its unnatural aspects. Malignant neoplasms, viral infections, gingivitis, acne, and hypertension are all ubiquitous phenomena. Yet medicine maintains a radically different stance toward these physical processes from that which it holds toward the so-called natural changes that occur during aging.

It might be argued that the processes denoted by the term *aging* do not fit the standard conception of disease operative in clinical medicine. However, in medical dictionaries, disease is almost always defined as any pathological change in the body. Pathological change is inevitably defined as constituting any morbid process in the body. And morbid processes are usually defined in terms of disease states of the body.[1] Regardless of the circularity surrounding this explication of the concept of somatic disease, aging would seem to have a prima facie claim to being counted as a disease. Pathological or morbid changes are often the sole criteria by which age is assessed in the human body. Coroners and medical examiners determine age by morbid changes and pathological alterations in a dead body.

What does seem to differentiate aging from other processes or states traditionally classified as diseases is the fact that aging is perceived as a natural or normal process. Medicine has traditionally viewed its role as that of ameliorating or combatting the abnormal, either through therapeutic interventions or prophylactic regimens. The natural and the normal, while not outside the sphere of medicine, are concepts that play key roles in licensing the intervention of the medical practitioner. For it is in response to or in anticipation of abnormality that physicians' activities are legitimated. And as E.A. Murphy, among many other doctors, has noted, "the clinician has tended to regard disease as that state in which the limits of the normal have been transgressed" (Murphy, 1966; Murphy, 1976, p. 122; Risse, 1978). Naturalness and normality have historically been used as baselines to determine the presence of disease and the necessity of medical activity.

In light of the powerful belief that the abnormal and unnatural are indicative of medicine's range of interest, it is easy to see why many biological processes are not thought to be the proper subject of medical intervention of therapy. Puberty, growth, and maturation *as processes in themselves* all appear to stand outside the sphere of medical concern since they are normal and natural occurrences among human beings. Similarly, it seems odd to think of sexuality or fertilization as possible disease states precisely because these states are commonly thought to be natural and normal components of the human condition.

Nonetheless, it is true that certain biological processes, such as contraception, pregnancy, and fertility, have been the subjects in recent years of heated debates as to their standing as possible disease states. The notions that it is natural and normal for only men and women to have sexual intercourse or for women to undergo menopause have been challenged in many quarters. The question arises as to whether the process of aging in itself can be classified as abnormal and unnatural in a way that will open the door for the reclassification of aging as a disease process and thus as a proper subject of medical attention, concern, and control.

Aging and Medical Intervention

The past few years have seen the rise of a powerful movement for the *right to die*. Some have even gone so far as to claim that physicians and health professionals have a moral obligation to play an active role in allowing patients to die under certain circumstances. To a great extent, the status of aging and dying as natural processes looms large in discussions about the *right to die* and *death with dignity*. Often those who debate the degree to which the medical profession should intervene in the process of dying disagree about the naturalness of the phenomena of aging and dying. If the alleged right to die is to be built on a conception of the naturalness of aging and dying, then the conceptual status of these terms vis-à-vis *naturalness* must be thoroughly examined.

The perception of biological events or processes as natural or unnatural is frequently decisive in determining whether physicians treat states or processes as diseases (Socarides, 1970; Illich, 1974; Goldberg, 1975). One need only think of the controversies that swirl around allegations concerning the biological naturalness of homosexuality or schizophrenia to see that this is so. This claim is further borne out by an argument that is frequently made by older physicians to new medical students.

Medical students often find it difficult to interact with or examine elderly patients. They may feel powerless when confronted with the seemingly irreversible debilities of old age. To overcome this reluctance, older physicians are likely to point out that aging and senescence are processes that happen to everyone, even young medical students. Aging is simply part of the human condition; it should hold no terror for a young doctor. Students are told that aging is natural and that, while there may be nothing they can do to alter the inevitable course of this process, they must learn to help patients cope with their aging as best they can. It is as if teaching physicians feel obligated to label the obviously debilitative and disease-like states of old age as natural in order to discourage the students' inclination to treat the elderly as sick or diseased.

What Is Aging?

What are the grounds on which this label is applied? Why do we think of aging as a natural process? The reason that comes immediately to mind is that aging is a common and normal process. It occurs with a statistical frequency of 100%. Inevitably and uniformly, bones become brittle, vision dims, joints stiffen, and muscles lose their tone. The obvious question that arises is whether commonality, familiarity, and inevitability are sufficient conditions for referring to certain biological states as natural. To answer this question, it is necessary to first draw a distinction between aging and chronological age.

In a trivial sense, given the existence of a chronological device, all bodies that exist can be said to age relative to the measurements provided by that device. But since physicians have little practical interest in making philosophical statements about the time-bound nature of existence, or empirical claims about the relativity of space and time, it is evident that they do not have this chronological sense in mind in speaking about the familiarity and inevitability of aging. In speaking of aging, physicians are interested in a particular set of biological changes that occur with respect to time. In the aged individual, cells manifest a high frequency of visible chromosomal aberrations. The nuclei of nerve cells become distorted by clumps of chromatin, and the surrounding cytoplasm contains fewer organelles, such as mitochondria. Collagen fibers become increasingly rigid and inflexible, as manifest in the familiar phenomenon of skin wrinkling. The aorta becomes wider and more tortuous. The immunological system weakens, and the elderly person becomes more susceptible to infections. Melanin pigment formation decreases and, consequently, hair begins to whiten (Hayflick, 1994).

Naturalness, Design, and Function

Changes of this kind, in association with aging, are universal and inevitable. Universality and inevitability do not, however, seem to be sufficient conditions for referring to a process as natural. Coronary atherosclerosis, neoplasms, high blood pressure, sore throats, colds, tooth decay, and depression are all nearly universal in their distribution and seemingly inevitable phenomena, and yet we would hardly agree to call any of these things natural processes or states. The inevitability of infection by microorganisms among all humans does not cause the physician to dismiss these infections as natural occurrences of no particular medical interest. The physician may not intervene, or even attempt to prevent such diseases, but such behavior is a result of a decision concerning an unnatural disease, not a natural process.

So, if universality and inevitability are not adequate conditions for naturalness, are any other criteria available by which naturalness can be assessed and used to drive a wedge between aging and disease? There is a further sense of *natural*[2] that may prove helpful in trying to understand why physicians are reluctant to label aging a disease, preferring to think of it as a natural process.

This sense of naturalness is rooted in the notions of design, purpose, and function. Axes are designed to serve as tools for cutting trees. Scalpels are meant to be used in cutting human tissue. It would seem most unnatural to use axes for surgery and scalpels for lumberjacking. In some sense, although a skillful surgeon might in fact be able to perform surgery with an axe, it would be unnatural to do so. Similarly, many bodily organs—the liver, spleen, blood vessels, kidneys, and many glands—can perform compensatory functions when certain other organic tissues are damaged or removed. But these are not the purposes or functions they were designed to perform. While the arteries of many organisms are capable of constricting to maintain blood pressure and reduce the flow of blood during hemorrhage-induced shock, the function of arteries is not to constrict in response to such circumstances. The presence of vasoconstriction in arteries is in fact an unnatural state that signals the physician that something has gone seriously awry in the body. It would seem that much of our willingness to accept aging as a natural process is parasitic upon this sense of natural function.

Two answers are commonly given to the question What is the function of aging? The first is a theological explanation. God, as a punishment for the sins of our ancestors in the (proverbial) garden of Eden, caused humans to age and die. On this view, people age because the Creator saw fit to design them that way for retribution or punishment. Aging serves as a reminder of our moral fallibility and weakness.

The second view, which is particularly widespread in scientific circles, is that the purpose or function of aging is to clear away the old to make way for the new for evolutionary reasons. This theory was first advanced by the German cytologist and evolutionary biologist August Weisman (1891). Weisman argued that aging and debilitation must be viewed as adaptational responses on the part of organisms to allow for new mutational and adaptive responses to fluctuating environments. Aging benefits the population by removing the superannuated to make room for the young. The function of aging is to ensure the death of organisms to allow evolutionary change and new adaptation to occur.

On both of these views, aging has an intended purpose or function. And it is from this quasi-Aristotelian attribution of a design that the concept of the naturalness of aging is often thought to arise (Kass, 2002).

The Concept of Biological Function

If the naturalness of aging resides in a functional interpretation, there is a rich and abundant literature on the subjects of function and purpose. However, rooting the source of the naturalness of biological processes in ideas of function or purpose also has its drawbacks, the primary problem being that philosophers have by no means reached anything even vaguely resembling a consensus about the meaning of such terms as *function* or *purpose*.

Fortunately, it is possible to avoid becoming bogged down in an analysis of functional or purposive statements in analyzing the function of aging. The only distinction required for understanding the function of aging is that between the aim of explaining the existence of a particular state, organ, or process and that of explaining how a state, organ, or process works in a particular system or organism. Functional or purposive statements are sometimes used to explain the existence of a trait or process historically. At other times, such statements are used mechanistically to explain how something works or operates. If we ask what is the function, or role, or purpose of the spleen in the human body, the question can be interpreted in two ways: How does the spleen work—what does it do in the body? or Why does the spleen exist in its present state in the human body— what is the historical story that explains why persons have spleens?[3]

It is this latter sense of function, the historical sense, that is relevant to the determination of the naturalness or unnaturalness of aging as a biological process. For while there is no shortage of theories purporting to explain how aging works or functions, these theories are not relevant to the historically motivated question about the function of aging. The determination of the naturalness of aging, if it is to be rooted in biology, will depend not on how the process of aging actually operates, but rather on the explanation one gives for the existence or presence of aging humans.[4] This is the sense of naturalness that Kass, Fukuyama, and others must rely upon to make their case that extending life by conquering aging is wrong because it is unnatural.

Does Aging Have a Function?

Two purported explanations—one theological, one scientific—of the function or purpose of aging have been given. Both are flawed. While the theological explanation of aging may carry great weight for numerous individuals, it will simply not do as a scientific explanation of why aging occurs in humans. Medical professionals may have to cope with their patients' advocacy of this explanation and their own religious feelings on the subject. But, from a scientific perspective, it will hardly do to claim that aging, as a result of God's vindictiveness, is a natural biological process and hence not a disease worthy of treatment.

More surprisingly, the scientific explanation of aging as serving an evolutionary role or purpose is also inadequate. It is simply not true that aging exists to serve any sort of evolutionary purpose or function. The claim that aging exists or occurs in individuals because it has a wider role or function in the evolutionary scheme of things rests on a faulty evolutionary analysis. There is nothing natural about aging and, contrary to the views of Kass, Fukuyama, and many others, aging is not a natural attribute of being human.

To assign a purpose to aging incorrectly assumes that it is possible for biological processes to exist that directly benefit or advance the evolutionary success of a species or population. In other words, it supposes that processes such as aging exist because they serve a function or purpose in the life history of a species—in this case, that of removing the old to make way for the new. However, evolutionary selection rarely acts to advance the prospects of an entire species or population. Selection acts on individual organisms and their phenotypic traits and properties. Some traits or properties confer advantages in certain environments on the organisms that possess them, and this fact increases the likelihood that the genes responsible for producing these traits will be passed on to future organisms.

Given that selective forces act on individuals and their genotypes and not on species, it makes no sense to speak of aging as serving an evolutionary function or purpose to benefit the species. How then do evolutionary biologists explain the existence of aging (Williams, 1966; Ghiselin, 1974)? Briefly, the explanation is that features, traits, or properties in individual organisms will be selected for if they confer a relative reproductive advantage on the individual, or his or her close kin. Any variation that increases inclusive reproductive fitness has a very high probability of being selected and maintained in the gene pool of a species. Selection, however, cannot look ahead to foresee the possible consequences of favoring certain traits at a given time; the environment selects for those traits and features that give an immediate return. An increased metabolic rate, for example, may prove advantageous early in life, in that it may provide more energy for seeking mates and avoiding predators; it may also result in early deterioration of the organism due to an increased accumulation of toxic wastes or genetic mutations in the body of an individual thus endowed (Herndon et al., 2002). Natural selection cannot foresee such delayed debilitating consequences.

Aging exists, then, as a consequence of lack of evolutionary foresight; it is simply a by-product of selective forces working to increase the chances of reproductive success in the life of an organism. Senescence has no function; it is simply the inadvertent subversion of organic function, later in life, in favor of maximizing reproductive advantage early in life.

The common belief that aging serves a function or purpose, if this belief is based on evolutionary theory, is mistaken. And, if this is so, it would seem that the common belief that aging is a natural process, as a consequence of the function or purpose it serves in the life of the species, is also mistaken. Consequently, unless it is possible to motivate the description on other grounds, it would seem that aging cannot be understood as a natural process. And if that is true, and if it is actually the case that what goes on during the aging process closely parallels the changes that occur during paradigmatic examples of disease,[5] then it would be unreasonable not to consider aging a disease.

Theories of Aging and the Concept of Disease

A consideration of the changes that constitute aging in human beings reinforces the similarities existing between aging and other clear-cut examples of somatic diseases. There is a set of external manifestations or symptoms: graying hair, increased susceptibility to infection, wrinkling skin, loss of muscular tone, and, frequently, loss of mental ability. These manifestations seem to be causally linked to a series of internal cellular and subcellular changes. The presence of symptoms and an underlying etiology closely parallels the standard paradigmatic examples of disease. If the analogy is pushed a bit further, the cause for considering aging a disease appears to become even stronger.

There are many theories as to what causes changes at the cellular and subcellular levels that produce the signs and symptoms associated with aging (Comfort, 1964, 1970; Hayflick, 1973). One view argues that aging is caused by an increase in the number of cross-linkages that exist in protein and nucleic acid molecules. Cross-linkages lower the biochemical efficiency and dependability of certain macromolecules involved in metabolism and other chemical reactions. Free radical by-products of metabolism are thought to accumulate in cells, thus allowing for an increase in available linkage sites for replicating nucleic acid strands and activating histone elements. This sort of cross-linkage is thought to be particularly important in the aging of collagen, the substance responsible for most of the overt symptoms we commonly associate with aging, such as wrinkled skin and loss of muscular flexibility.

Another view holds that aging results from an accumulation of genetic mutations in the chromosomes of cells in the body. The idea underlying this theory is that chromosomes are exposed over time to a steady stream of radiation and other mutagenic agents. The accumulation of mutational hits on the genes lying on the chromosomes results in the progressive inactivation of these genes (Herndon et al., 2002). The evidence of a higher incidence of chromosomal breaks and aberrations in the aged is consistent with this mutational theory of aging.

Along with the cross-linkage and mutational theories, there is one other important hypothesis concerning the cause of aging. The autoimmune theory holds that, as time passes and the chromosomes of cells in the human body accumulate more mutations, certain key tissues begin to synthesize antibodies that can no longer distinguish between self and foreign material. Thus, a number of autoimmune reactions occur in the body as the immunological system begins to turn against the individual it was *designed* to protect. Arthritis and pernicious anemia are symptomatic of the sorts of debilities resulting from the malfunction of the immunological system. While this theory is closely allied to the mutation theory, the autoimmune view of aging holds that accumulated mutations do not simply result in deterioration of cellular activity but, rather, produce lethal cellular end products that consume and destroy healthy tissue.

It would be rash to hold that any of the three hypotheses cited— the cross-linkage, mutational, or autoimmune hypotheses—will, in the end, turn out to be the correct explanation of aging. All three views are, in fact, closely related in that cross-linkages can result from periodic exposure to mutagenic agents and can, in turn, produce genetic aberrations that eventuate in cellular dysfunction or even autoimmunological reactions. What is important, however, is not whether one of these theories or *any* of them is in fact the correct theory of aging, but that all of them postulate mechanisms that are closely analogous to those mechanisms cited by clinicians in describing disease processes in the body.

The concept of disease is, without doubt, a slippery and evasive notion in medicine (Veatch, 1973). Once one moves away from what can be termed *paradigmatic* examples of disease, such as tuberculosis or diphtheria, toward more nebulous examples, such as acne or jittery nerves, it becomes difficult to say exactly what are the criteria requisite for labeling a condition a somatic disease. However, even though it is notoriously difficult to concoct a set of necessary and sufficient conditions for employing the term *organic disease*, it is possible to cite a list of general criteria that seem relevant in attempting to decide whether a bodily state or process is appropriately labeled a disease.

One criterion is that the state or process produces discomfort or suffering. A second is that the process or state can be traced back to a specific cause, event, or circumstance. A third is that there is a set of clear-cut structural changes, both macroscopic and microscopic, that follow in a uniform, sequential manner subsequent to the initial precipitating or causal event. A fourth is that there is a set of clinical symptoms or manifestations (headache, pain in the chest, rapid pulse, shortness of breath) commonly associated with the observed physiological alterations in structure. Finally, there is usually some sort of impairment in the functions, behavior, or activity of a person thought to be diseased (Boorse, 1975). Not all diseases will satisfy all or any of the criteria I have suggested. One need only consider the arguments surrounding the classification of astigmatism, alcoholism, drug addiction, gambling, and hyperactivity to realize the inadequacy of these criteria as necessary and sufficient conditions for the determination of disease. But that the suggested criteria are relevant to such determination is shown by the fact that advocates of all persuasions regarding controversial states and processes commonly resort to considerations of causation, clinical manifestations, etiology, functional impairment, and suffering in arguing the merits of their various views concerning the status of controversial cases.

With respect to the conceptual ambiguity surrounding the notion of disease, it is important to remember that medicine is by no means unique in being saddled with what might be termed *fuzzy-edged* concepts. One need only consider the status of terms such as *species, adaptation,* and *mutation* in biology, or *stimulus, behavior,* and *instinct* in psychology, to realize that medicine is not alone in the ambiguity of its key terms. It is also true that, just as the biologist is able to use biological theory to aid in the determination of relevant criteria for a concept, the physician is able to use his or her knowledge of the structure and function of the body to decide on relevant criteria for the determination of disease. If one accepts the relevance of the five suggested criteria, aging as a biological process is seen to possess all the key properties of a disease. Unlike astigmatism or nervousness, aging possesses a definitive group of clinical manifestations or symptoms; a clear-cut etiology of structural changes at both the macroscopic and microscopic levels; a significant measure of impairment, discomfort, and suffering; and, if we are willing to grant the same tolerance to current theories of aging as we grant to theories in other domains of medicine, an explicit set of precipitating factors. Aging has all the relevant markings of a disease process. It has none of the attributes of a functional process. The explanation of why aging occurs has many of the attributes of a stochastic or chance phenomenon. And this makes aging unnatural and in no way an intrinsic part of human nature.

As such, there is no reason why it is intrinsically wrong to try to reverse or cure aging. There may be external reasons—cost, inequity, or even a fear that the overall quality of life will diminish—but those who want to make the case against treating aging as a disease must show why human beings are not capable of solving the challenges that a longer life expectancy would create.

Notes

1. See, for example, *Dorland's Illustrated Medical Dictionary*, 25th ed. (Philadelphia: W.B. Saunders, 1974).

2. Cf. D.B. Hausman, "What is Natural?," *Perspectives in Biology and Medicine*, 19 (1975), 92–101, for an illuminating discussion of the concept.

3. For a sample of the extant explications of the concept of function see L. Wright, "Functions," *Philosophical Review*, 82 (1973), 139–168; R. Cummins, "Functional Analysis," *Journal of Philosophy*, 72 (1975), 741–765; and M.A. Boden, *Purposive Explanation in Psychology* (Cambridge, MA: Harvard, 1972). See also E. Nagel, *Teleology Revisited* (New York: Columbia University Press, 1979).

4. Further discussion of the distinction between explaining the operation of a trait or feature and explaining the origin and presence of a trait or feature can be found in A.L. Caplan, "Evolution, Ethics and the Milk of Human Kindness," *Hastings Center Report*, 6(2), (1976), 20–26.

5. For an interesting attempt to analyze the concepts of illness and disease, see C. Boorse, "On the Distinction Between Illness and Disease," *Philosophy and Public Affairs*, 5(1), (1975), 49–68.

References

Barlow, R. (2002, November 14). Ethicist questions quest to extend life. *Boston Globe*, p. 2.

Boorse, C. (1975). On the distinction between illness and disease. *Philosophy and Public Affairs*, 5(1), 49–68.

Callahan, D. (1995). *What Kind of Life? The Limits of Medical Progress.* Washington, DC: Georgetown University Press.

Comfort, A. (1964). *Aging: The Biology of Senescence.* New York: Holt, Rinehart & Winston.

Comfort, A. (1970). Biological theories of aging. *Human Development*, 13, 127–139.

Fukuyama, F. (2002). *Our Posthuman Future: Consequences of the Biotechnology Revolution.* New York: Farrar, Straus & Giroux.

Ghiselin, M.T. (1974). *The Economy of Nature and the Evolution of Sex.* Berkeley: University of California Press.

Goldberg, S. (1975). What is "normal"?: Logical aspects of the question of homosexual behavior. *Psychiatry*, 38, 227–242.

Hayflick, L. (1973). *How and Why We Age.* New York: Ballantine Books?

Hayflick, L. (1994). The strategy of senescence. *Gerontologist*, 37–45.

Herndon, L.A., Schmeissner, P.J., Dudaronek, J.M., Brown, P.A., Listner, K.M., Sakano, Y., Paupard, M.C., Hall, D.H., and Driscoll, M. (2002). Stochastic and genetic factors influence tissue-specific decline in aging *C. elegans. Nature*, 419, 808–814.

Illich, I. (1974). The political uses of natural death. *Hastings Center Studies*, 2, 3–20.

Kass, L.R. (2002). *Life, Liberty and the Defense of Dignity*. Encounter Books. San Francisco, CA:

Kristol, W. and Cohen, E. (Eds.). (2002). *The Future Is Now: America Confronts the New Genetics*. Lanham, MD: Rowman & Littlefield.

Meilander, G. (2002). Genes as Resources. *Hedgehog Review*, 4(3), 66–79.

Murphy, E.A. (1966). A scientific viewpoint on normalcy. *Perspectives in Biology and Medicine*, 9(3), 333–348.

Murphy, E.A. (1976). *The Logic of Medicine*. Baltimore: Johns Hopkins University Press.

Risse, G.B. (1978). Health and disease: History of the concepts. In: Reich, W.T., ed. *Encyclopedia of Bioethics*. New York: Free Press, 579–585.

Socarides, C. (1970). Homosexuality and medicine. *Journal of the American Medical Association*, 212(7), 1199–1202.

Veatch, R.M. (1973). The medical model: Its nature and problems. *Hastings Center Studies*, 1(3), 59–76.

Weisman, A. (1891). *Essays Upon Heredity and Kindred Biological Problems*. Oxford: Clarendon Press.

Williams, G.C. (1966). *Adaptation and Natural Selection*. Princeton, NJ: Princeton University Press.

13

Longevity, Identity, and Moral Character: A Feminist Approach

Christine Overall

*I*ncreases in human life expectancy over the past century and the possibility of growth in the total human life span raise empirical questions about the differences that greater longevity is making and will make in how we human beings live our lives, how we think of ourselves, and how we relate to each other. They raise factual questions about what human beings have and will have time to learn, to do, to experience, and to become habituated to, whether individually or collectively. However, the significant ethical question is normative: in a context of increasing longevity, how *ought* we to live our lives, think of ourselves, and relate to each other?

Life expectancy refers to the average number of years an individual will live; this figure varies by sex, race, and socioeconomic class. *Life span* refers to the maximum amount of time actually lived by any human being, a figure that now stands at around 120 years. There is indisputable evidence that, because of better living conditions and improved medical care, life expectancies have improved markedly over the past century and a half and are likely to continue to do so in the developing nations as well as in the West. There is, however, no scientific consensus as to whether significant increases in maximum life span are attainable. I will nonetheless assume that life span extension is also possible.

In my book (Overall, 2003), I explore a wide range of arguments for and against the value for human beings of an extended life. I will not recapitulate the details of those arguments here. Instead I assume that, other things being equal, a longer life is a better one, provided that one is in a minimally good state of health. The main reason, simply stated, is that a longer life is the prerequisite for almost everything else that one might want. "For anyone who has desires about future states requiring his own existence, it is rational that he regret the anticipation of his nonexistence" (Veatch, 1989, p. 236). The case for valuing longer life is based not on any allegation about the supposed intrinsic value of longevity, of life itself, or of human lives. Instead, it is founded on a genuine appreciation of human potential, of what people want in their lives and are capable of doing and experiencing when given more opportunities. An increased life span gives human beings the chance for activities and experiences that they would not otherwise have enjoyed. Collectively, extending average life expectancy provides for the society in which it occurs the value of increased experience, know-how, labor, loving relationships, and so on—that is, whatever healthy old(er) people can contribute.[1]

I therefore take for granted that increases in life expectancy and life span are worth seeking and, in particular, that society should follow a policy that I call *affirmative prolongevitism* (Overall, 2003), in which efforts are made to increase the life expectancy of members of disadvantaged groups such as poor people, native people, and people of color, whose current life expectancy is lower than that of more privileged white people. In this chapter, I consider not what the value of longer life is to the individual and to society, but rather what longer life implies for the values that we learn, promulgate, and adhere to, both individually and collectively. My focus here is not on what future moralities will be like. That is, I am not trying to make predictions about the future of moral change. Instead, I am making a case for not just the possibility but also the desirability of moral change, both individually and collectively, given the fact that lives are getting longer. In a context of increasing length of life, what kinds of persons should we be and strive to become, and what ought our responsibilities and values to be? I shall try to delineate, from a feminist philosophical perspective, why this problem arises and is important. I shall also propose a theoretical framework from which these normative questions can best be answered.[2]

The Problem and Its Importance

If human lives become significantly longer, we might be tempted to believe that we human beings can just go on in the same way that we have in the past, and that no moral changes are necessary. Daniel Callahan, who for 25 years has argued against increasing either the human life span or human life expectancy, states that there is no good case to show that a longer life would be better, for, he says, "More of the same is not, by itself, a very good argument" (Callahan, 1977, p. 37).[3] Callahan claims that those who seek longer lives want "the clock of the life cycle stopped at a particular point" (1998, pp. 131–132). The realization of this wish, he says, would result in "boredom and ennui, with the possibility of significant change arrested and frozen" (1998, p. 132). Indeed, he suggests that there is no reason to believe that an increased life expectancy would lead to "a better family life, greater economic productivity, a richer cultural and scientific life, or a generally higher standard of collective happiness and sense of well-being" (1998, p. 134).

But Callahan fails to offer arguments to show that longer life would necessarily be "more of the same." The empirical evidence from the distant and near past provides strong evidence both of the capacity of human beings to adapt to and change with the opportunities afforded by increasing age, and of the difficulty, if not the impossibility, of resisting social and technological changes and carrying on in the same way. The accelerating pace of transformation, especially since the Industrial Revolution, indicates that there will be even more to which we must adjust. Even if there can reasonably be said to be a fixed human nature, it nonetheless possesses sufficient plasticity and versatility to allow considerable adaptation to changing conditions, conditions created both through human volition and independent of it. Contrary to Aristotle, human character is not unchangeable, and the plasticity of human nature is not mere passivity to being shaped but the product of active choices in interaction with social and nonsocial environments.

Biomedical ethicists who oppose increasing human life argue that with current life expectancies, individuals already are able to live a full life, so that its ending at the current life expectancy is not an evil (Callahan, 1977, p. 37; 1987, pp. 66–67; 1998, pp. 130–135; see also Hardwig, 2000). But what is a full life? Callahan claims that it is an existence in which "one's life possibilities have on the whole been accomplished" (1987, p. 66). Yet one's life possibilities might well mean one thing under the current life expectancy and something else rather different with a longer life expectancy and a greater maximum life span.

Today, our "life possibilities" are defined and understood within contemporary strictures, not by reference to potentially greater longevity. For example, Callahan says that a "natural death" arrives when, among other conditions, "one's life work has been accomplished" and "one's moral obligations to those for whom one has had responsibility have been discharged" (1977, p. 33; 1987, p. 66). But notice that if our lives become increasingly long, then the concepts of "one's life work" and "one's moral obligations" are likely to change and their dimensions to expand. It is an error, the fallacy of begging the question, to make use of the limited parameters set by current life expectancies in order to argue against increasing human longevity.

For Callahan, one's life's work means "primarily one's vocational or professional work" (1977, p. 33). Even setting aside the possible limitations on or lack of clarity in this definition (does it include familial work, domestic work, volunteer work, hobbies and avocations?), it is also likely that as lives get longer, the scope of individuals' goals will become greater, and people will play a variety of working roles during their lifetimes. Generally, our ideas of what we are capable of taking on will evolve and develop. As they do today, people will undertake new tasks, projects, and interests at different life stages, but if those life stages are longer, then the range of tasks, projects, and interests can become broader.

In addition, our moral obligations may change and grow. As longevity increases, the number of relationships in which one engages and the number of people for whom one has moral responsibility may enlarge. Responsibilities may last longer; the nature of the responsibilities may change; and one may acquire and then discharge responsibilities at various points in a longer life. Once again, to assume that current social and moral exigencies—defined by Callahan in a limited fashion as responsibility for one's immediate biological children (1987, p. 69)—delineate the outward limits of what human beings should expect and do is to beg the question.

The future itself will mean something quite different when there is, reliably, more of it for the average individual. Short lives such as those that prevailed in much of the past and still prevail in poverty-stricken areas of the world must necessarily be more concerned with the basics of physical survival and social reproduction than with education, investigation, creativity, and personal and social development. By contrast, a longer life can be concerned not only with physical maturation but also with individual and cultural maturity and the living of an *optimal life*, a life of fulfillment or meaningfulness (Baier, 1974, pp. 4–5). A society in which lives are longer can aim at the enrichment and enhancement of citizens' lives. I therefore suggest that with increases in longevity, we should not expect more of the same, and we should prepare for and see the necessity of moral change.

It might be objected that, just as individuals ought not to be expected to have different values and responsibilities because of their gender or race, so also is it an error to attribute different values and responsibilities to people because of their age. To ascribe moral responsibilities on the basis of gender or race is to fall prey to sexism and racism, the stereotyping of people, respectively, on the basis of gender and racialization. Therefore, the objection goes, it is an error to suppose that age, even the possibly much greater age that might be achieved through socially steered research and policies to extend life expectancy and life span, should make a difference to one's moral values and responsibilities.

However, my point is not that merely getting older demands new values and responsibilities. My point is that greater longevity, as a widespread social phenomenon, requires the development of new moral systems. The reason is that as the human life span increases, different stages of life are being and will continue to be redefined. I contend that this redefinition of life stages will, unlike gender and racial identities, necessitate moral change. The evidence already shows that increasing longevity creates opportunities for new ways of living (Goddard, 1982, p. 152). For example:

- The enormous growth in research and technology and the concomitant expansion of the knowledge and skills required for many jobs and occupations will have two effects. First, they will continue to increase the time during which offspring are financially dependent or obtaining formal education and are considered to be children and young adults. Thus, what it means to be a child and a young adult will be redefined. Second, the growth in research and technology and the concomitant expansion of knowledge and skills will continue to make it necessary for individuals to move into and out of educational institutions and training environments at a variety of points during their lives. *Lifelong learning* in the form of formal and informal schooling will permit people to continue to acquire skills, information, and understanding as need and interest dictate. Thus, what *schooling* and *education* mean will be redefined.

- Familial, romantic, and amical relationships could last longer. In addition, there would be opportunities for more relationships at various points during the longer life. There may be an increase in the current trend of postponing decisions to enter into permanent and/or legally sanctioned relationships such as marriage. For many, it might be normal and unsurprising to have several legal or common-law marriages or other intimate relationships during one's life, along with divorces and breakups. Moreover, since sexual orientation and gender are becoming more fluid in some people, there may be more variations in sexual and gender identities. Thus, what *marriage, partnership, friendship, sexuality,* and *gender* mean will be redefined.

- Better health and increasing technological control over conception, contraception, gestation, and birth make it possible not only to change the period of time that women devote to reproductive behaviors, but also to have children later in life. Extended or intermittent periods of childbearing and childrearing could be aided by adoption both within and outside national borders, and by the use of new reproductive technologies and practices, whether or not they are legally sanctioned, including sperm donation, in vitro fertilization, contract motherhood, and cloning. One would have much more of a chance not only to raise one's children but to know them well past what we now call middle age. The ideas of, and the length of time committed to, parenthood and childrearing could change as the relationship of parent to child becomes ever longer. We would live to see our great-grandchildren and even our great-great-grandchildren grow to adulthood, and large multigenerational extended families, not necessarily all living in the same place or even the same country, would be possible. Changes in family configurations would include more single parents, blended families, gay couples, and lesbian couples. Thus, *father, mother, parent, grandparent,* and *family* will be redefined.

- With the evolution of technology, changes in resources, and growth in knowledge, there will also be changes to work, work lives, and the number of jobs or careers that an individual may hold (for all of these, see Madigan, 1999, p. 43). Longer lives and the rapid pace of change provide the opportunity and even the necessity of engaging in several careers during one lifetime, and of both self-employment and moving from one employer to another rather than working for a single institution for all one's working days. With changes in access to employment and work, there will be changes in material security, living environments, and mobility. The life stage called *retirement,* when individuals with adequate financial means can be relieved of all or most paid work, engage in leisure activities, and enjoy relatively good health for a longer period of time is becoming a reality for many in the West. The age of retirement may change, becoming more flexible, and work sabbaticals may be available. *Work, job, career,* and *retirement* will therefore be redefined.

In enumerating these possible changes to life stages, I am not suggesting that they are all unavoidable, or that they are necessarily all desirable and good. My point is just that as human longevity increases, life stages will be re-created and reinterpreted; we will adopt new roles and new identities. Even within current life spans, we can see that some human beings are capable of changing their lives, of making new beginnings, of virtually becoming different selves (Overall, 2003). The religious convert, the reformed alcoholic, the dedicated first-time parent, the newly disabled individual, the immigrant to a different society, the recently released prisoner, and the adult who learns to read at the age of 40 are all persons who are engaged in processes of re-creating themselves. Given the resources and the opportunities, human beings are capable of changing their lives, often even in the face of oppressive or debilitating circumstances.

Many human beings today, perhaps the vast majority, never have the chance fully to explore and express all of their potential as physical/emotional/moral/intellectual beings. What type of person we can reasonably want and intend to be depends in part on what our social and environmental context permits, forbids, or encourages.

A more prolonged life would provide at least some of that missed opportunity. With new and redefined life stages, human beings will have the prospect of taking up new values and responsibilities. What type of person we *ought* to be depends on what kind of person we can be. When we get a glimpse of how our identities—who we are—may change as a result of increasing years, we may also see in what ways our character—who we ought to be—should change.

Rethinking Morality

To answer the question of how we should live in the context of extended life expectancies and life spans, I propose a feminist virtue ethics approach. The word *virtue* has acquired, within the past century, a connotation of chastity, especially women's chastity and sexual purity. This association is unfortunate. In its older sense, *virtue* meant "moral excellence," and this is the sense in which it is used within virtue ethics. In general, virtue ethics is less concerned with the modern ethical questions "What are my moral obligations?" and "What is my duty?" than with problems that are both ancient and yet enduring: "How should I live?" and "What kind of person should I be?"

In virtue ethics, the unit of ethical appraisal and judgment is not an action or a class of actions, but the character and life of an individual. Although it is "neither desirable nor feasible" entirely to separate actions from agents (Tong, 1998, p. 136), the focus of virtue ethics is on the individual agent and his or her character, from which actions flow. Thus, morality is rooted more in persons and their characters than in acts or rules. What is foundational is not right and wrong action alone, but rather good and bad character, which predispose one to right or wrong action. Character is a "complex disposition" to act in certain ways (S. Leighton, personal communication); one's character is the composite of the psychological qualities, both mental and moral, that make one a distinct person.

Virtue theorists believe there is an important connection between virtue and human flourishing. Virtues may be variously other-regarding and self-regarding, and possessing moral virtues, being morally virtuous, benefits both other people and oneself. Thus, becoming a good person and cultivating moral virtues is closely tied to the creation of good both for oneself and for others. In the words of Rosalind Hursthouse, "A virtuous agent is one who acts virtuously, that is, one who has and exercises the virtues" (1996, p. 23), and "An action is right iff [if and only if] it is what a virtuous agent would characteristically (i.e., acting in character) do in the circumstances" (p. 22). Asking oneself what a virtuous person would do in a given case need not generate hard and fast rules; virtue is not a fixed feature, but something that one repeatedly chooses and expresses in action. The virtuous person has moral knowledge that enables him or her to choose the appropriate actions within ethical contexts; he or she is a moral role model whose behavior is a guide to a moral way of life.

What distinguishes feminist from nonfeminist ethics? What would make virtue ethics feminist? I shall describe three main characteristics of feminist virtue ethics, characteristics that demonstrate, I think, how well suited virtue ethics is to being the morality for increased human longevity.

Personal and Social Context

Modern Western philosophy advocates impartial reasoning as the method for moral decisionmaking. However, "in requiring the absence of bias toward or against any subjective interests, impartiality thereby demands that the moral agent reason in detachment from her own loyalties, projects, and emotions. These forms of detachment . . . are inimical to what is required for the maintenance of close personal relationships" (Friedman, 1998, p. 394). Moreover, "[I]mpartiality requires that persons and situations be conceptualized in terms of generalizable categories. This approach ignores the rich contextual detail of particular situations" (1998, p. 397). By contrast, feminism advocates what Alisa Carse calls "qualified particularism," which "highlight[s] concrete and nuanced perception and understanding— including an attunement to the reality of other people and to the actual relational contexts we find ourselves in" (Carse, quoted in Tong, 1998, p. 134). We are not just individual moral actors, but also workers, children, parents, friends, colleagues, creators, consumers, and citizens. We are situated, and we live within relationships. Feminist virtue ethics therefore bids moral actors and appraisers to take personal and social contexts into account when making moral decisions and judgments. Virtues (and vices) do not develop in a social vacuum, and the expression of good character involves connections and interactions with other human beings. As Sarah Conly acknowledges, virtue ethics emphasizes "the personal nature of moral life"; it implies that "our personal commitments should inform our moral choices" (Conly, 2001, p. 12).

Feminist virtue ethics allows for the possibility that appropriate and genuine virtues may be defined in relation to the specific communities in which they are needed and valued (Blum, 1996, p. 233). For example, a community whose existence depends on agriculture in an unstable climate may require of many of its members the characteristics of patience, stoicism, versatility, and acceptance. A community that is under constant attack from hostile neighbors may require the characteristics of courage, strength, and endurance. Some virtues, then, are both generated by and also function to sustain the communities within which they exist (Blum, 1996, p. 234). This is not to say that patience, versatility, courage, and so on are not virtues outside of those communities, or that they may not be needed in other communities with different characteristics and in different environments. I am not advocating ethical relativism. It is merely to emphasize that the pragmatic salience of certain virtues can ebb and flow, and that some virtues may be of greater value for the flourishing of some communities, and of individuals in those communities, than for others.

Since feminist ethics emphasizes the importance of personal and social contexts both in shaping moral challenges and in providing the data for responding to them, it requires us to be aware of contexts of aging and of increasing longevity. Philosophical sensitivity to the ways social contexts affect ethics and morality must be extended to take into account the increasing length of human lives. Some virtues, like honesty and truthfulness, may be important for a lifetime, while others, such as receptiveness or assertiveness, may be more useful at some life stages than at others. As communities change and evolve, in part because people live longer and have different and wider opportunities, the nature of the virtues that are relevant to life within those communities may change, requiring, for example, versatility, resilience, tolerance, compassion, courage, and openness to differences and diversity.

The Influence of Oppression and Marginalization on Morality

So feminists insist that the individual and cultural contexts of moral characteristics, problems, and judgments must be acknowledged. As Margaret Urban Walker puts it, "moral knowledge like other knowledge is situated (that is, it is made possible and is limited by where it comes from and how it is achieved)" (Walker, 1998, p. 6). Ethicists ought not to make moral evaluations or construct moral theory within a vacuum. Morality and moral systems cannot be analyzed and assessed without attention to the social context in which moral values are transmitted and moral decisions are made. Ethicists and policy makers must take into account the effects and implications of cultural categories such as gender, race, class, sexual orientation, ability, and age, and their attendant belief systems and stereotypes.

Feminism helps us to consider how these assigned and acquired identities influence what kinds of persons we choose to become and are shaped to be. It alerts us to the significance of systematic forms of oppression such as sexism, racism, classism, ableism, and heterosexism, which differentially advantage and disadvantage members of different groups, shape social images of what different groups are like and should be like, and constrain people's lives in order to force them to conform to norms derived not from their best interests but from presumptions about their place in society. Individual communities, even small ones, are not monocultures, and some of the differences within a community come from the inequities they encompass and the relationships of dominance and subordination that prevail between different subgroups.

Feminists also draw attention to the influence of ageism and age categories on personal identities and social interactions (e.g., Copper, 1988; Macdonald, 1991; Walker, 1999). Western society is rife with stereotyping on the basis of age, stereotyping that is empirically and morally unjustified:

> Old people in American society constitute a minority group whose members are victims of ageism. For decades, there has been widespread acceptance of negative stereotypes about the aged involving references to their intellectual decline, conservatism, sexual decline, lack of productivity, and preference for disengagement. Though most such images are based on half-truths or outright falsities, they continue to be used to justify the maltreatment of the aged by American society.
>
> (Levin and Levin, 1980, p. 95)

For, as Phillida Salmon points out, contrary to ageist biases, it is "supremely improbable that a person's age should define her better than anything else about her—that the mere passage of time should tell us all we need to know of her. It might even be said that a standardized, age-governed view is less and less appropriate as people get older. . . . [I]t may be that the person becomes more themselves and less like anyone else, the further they advance through life" (Salmon, 1985, p. 41). Contrary to ageist stereotypes about aging people, the potential to adapt and change is a fundamental characteristic of all human beings at all ages. Hence, as human lives get longer, it will be essential to be critical of categories such as *the elderly*, *the aging*, and *senior citizens*. We would have to give up, once and for all, the unthinking assumption that adulthood is the apex of life, for which childhood is the preparation and from which old age is merely the decline and downward deterioration (Salmon, 1985, pp. 3–4).

Feminists point out that many of our present moral categories, concepts, and expectations are tainted by prevailing conditions of inequality, marginalization, and injustice. Feminist ethicists argue that traditional philosophical concepts of personhood, autonomy, obligation, rules, and the nature of morality itself, purported to be objective and neutral, have been skewed by philosophers' failure to be critical of these social categories and their implications. As Walker puts it, "moral theories end up encoding specific social positions and cultural assumptions in highly idealized forms" (Walker, 1998, p. x). "These theories idealize relations of nonintimate, mutually independent peers seeking to preserve autonomy or enhance self-interest in rule- (or role-) bound voluntary interactions. They mirror spheres of activity, social roles, and character ideals associated with socially advantaged men" (Walker, 1998, p. 20).

Feminist virtue ethics is founded upon this critical analysis of subordinated identities and the necessity of a politically grounded evaluation of moral systems. Prevailing concepts of moral goodness and virtue are not immune to cultural influence and must be subjected to evaluation. Persons of different sexes, races, classes, and so on learn different sorts of virtues and come to ascribe moral value to different activities and goals. Many virtues are gendered, racialized, and reflective of other categories such as class. In the past, for example, the virtues expected from the slave were not the same as the virtues expected from the free man. The virtuous child was not supposed to act in the same ways as the virtuous adult. Being good was different for a *lady* than for a more *common* woman. Because slavery is wrong, we must be critical of the virtues assigned to slaves and to their masters. If the social categories of lady and of the common woman demean women and limit their potential, then we must also consider how the virtues associated with these categories uphold marginalization. And if children have traditionally been treated as chattels or commodities, then we must investigate how the virtues assigned to children may uphold their status as object and prevent them from being recognized as developing persons.

Moreover, just as the virtues traditionally attributed to women both arose from and helped to sustain the sexism that kept women down, so also, as Sara Ruddick points out, "[T]he alleged virtues of age often mirror the values responsible for ageism" (Ruddick, 1999, p. 45). Feminist virtue ethics casts a critical eye upon the supposed virtues typically assigned to the aged. In the not so far off past, old people were expected to be quiet, complaisant, cooperative, and helpful. More recently, aging people have been expected to be cheery, active, and independent. Both prescriptions appear designed to counteract the supposed weaknesses and moral failings of elderly people. That is, they both arise from and reinforce invidious stereotypes of elderly people. They also serve an oppressive function: as Ruddick comments, prescriptive "portraits of productive and plucky 'good elderly' " may intimidate people who are already dealing with exhaustion, sadness, and fear (Ruddick, 1999, p. 46).

With increasing longevity, it becomes even more important to be cognizant of how ageism and age categories influence morality and moral theory, and to consider how morality might justifiably change if an anti-ageist stance is taken. Feminist virtue ethics mandates political assessment of existing ideas about the virtues of aging, old people, and great longevity.

Unacknowledged Moral Virtues

The perspective of feminist virtue ethics also helps us to see that members of oppressed groups cultivate and possess genuinely valuable virtues, sometimes partly as a result of coping with and responding to the subordinated position assigned to them. Yet these virtues under oppression are often unrecognized, actively shunned, or perceived as being not appropriate for more privileged persons. For example, Susan Moller Okin talks about the virtues women have historically needed to sustain and care for other human beings, such characteristics as "the capacity to nurture, patience, the ability to listen carefully and to teach (sometimes mundane things) well, and the readiness to give up or postpone one's own projects in order to pay attention to the needs or projects of others" (Okin, 1996, pp. 227–228). Because the kind of labor that is sustained by these capacities is not always recognized as true work or as truly valuable, the capacities themselves have not always been acknowledged as virtues, yet they deserve to be recognized. The cultivation of traditional "women's" virtues such as caring and sympathy seems to "promise a more humane, benevolent world than does mere action according to duty" (Conly, 2001, p. 12).

Therefore, when we think about the kinds of virtues needed for extended life, we should not simply adhere to traditional notions of middle-class, white, masculine, and youthful (or age-neutral) virtue. We should recognize that many of the characteristics actually acquired by aging people and people gifted with unusual longevity could be genuine virtues and would be genuinely beneficial for other members of the community to cultivate. These might include reflective thought, caring, innovativeness, determination, and a commitment to (some forms of) continued independence, along with the recognition that (some forms of) dependence may be inevitable. Ruddick lists as virtues of old people "curiosity; a capacity for pleasure and delight; concern for near and distant others; capacities to forgive and let go, to accept, adjust, and appreciate; and 'wise independence,' which includes not only the ability to plan and control one's life but also the ability to acknowledge one's limitations and accept help in ways that are gratifying to the helper" (Ruddick, 1999, p. 50). Although it's likely that developing many of these characteristics requires, as a necessary condition, maturity and years of living, the claim is not that all elderly people possess them. The point is that they are significant virtues, recognizable as such through the anti-ageist political analysis afforded by feminist virtue ethics. If ageism inhibits us from recognizing the virtues of aging long and well, feminist virtue ethics provides a remedy.

Feminist Virtue Ethics and Extended Lives

As I suggested earlier, the extension of human life is of significant value because it provides human beings with opportunities for engaging in activities and seeking experiences that they would not otherwise have enjoyed if their lives had ended sooner. This is not to say that any experience or any activity is necessarily valuable. Nor is it to assume that every prolonged life is necessarily better, that no one may ever rationally reject a longer life, or that all persons will inevitably make good use of the years they have. But it is to say that what is deeply evil about death, especially a death that is earlier than necessary, is that it terminates all possibilities for anything more.

A longer life provides a greater chance for human flourishing, for learning virtues, and for living a good life. The person who seeks to foster in herself the appropriate virtues and who is successful to at least some degree is the person who will best be able to adapt to a changing environment, who will be more likely to transform herself, and who will be able to flourish within the context of a longer life. I suggest that if, within the context of increasing longevity, we adopt feminist virtue ethics, we will find ourselves reflecting about not just what kind of person we should be, but what kind of person we should *become.* We will need to ask ourselves not just what kind of life we should *lead,* but also what kind of life we should *leave*—that is, what aspects of ourselves we should voluntarily choose to abandon because they no longer contribute to individual or collective well-being. Moreover, in a world in which people are able to enjoy extended life-times, our moral lives will not, and probably cannot and should not, be monolithic. Salmon comments, "We all carry within us, encompass within ourselves, something of the people we have been. It is to these people, intimately familiar, though partly 'other,' that we constantly turn" (Salmon, 1985, p. 15). By the same token, by living longer, we acquire many more people to whom we can turn.

Conly, however, objects that virtue ethics, including feminist appropriations of it, has a fundamental flaw: because virtue ethics is concerned with "our whole internal orientation—our emotions, our commitments, our attitudes towards others, our whole psychology"—it is highly intrusive. It makes ethics inescapable; no area of one's life is immune to it: "The cultivation of virtue is a moral task from which there is no respite" (Conly, 2001, p. 13). Moreover, because it is concerned with one's character, with who one fundamentally is, attempts to adopt virtue ethics will produce personal fragmentation when the demands of different virtues conflict with each other, as they inevitably will. Hence, "[t]he problem [with virtue ethics] is not that living virtuously may make one unhappy . . . but that it promotes a condition in which the very goal we want to achieve, a unified and integrated character, becomes impossible" (Conly, 2001, p. 14).

I think this objection is founded upon an error, and that error becomes even more obvious if we contemplate adopting virtue ethics within the context of lengthening human lives. Conly assumes that a "unified and integrated character" is necessarily a goal for those who hope to live good lives. She fears the development of "an unacceptable fragmentation into incoherent parts, each pulling in a different direction, with no mediating principle" (Conly, 2001, p. 14). But the idea of a unified self is something of an illusion, born precisely of the modernist tendency to see the self as the contained, independent, nonrelational individual that feminism has criticized. Attention to the relational nature of human social life makes it clear that a human person is a composite of many identities, roles, characteristics, skills, relationships, desires, and needs. Moreover, this composite self, far from being pathological, is a highly adaptive means of handling the variegated demands of postindustrial human life. Within an extended life we will more and more be asking ourselves not just what kind of *life* we should lead, but also what kind of *lives* we should lead. Longer life provides the potential for an extended learning process, for more experience and activities, and for opportunities to develop one's character. Within an extended life we will play more roles: son or daughter, parent, student, friend, worker, employer, role model, leader, grandparent, volunteer, caregiver, partner, great-grandparent, colleague, owner, consumer, citizen, voter, artist, athlete, business person, hobbyist, lobbyist. These new roles will generate moral questions about cultivating and changing one's character and one's community that are best handled through feminist virtue ethics. With its emphasis on personal and social contexts, its awareness of the effects of stereotyped identities and forms of oppression such as ageism, and its attention to the virtues of aging and longevity, feminist virtue ethics suggests ways of reforming morality as the human life span and life expectancies become longer.

My goal in this chapter has not been to establish that feminist virtue ethics is the best approach to ethics in general but, somewhat more modestly, to show that feminist virtue ethics is ideally suited to the challenges posed by increasing human longevity. My aim is not moral prescription or the promotion of moral uniformity, but rather to make plausible the theoretical point that feminist virtue ethics provides a general framework for thinking about our future moral lives. While I have named what I think are some important virtues, I offer here no definitive answers to questions about the specific characteristics that should be cultivated within the context of longer lives.[4] Elderly people "are neither more nor less virtuous than people of other age groups" (Ruddick, 1999, p. 47). Yet the virtues needed for longevity may be found in the characters of people who live longer and age well, who acquire them through the experiences and activities of flourishing within an extended lifetime.

Acknowledgments

I am grateful to Steven Leighton for his assistance in understanding early philosophical concepts of virtue and to Carlos Prado for providing me with several books relevant to this chapter.

Notes

1. Within a longer life there is more time to acquire moral wisdom and insight, although, of course, there's nothing inevitable about that. I do not want to romanticize old age or what can be learned or experienced by living long. That is why the question of how to live as lives become longer is a normative issue, not an empirical one. In this chapter I am not concerned with what people do achieve, acquire, experience, or learn, but rather with the prospects for what they both can and ought to do.

2. This discussion is based upon two further assumptions. First, I assume a secular context for the discussion. I shall not make use of specifically religious values (although some values advocated by some religions may well be relevant to the discussion), and I shall not assume the existence of an omnipotent, omniscient god. Therefore, second, I assume that ethical issues generated by the prospect of longer human life arise in the context of existence here on earth, not in connection with any purported afterlife, whether in heaven or in the form of a reincarnated state of existence.

3. Callahan fails to provide an argument showing why more of the same cannot be good. One could reasonably say that whether or not more of the same is good depends on what one's life has already been like. If more of same includes additional fulfilling relationships, interesting activities, and personal challenges, then more of the same sounds desirable to me.

4. Some questions about the virtues needed for greater longevity are self-reflexive. For example, what should our moral attitude toward future generations be? Should we cultivate a disposition to increase human lives?

References

Baier, K. (1974). The sanctity of life. *Journal of Social Philosophy,* 5(2), 1–6.
Blum, L. (1996). Community and virtue. In: Crisp, R., ed. *How Should One Live? Essays on the Virtues,* Oxford: Clarendon Press, pp. 231–250.

Callahan, D. (1977). On defining a "natural death." *The Hastings Center Report*, 7(3), 32–37.

Callahan, D. (1987). *Setting Limits: Medical Goals in an Aging Society*. New York: Simon & Schuster.

Callahan, D. (1998). *False Hopes: Why America's Quest for Perfect Health is a Recipe for Failure*. New York: Simon & Schuster.

Conly, S. (2001). Why feminists should oppose feminist virtue ethics. *Philosophy Now*, no. 33, 12–14.

Copper, B. (1988). *Over the Hill: Reflections on Ageism Between Women*. Freedom, CA: Crossing Press.

Friedman, M. (1998). Impartiality. In: Jaggar, A.M. and Young, I.M., eds. *A Companion to Feminist Philosophy*. Malden, MA: Blackwell, pp. 393–401.

Goddard, J.L. (1982). Extension of the life span: A national goal? In: McKee, P.L., ed. *Philosophical Foundations of Gerontology*. New York: Human Sciences Press, pp. 137–154.

Hardwig, J. (2000). *Is There a Duty to Die? And Other Essays in Medical Ethics*. New York: Routledge.

Hursthouse, R. (1996). Normative virtue ethics. In: Crisp, R., ed. *How Should One Live? Essays on the Virtues*. Oxford: Clarendon Press, pp. 19–36.

Levin, J. and Levin, W.C. (1980). *Ageism: Prejudice and Discrimination Against the Elderly*. Belmont, CA: Wadsworth.

Macdonald, B. with Rich, C. (1991). *Look Me in the Eye: Old Women, Aging and Ageism*, expanded ed. Minneapolis: Spinsters Ink.

Madigan, T.J. (1999). Forward to Methusaleh: Do we really want to live a long, long time?" *Free Inquiry*, 19(4), 42–43.

Okin, S.M. (1996). Feminism, moral development, and the virtues. In: Crisp, R., ed. *How Should One Live? Essays on the Virtues*. Oxford: Clarendon Press, pp. 211–229.

Overall, C. (2003). *Aging, Death, and Human Longevity: A Philosophical Inquiry*. Berkeley: University of California Press.

Ruddick, S. (1999). Virtues and age. In: Walker, M.U., ed. *Mother Time: Women, Aging, and Ethics*. Lanham, MD: Roman & Littlefield, pp. 45–60.

Salmon, P. (1985). *Living in Time: A New Look at Personal Development*. London: J.M. Dent.

Tong, R. (1998). The ethics of care: A feminist virtue ethics of care for healthcare practitioners. *Journal of Medicine and Philosophy*, 23(2), 131–152.

Veatch, R. (1989). *Death, Dying and the Biological Revolution: Our Last Quest for Responsibility*, rev. ed. New Haven, CT: Yale University Press.

Walker, M.U. (1998). *Moral Understandings: A Feminist Study in Ethics*. New York: Routledge.

Walker, M.U. (Ed.). (1999). *Mother Time: Women, Aging, and Ethics*. Lanham, MD: Roman & Littlefield.

14

L'Chaim and Its Limits: Why Not Immortality?

Leon R. Kass

You don't have to be Jewish to drink *L'Chaim*, to lift a glass "To Life." Everyone in his right mind believes that life is good and that death is bad. But Jews have always had an unusually keen appreciation of life, and not only because it has been stolen from them so often and so cruelly. The celebration of life—of *this* life, not the next one—has from the beginning been central to Jewish ethical and religious sensibilities. In the Torah, "Be fruitful and multiply" is God's first blessing and first command. Judaism from its inception rejected child-sacrifice and regarded long life as a fitting divine reward for righteous living. At the same time, Judaism embraces medicine and the human activity of healing the sick; from the Torah the rabbis deduced not only permission for doctors to heal, but also the positive obligation to do so. Indeed, so strong is this reverence for life that the duty of *pikuah nefesh* requires that Jews violate the holy Shabbat in order to save a life. Not by accident do we Jews raise our glasses "*L'Chaim.*"

Neither is it accidental that Jews have been enthusiastic boosters of modern medicine and modern biomedical science. Vastly out of proportion to their numbers, they build hospitals and laboratories, support medical research, and see their sons and daughters in the vanguard wherever new scientific discoveries are to be made and new remedies to be found. Yet this beloved biomedical project, for all its blessings, now raises for Jews and for all humanity a plethora of serious and often unprecedented moral challenges. Laboratory-assisted reproduction, artificial organs, genetic manipulation, psychoactive drugs, computer implants in the brain, and techniques to conquer aging—these and other present and projected techniques for altering our bodies and minds pose challenges to the very meaning of our humanity. Our growing power to control human life may require us to consider possible limits to the principle of *L'Chaim.*

One well-known set of challenges results from undesired consequences of medical success in sustaining life, as more and more people are kept alive by artificial means in greatly debilitated and degraded conditions. When, if ever, is it permissible for doctors to withhold antibiotics, discontinue a respirator, remove a feeding tube, or even assist in suicide or perform euthanasia?

A second set of challenges concerns the morality of means used to seek the cure of disease or the creation of life. Is it ethical to create living human embryos for the sole purpose of experimenting on them? To conceive a child in order that it may become a compatible bone marrow donor for an afflicted "sibling?" Is it ethical to practice human cloning to provide a child for an infertile couple?

Third, we may soon face challenges concerning the goal itself: Should we, partisans of life, welcome efforts to increase not just the average but also the maximum human life span, by conquering aging, decay, and ultimately mortality itself?

In the debates taking place in the United States, Jewish commentators on these and related medical ethical topics nearly always come down strongly in favor of medical progress and on the side of life—more life, longer life, new life. They treat the cure of disease, the prevention of death, and the prolongation of life as near-absolute values, trumping most if not all other moral objections. Unlike, say, Roman Catholic moralists who hold to certain natural law teachings that set limits on what are considered permissible practices, the Jewish commentators, even if they acknowledge difficulties, ultimately wind up saying that life and health are good, and that therefore whatever serves more of each and both is better.

Let me give two examples from of my own experience. Four years ago, when I gave testimony on the ethics of human cloning before the National Bioethics Advisory Commission, I was surprised to discover that the two experts who had been invited to testify on the Jewish point of view were not especially troubled by the prospect. The Orthodox rabbi, invoking the goodness of life and the injunction to be fruitful and multiply, held that cloning of the husband or the wife to provide a child for an infertile couple was utterly unobjectionable according to Jewish law. The Conservative rabbi, while acknowledging certain worries, concluded: "If cloning human beings is intended to advance medical research or cure infertility, it has a proper place in God's scheme of things, as understood in the Jewish tradition." Let someone else worry about Brave-New-Worldly turning procreation into manufacture or the meaning of replacing heterosexual procreation by asexual propagation. Prospective cures for diseases and children for infertile couples suffice to legitimate human cloning—and, by extension, will legitimate farming human embryos for spare body parts or even creating babies in bottles when that becomes feasible.

The second example. At a meeting in March 2000 on "Extended Life, Eternal Life," scientists and theologians were invited to discuss the desirability of increasing the maximum human life span and, more radically, of treating death itself as a disease to be conquered. The major Jewish speaker, a professor at a leading rabbinical seminary, embraced the project—you should excuse me—whole hog. Gently needling his Christian colleagues by asserting that, for Jews, God is Life, rather than Love, he used this principle to justify any and all life-preserving and life-extending technologies, including those that might yield massive increases in the maximum human life expectancy. When I pressed him in discussion to see if he had any objections to the biomedical pursuit of immortality, he responded that Judaism would only welcome such a project.

I am prepared to accept the view that traditional Jewish sources may be silent on these matters, given that the halakhah could know nothing about test-tube babies, cloning, or the campaign to conquer aging. But, in my opinion, such unqualified endorsement of medical progress and the unlimited pursuit of longevity cannot be the counsel of wisdom, and, therefore, should not be the counsel of Jewish wisdom. *L'Chaim*, but with limits.

Let us address the question of *L'Chaim* and its limits in its starkest and most radical form: If life is good and more is better, should we not regard death as a disease and try to cure it? Although this formulation of the question may seem too futuristic or far-fetched, there are several reasons for taking it up and treating it seriously.

First, reputable scientists are today answering the question in the affirmative and are already making large efforts toward bringing about a cure. Three kinds of research, still in their infancy, are attracting new attention and energies. First is the use of hormones, especially human growth hormone (hGH), to restore and enhance youthful bodily vigor. In the United States, over ten thousand people—including many physicians—are already injecting themselves daily with hGH for anti-aging purposes, with apparently remarkable improvements in bodily fitness and performance, though there is still no evidence that the hormones yield any increase in life expectancy. When the patent on hGH expires in 2002 and the cost comes down from its current $1,000 per month, many more people are almost certainly going to be injecting themselves from the hormonal fountain of youth.

Second is research on stem cells, those omnicompetent primordial cells that, on different signals, turn into all the tissues of the body—liver, heart, kidney, brain, etc. Stem cell technologies—combined with techniques of cloning—hold out the promise of an indefinite supply of replacement tissues and organs for any and all worn-out body parts. This is a booming area in commercial biotechnology, and one of the leading biotech entrepreneurs has been touting his company's research as promising indefinite prolongation of life.

Third, there is research into the genetic switches that control the biological processes of aging. The maximum life span for each species—roughly one hundred years for human beings—is almost certainly under genetic control. In a startling recent discovery, fruitfly geneticists have shown that mutations in a *single* gene produce a 50 percent increase in the natural lifetime of the flies. Once the genes involved in regulating the human life cycle and setting the midnight hour are identified, scientists predict that they will be able to increase the human maximum age well beyond its natural limit. Quite frankly, I find some of the claims and predictions to be overblown, but it would be foolhardy to bet against scientific and technical progress along these lines.

But even if cures for aging and death are a long way off, there is a second and more fundamental reason for inquiring into the radical question of the desirability of gaining a cure for death. For truth to tell, victory over mortality is the unstated but implicit goal of modern medical science, indeed of the entire modern scientific project, to which mankind was summoned almost four hundred years ago by Francis Bacon and Rene Descartes. They quite consciously trumpeted the conquest of nature for the relief of the man's estate, and they founded a science whose explicit purpose was to reverse the curse laid on Adam and Eve, and especially to restore the tree of life, by means of the tree of (scientific) knowledge. With medicine's increasing successes, realized mainly in the past half century, every death is increasingly regarded as premature, a failure of today's medicine that future research will prevent. In parallel with medical progress, a new moral sensibility has developed that serves precisely medicine's crusade against mortality: anything is permitted if it saves life, cures disease, prevents death. Regardless, therefore, of the imminence of anti-aging remedies, it is most worthwhile to reexamine the assumption upon which we have been operating: that everything should be done to preserve health and prolong life as much as possible, and that all other values must bow before the biomedical gods of better health, greater vigor, and longer life.

Recent proposals that we should conquer aging and death have not been without their critics. The criticism takes two forms: predictions of bad social consequences and complaints about distributive justice. Regarding the former, there are concerns about the effect on the size and age distributions of the population. How will growing numbers and percentages of people living well past one hundred affect, for example, work opportunities, retirement plans, hiring and promotion, cultural attitudes and beliefs, the structure of family life, relations between the generations, or the locus of rule and authority in government, business, and the professions? Even the most cursory examination of these matters suggests that the cumulative results of aggregated decisions for longer and more vigorous life could be highly disruptive and undesirable, even to the point that many individuals would be *worse off* through most of their lives, and worse off enough to offset the benefits of better health afforded them near the end of life. Indeed, several people have predicted that retardation of aging will present a classic instance of the Tragedy of the Commons, in which genuine and sought-for gains to individuals are nullified or worse, owing to the social consequences of granting them to everyone.

But other critics worry that technology's gift of long or immortal life will not be granted to everyone, especially if, as is likely, the treatments turn out to be expensive. Would it not be the ultimate injustice if only some people could afford a deathless existence, if the world were divided not only into rich and poor but into mortal and immortal?

Against these critics, the proponents of immortality research answer confidently that we will gradually figure out a way to solve these problems. We can handle any adverse social consequences through careful planning; we can overcome the inequities through cheaper technologies. Though I think these optimists woefully naive, let me for the moment grant their view regarding these issues. For both the proponents and their critics have yet to address thoughtfully the heart of the matter, the question of the goodness of the goal. The core question is this: Is it really true that longer life for individuals is an unqualified good?

How *much* longer life is a blessing for an individual? Ignoring now the possible harms flowing back to individuals from adverse social consequences, how much more life is good for us as individuals, other things being equal? How much more life do we want, assuming it to be healthy and vigorous? Assuming that it were up to us to set the human life span, where would or should we set the limit and why?

The simple answer is that no limit should be set. Life is good, and death is bad. Therefore, the more life the better, provided, of course, that we remain fit and our friends do, too.

This answer has the virtues of clarity and honesty. But most public advocates of conquering aging deny any such greediness. They hope not for immortality, but for something reasonable—just a few more years.

How many years are reasonably few? Let us start with ten. Which of us would find unreasonable or unwelcome the addition of ten healthy and vigorous years to his or her life, years like those between ages thirty and forty? We could learn more, earn more, see more, do more. Maybe we should ask for five years on top of that? Or ten? Why not fifteen, or twenty, or more?

If we can't immediately land on the reasonable number of added years, perhaps we can locate the principle. What is the principle of reasonableness? Time needed for our plans and projects yet to be completed? Some multiple of the age of a generation, say, so that we might live to see our great-grandchildren fully grown? Some notion—traditional, natural, revealed—of the proper life span for beings such as man? We have no answer to this question. We do not even know how to choose among the principles for setting our new life span.

Under such circumstances, lacking a standard of reasonable-ness, we fall back on our wants and desires. Under liberal democracy, this means the desires of the majority, for whom the attachment to life—or the fear of death—knows no limits. It turns out that the simple answer is the best: we want to live and live, and not to wither and not to die. For most of us, especially under modern secular conditions in which more and more people believe that this is the only life they have, the desire to prolong the life span (even modestly) must be seen as expressing a desire *never* to grow old and die. However naive their counsel, those who propose immortality deserve credit: they honestly and shamelessly expose this desire.

Some, of course, eschew any desire for longer life. They seek not adding years to life, but life to years. For them, the ideal life span would be our natural (once thought three-, now known to be) fourscore and ten, or if by reason of strength, fivescore, lived with full powers right up to death, which could come rather suddenly, painlessly, at the maximal age.

This has much to recommend it. Who would not want to avoid senility, crippling arthritis, the need for hearing aids and dentures, and the degrading dependencies of old age? But, in the absence of these degenerations, would we remain content to spurn longer life? Would we not become even more disinclined to exit? Would not death become even more of an affront? Would not the fear and loathing of death increase in the absence of its harbingers? We could no longer comfort the widow by pointing out that her husband was delivered from his suffering. Death would always be untimely, unpre-pared for, shocking.

Montaigne saw it clearly:

> I notice that in proportion as I sink into sickness, I naturally enter into a certain disdain for life. I find that I have much more trouble digesting this resolution when I am in health than when I have a fever. Inasmuch as I no longer cling so hard to the good things of life when I begin to lose the use and pleasure of them, I come to view death with much less frightened eyes. This makes me hope that the farther I get from life and the nearer to death, the more easily I shall accept the exchange. . . .
> If we fell into such a change [decrepitude] suddenly, I don't think we could endure it. But when we are led by Nature's hand down a gentle and virtually imperceptible slope, bit by bit, one

step at a time, she rolls us into this wretched state and makes us familiar with it; so that we find no shock when youth dies within us, which in essence and in truth is a harder death than the complete death of a languishing life or the death of old age; inasmuch as the leap is not so cruel from a painful life as from a sweet and flourishing life to a grievous and painful one.

Thus it is highly likely that even a modest prolongation of life with vigor or even only a preservation of youthfulness with no increase in longevity would make death less acceptable and exacerbate the desire to keep pushing it away—unless, for some reason, such life could also prove less satisfying.

Could longer, healthier life be less satisfying? How could it be, if life is good and death is bad? Perhaps the simple view is in error. Perhaps mortality is not simply an evil, perhaps it is even a blessing—not only for the welfare of the community, but even for us as individuals. How could this be?

I wish to make the case for the virtues of mortality. Against my own strong love of life, and against my even stronger wish that no more of my loved ones should die, I aspire to speak truth to my desires by showing that the finitude of human life is a blessing for every human individual, whether he knows it or not.

I know I won't persuade many people to accept my position. But I do hope I can convince readers of the gravity—I would say, the unique gravity—of this question. We are not talking about some minor new innovation with ethical wrinkles about which we may chatter or regulate as usual. Conquering death is not something that we can try for a while and then decide whether the results are better or worse—according to, God only knows, what standard. On the contrary, this is a question in which our very humanity is at stake, not only in the consequences but also in the very meaning of the choice. For to argue that human life would be better without death is, I submit, to argue that human life would be better being something other than human. To be immortal would not be just to continue life as we mortals now know it, only forever. The new immortals, in the decisive sense, would not be like us at all. If this is true, a human choice for bodily immortality would suffer from the deep confusion of choosing to have some great good only on the condition of turning into someone else. Moreover, such an immortal someone else, in my view, will be less well off than we mortals are now, thanks indeed to our mortality.

It goes without saying that there is no virtue in the death of a child or a young adult, or the untimely or premature death of anyone, before he or she had attained the measure of man's days. I do not mean to imply that there is virtue in the particular *event* of death for anyone. Nor am I suggesting that separation through death is not painful for the survivors, those for whom the deceased was an integral part of their lives. Instead, my question concerns the fact of our finitude, the fact of our mortality—the fact *that we must die,* the fact that a full life for a human being has a biological built-in limit, one that has evolved as part of our nature. Does this fact also have value? Is our finitude good for us—as individuals? (I intend this question entirely in the realm of natural reason and apart from any question about a life after death.)

To praise mortality must seem to be madness. If mortality is a blessing, it surely is not widely regarded as such. Life seeks to live, and rightly suspects all counsels of finitude. "Better to be a slave on earth than the king over all the dead," says Achilles in Hades to the visiting Odysseus, in apparent regret for his prior choice of the short but glorious life. Moreover, though some cultures—such as the Eskimo—can instruct and moderate somewhat the lust for life, liberal Western society gives it free rein, beginning with a political philosophy founded on a fear of violent death, and reaching to our current cults of youth and novelty, the cosmetic replastering of the wrinkles of age, and the widespread anxiety about disease and survival. Finally, the virtues of finitude—if there are any—may never be widely appreciated in any age or culture if appreciation depends on a certain wisdom, if wisdom requires a certain detachment from the love of oneself and one's own, and if the possibility of such detachment is given only to the few. Still, if it is wisdom, the rest of us should hearken, for we may learn something of value for ourselves.

How, then, might our finitude be good for us? I offer four benefits, first among which is *interest and engagement.* If the human life span were increased even by only twenty years, would the pleasures of life increase proportionately? Would professional tennis players really enjoy playing 25 percent more games of tennis? Would the Don Juans of our world feel better for having seduced 1250 women rather than 1000? Having experienced the joys and tribulations of raising a family until the last had left for college, how many parents would like to extend the experience by another ten years? Likewise, those whose satisfaction comes from climbing the career ladder might well ask what there would be to do for fifteen years after one had been CEO of Microsoft, a member of Congress, or the president of Harvard for a quarter of a century. Even less clear are the additions to personal happiness from more of the same of the less pleasant and less fulfilling activities in which so many of us are engaged so much of the time. It seems to be as the poet says: "We move and ever spend our lives amid the same things, and not by any length of life is any new pleasure hammered out."

Second, *seriousness and aspiration.* Could life be serious or meaningful without the limit of mortality? Is not the limit on our time the ground of our taking life seriously and living it passionately? To know and to feel that one goes around only once, and that the deadline is not out of sight, is for many people the necessary spur to the pursuit of something worthwhile. "Teach us to number our days," says the Psalmist, "that we may get a heart of wisdom." To number our days is the condition for making them count. Homer's immortals— Zeus and Hera, Apollo and Athena—for all their eternal beauty and youthfulness, live shallow and rather frivolous lives, their passions only transiently engaged, in first this and then that. They live as spectators of the mortals, who by comparison have depth, aspiration, genuine feeling, and hence a real center in their lives. Mortality makes life matter.

There may be some activities, especially in some human beings, that do not require finitude as a spur. A powerful desire for understanding can do without external proddings, let alone one related to mortality; and as there is never too much time to learn and to understand, longer, more vigorous life might be simply a boon. The best sorts of friendship, too, seem capable of indefinite growth, especially where growth is somehow tied to learning—though one may wonder whether real friendship doesn't depend in part on the shared perceptions of a common fate. But, in any case, I suspect that these are among the rare exceptions. For most activities, and for most of us, I think it is crucial that we recognize and feel the force of not having world enough and time.

A third matter, *beauty and love.* Death, says Wallace Stevens, is the mother of beauty. What he means is not easy to say. Perhaps he means that only a mortal being, aware of his mortality and the transience and vulnerability of all natural things, is moved to make beautiful artifacts, objects that will last, objects whose order will be immune to decay as their maker is not, beautiful objects that will bespeak and beautify a world that needs beautification, beautiful objects for other mortal beings who can appreciate what they cannot themselves make because of a taste for the beautiful, a taste perhaps connected to awareness of the ugliness of decay.

Perhaps the poet means to speak of natural beauty as well, which beauty—unlike that of objects of art—depends on its *im*permanence. Could the beauty of flowers depend on the fact that they will soon wither? Does the beauty of spring warblers depend on the fall drabness that precedes and follows? What about the fading, late afternoon winter light or the spreading sunset? Is the beautiful necessarily fleeting, a peak that cannot be sustained? Or does the poet mean not that the beautiful is beautiful because mortal, but that our appreciation of its beauty depends on our appreciation of mortality—in us and in the beautiful? Does not love swell before the beautiful precisely on recognizing that it (and we) will not always be? Is not our mortality the cause of our enhanced appreciation of the beautiful and the worthy, and of our treasuring and loving them? How deeply could one deathless "human" being love another?

Fourth, there is the peculiarly human beauty of character, *virtue and moral excellence.* To be mortal means that it is possible to give one's life, not only in one moment, say, on the field of battle, but also in the many other ways in which we are able in action to rise above attachment to survival. Through moral courage, endurance, greatness of soul, generosity, devotion to justice—in acts great and small—we rise above our mere creatureliness, spending the precious coinage of the time of our lives for the sake of the noble and the good and the holy. We free ourselves from fear, from bodily pleasures, or from attachments to wealth—all largely connected with survival—and in doing virtuous deeds overcome the weight of our neediness; yet for this nobility, vulnerability and mortality are the necessary conditions. The immortals cannot be noble.

Of this, too, the poets teach. Odysseus, long suffering, has already heard the shade of Achilles' testimony in praise of life when he is offered immortal life by the nymph Calypso. She is a beautiful goddess, attractive, kind, yielding; she sings sweetly and weaves on a golden loom; her island is well ordered and lovely, free of hardships and suffering. Says the poet, "Even a god who came into that place would have admired what he saw, the heart delighted within him." Yet Odysseus turns down the offer to be lord of her household and immortal:

Goddess and queen, do not be angry with me. I myself know that all you say is true and that circumspect Penelope can never match the impression you make for beauty and stature. She is mortal after all, and you are immortal and ageless. But even so, what I want and all my days I pine for is to go back to my house and see that day of my homecoming. And if some god batters me far out on the wine-blue water, I will endure it, keeping a stubborn spirit inside me, for already I have suffered much and done much hard work on the waves and in the fighting.

To suffer, to endure, to trouble oneself for the sake of home, family, community, and genuine friendship, is truly to live, and is the clear choice of this exemplary mortal. This choice is both the mark of one's excellence and the basis for the visible display of one's excellence in deeds noble and just. Immortality is a kind of oblivion—like death itself.

But, someone might reasonably object, if mortality is such a blessing, why do so few cultures recognize it as such? Why do so many teach the promise of life after death, of something eternal, of something imperishable? This takes us to the heart of the matter.

What is the meaning of this concern with immortality? *Why* do we human beings seek immortality? Why do we want to live longer or forever? Is it really first and most because we do not want to die, because we do not want to leave this embodied life on earth or give up our earthly pastimes, because we want to see more and do more? I do not think so. This may be what we say, but it is not what we finally mean. Mortality as such is not our defect, nor bodily immortality our goal. Rather, mortality is at most a pointer, a derivative manifestation, or an accompaniment of some deeper deficiency. The promise of immortality and eternity answers rather to a deep truth about the human soul: the human soul yearns for, longs for, aspires to some condition, some state, some goal toward which our earthly activities are directed but that cannot be attained in earthly life. Our soul's reach exceeds our grasp; it seeks more than continuance; it reaches for something beyond us, something that for the most part eludes us. Our distress with mortality is the derivative manifestation of the conflict between the transcendent longings of the soul and the all-too-finite powers and fleshly concerns of the body.

What is it that we lack and long for, but cannot reach? One possibility is completion in another person. For example, Plato's Aristophanes says that we seek wholeness through complete and permanent bodily and psychic union with a unique human being whom we love, our "missing other half." Plato's Socrates, in contrast, says that it is rather wholeness through wisdom, through comprehensive knowledge of the beautiful truth about the whole, that which philosophy seeks but can never attain. Yet again, biblical religion says that we seek wholeness by dwelling in God's presence, love, and redemption— a restoration of innocent wholeheartedness lost in the Garden of Eden. But, please note, these and many other such accounts of human aspiration, despite their differences, all agree on this crucial point: humanity longs not so much for deathlessness as for wholeness, wisdom, goodness, and godliness—longings that cannot be satisfied fully in our embodied earthly life, the only life, by natural reason, we know we have. Hence the attractiveness of any prospect or promise of a different and thereby fulfilling life hereafter. The decisive inference is clear: none of these longings can be satisfied by prolonging earthly life. Not even an unlimited amount of "more of the same" will satisfy our deepest aspirations.

If this is correct, here follows a decisive corollary regarding the battle against death. The human taste for immortality, for the imperishable and the eternal, is not a taste that biomedical conquest of death can satisfy. We would still be incomplete; we would still lack wisdom; we would still lack God's presence and redemption. Mere continuance will not buy fulfillment. Worse, its pursuit threatens—already threatens—human happiness by distracting us from the goals toward which our souls naturally point. By diverting our aim, by misdirecting so much individual and social energy toward the goal of bodily immortality, we may seriously undermine our chances for living as well as we can and for satisfying to some extent, however incompletely, our deepest longings for what is best. The implication for human life is hardly nihilistic: once we acknowledge and accept our finitude, we can concern ourselves with living *well,* and care first and most for the *well-being* of our souls, and not so much for their mere existence.

But perhaps this is all a mistake. Perhaps there is no such longing of the soul. Perhaps there is no soul. Certainly modern science doesn't speak about the soul; neither does medicine or even our *psy*chiatrists, whose name means "healers of the soul." Perhaps we are just animals, complex ones to be sure, but animals nonetheless, content just to be here, frightened in the face of danger, avoiding pain, seeking pleasure.

Curiously, however, biology has its own view of our nature and its inclinations. Biology also teaches about transcendence, though it eschews talk about the soul. Biology has long shown us a feasible way to rise above our finitude and to participate in something permanent and eternal: I refer not to stem cells, but to procreation—the bearing and caring for offspring, for the sake of which many animals risk and even sacrifice their lives. Indeed, in all higher animals, reproduction *as such* implies both the acceptance of the death of self and participation in its transcendence. The salmon, willingly swimming upstream to spawn and die, makes vivid this universal truth.

But man is natured for more than spawning. Human biology teaches how our life points beyond itself—to our offspring, to our community, to our species. Like the other animals, man is built for reproduction. More than the other animals, man is also built for sociality. And, alone among the animals, man is also built for culture— not only though capacities to transmit and receive skills and techniques, but also through capacities for shared beliefs, opinions, rituals, and traditions. We are built with leanings toward, and capacities for, perpetuation. Is it not possible that aging and mortality are part of this construction, and that the rate of aging and the human life span have been selected for their usefulness to the task of perpetuation? Could not extending the human life span place a great strain on our nature, jeopardizing our project and depriving us of success? Interestingly, perpetuation is a goal that *is* attainable, a transcendence of self that *is* (largely) realizable. Here is a form of participating in the enduring that is open to us, without qualification—provided, that is, that we remain open to it.

Biological considerations aside, simply to covet a prolonged life span for ourselves is both a sign and a cause of our failure to open ourselves to procreation and to any higher purpose. It is probably no accident that it is a generation whose intelligentsia proclaim the death of God and the meaninglessness of life that embarks on life's indefinite prolongation and that seeks to cure the emptiness of life by extending it forever. For the desire to prolong youthfulness is not only a childish desire to eat one's life and keep it; it is also an expression of a childish and narcissistic wish incompatible with devotion to posterity. It seeks an endless present, isolated from anything truly eternal, and severed from any true continuity with past and future. It is in principle hostile to children, because children, those who come after, are those who will take one's place; *they* are life's answer to mortality, and their presence in one's house is a constant reminder that one no longer belongs to the frontier generation. One cannot pursue agelessness for oneself and remain faithful to the spirit and meaning of perpetuation.

In perpetuation, we send forth not just the seed of our bodies, but also the bearer of our hopes, our truths, and those of our tradition. If our children are to flower, we need to sow them well and nurture them, cultivate them in rich and wholesome soil, clothe them in fine and decent opinions and mores, and direct them toward the highest light, to grow straight and tall—that they may take our place as we took that of those who planted us and made way for us, so that in time they, too, may make way and plant. But if they are truly to flower, we must go to seed; we must wither and give ground.

Against these considerations, the clever ones will propose that if we could do away with death, we would do away with the need for posterity. But that is a self-serving and shallow answer, one that thinks of life and aging solely in terms of the state of the body. It ignores the psychological effects simply of the passage of time—of experiencing and learning about the way things are. After a while, no matter how healthy we are, no matter how respected and well placed we are socially, most of us cease to look upon the world with fresh eyes. Little surprises us, nothing shocks us, righteous indignation at injustice dies out. We have seen it all already, seen it all. We have often been deceived, we have made many mistakes of our own. Many of us become small-souled, having been humbled not by bodily decline or the loss of loved ones but by life itself. So our ambition also begins to flag, or at least our noblest ambitions. As we grow older, Aristotle already noted, we "aspire to nothing great and exalted and crave the mere necessities and comforts of existence." At some point, most of us turn and say to our intimates, Is this all there is? We settle, we accept our situation—if we are lucky enough to be able to accept it. In many ways, perhaps in the most profound ways, most of us go to sleep long before our deaths—and we might even do so earlier in life if death no longer spurred us to make something of ourselves.

In contrast, it is in the young that aspiration, hope, freshness, boldness, and openness spring anew—even when they take the form of overturning our monuments. Immortality for oneself through children may be a delusion, but participating in the natural and eternal renewal of human possibility through children is not—not even in today's world.

For it still stands as it did when Homer made Glaukos say to Diomedes:

> As is the generation of leaves, so is that of humanity. The wind scatters the leaves to the ground, but the live timber burgeons with leaves again in the season of spring returning. So one generation of man will grow while another dies.

And yet it also still stands, as this very insight of Homer's itself reveals, that human beings are in another respect unlike the leaves; that the eternal renewal of human beings embraces also the eternally human possibility of learning and self-awareness; that we, too, here and now, may participate with Homer, with Plato, with the Bible, yes with Descartes and Bacon, in catching at least some glimpse of the enduring truths about nature, God, and human affairs; and that we, too, may hand down and perpetuate this pursuit of wisdom and goodness in our children and our children's children. Children and their education, not growth hormone and perpetual organ replacement, are life's—and wisdom's—answer to mortality.

This ancient Homeric wisdom is, in fact, not so far from traditional Jewish wisdom. For although we believe that life is good and long life is better, we hold something higher than life itself to be best. We violate one Shabbat so that the person whose life is saved may observe many Shabbatoth. We are obliged to accept death rather than commit idolatry, murder, or sexual outrage. Though we love life and drink *L'Chaim*, we have been taught of old to love wisdom and justice and godliness more; among Jews, at least until recently, teachers were more revered than doctors. Regarding immortality, God Himself declares—in the Garden of Eden story—that human beings, once they have attained the burdensome knowledge of good and bad, should not have access to the tree of life. Instead, they are to cleave to the Torah as a tree of life, a life-perfecting path to righteousness and holiness. Unlike the death-defying Egyptians, those ancient precursors of the quest for bodily immortality, the Children of Israel do not mummify or embalm their dead; we bury our ancestors but keep them alive in memory, and, accepting our mortality, we look forward to the next generation. Indeed, the mitzvah to be fruitful and multiply, when rightly understood, celebrates not the life we have and selfishly would cling to, but the life that replaces us.

Confronted with the growing moral challenges posed by bio-medical technology, let us resist the siren song of the conquest of aging and death. Let us cleave to our ancient wisdom and lift our voices and properly toast *L'Chaim*, to life beyond our own, to the life of our grandchildren and their grandchildren. May they, God willing, know health and long life, but especially so that they may also know the pursuit of truth and righteousness and holiness. And may they hand down and perpetuate this pursuit of what is humanly finest to succeeding generations for all time to come.

Acknowledgments

This chapter appeared previously under the same title in the journal *First Things*, No. 113 (2001), 17–24.

15

Anti-Aging Research and the Limits of Medicine

Eric T. Juengst

According to the *AMA News*, 2500 physicians have established specialty practices devoted to *longevity medicine* in the past decade, and an American Academy of Anti-Aging Medicine (A4M) already boasts 11,000 members. The goal of this clinical community is to extend the time its patients can live without the morbidities of the aging process: "memory loss, muscle loss, visual impairment, slowed gait and speech, wrinkling of the skin, hardening of the arteries and all the other maladies we call aging" (Shelton, 2000, p. 25). At the moment, there is little the practitioners of anti-aging medicine can prescribe that has any scientific validation (Butler et al., 2002; Olshansky et al., 2002). But the basic scientists who study the biology of human aging, the *biogerontologists*, are slowly making headway (see Chapter 1), and a central research agenda for that community is to provide clinicians with the tools they require to make anti-aging medicine a reality (Juengst et. al., 2003). This prospect raises a philosophical problem for the medical profession with important ethical implications: is human aging an appropriate target for medical intervention? If they could intervene to slow the aging process, would anti-aging clinicians be practicing health care, or would they simply using the mantle of medicine to do something else entirely?

This chapter will begin by arguing that the most obvious approach to the issue—deciding whether the aging process itself should be considered a disease—will not take the analysis very far. Drawing such lines seems important, since if there is nothing pathological about the aging processes, there is no obvious rationale for health professionals to attempt to control them. But determining whether anti-aging interventions could ever count as medically necessary treatments or whether they should be interpreted as, at best, elective enhancements like cosmetic surgery is a task that faces a basic conceptual difficulty. Almost any intervention that would postpone specific milestones of normal aging would also help prevent the more obvious health problems to which those milestones make one susceptible. As long as decelerated aging and disease prevention are two sides of the same coin, the life-extending effects of such interventions will always be eclipsed by the medical obligation to prevent disease, effectively deciding the question of the intervention's medical appropriateness.

Because of this difficulty, other arguments will have to be mounted if one seeks to claim that anti-aging interventions go beyond the appropriate limits of medicine. The second part of the chapter describes three of these arguments and their implications for practice. The first is the argument that anti-aging interventions cannot be part of *human* health care, because aging is constitutive of what it is to be human. On this view, anti-aging interventions may well address health problems, but they cannot do so without sacrificing patients' identity as authentic human beings (Kass, 2001). A second argument is that while anti-aging interventions may benefit individuals, the individual is not the proper unit of analysis to use in assessing their medical merits. Instead, anti-aging interventions, like public health interventions, can be responsibly assessed only in terms of their impact on families and communities (Hackler, 2001–2002). While it is in no one's best interests to be quarantined, quarantine is not an intervention that is assessed at the individual level. Similarly, the argument goes, while it may be in some one's best interest to have the aging processes decelerated, doing so would have important effects on the web of relationships in which individual patients live and is best assessed as health care at that level. Finally, a third argument that bears scrutiny is the argument that, while anti-aging interventions could be used to forestall genuine health problems, they can do so only by creating and exacerbating fundamental social injustices, and for that reason fall beyond the realm of respon- sible health care. Here, the claim is that the anti-aging enterprise is complicitous with prejudicial social attitudes toward aging and the elderly, and would feed discrimination against those who do age nor- mally. On this view, an anti-aging ideology within medicine could be just as pernicious as medical racism and sexism and should be simi- larly eschewed as a professional perversion (Hayflick, 2001–2002). While none of these arguments succeed as well as their proponents might like, all three expose neglected questions about the medical profession's moral commitments that will need to be addressed as anti-aging technologies emerge from the laboratory.

Preventive Medicine and the Compression of Morbidity

One common way to draw the moral boundaries of medicine is to begin with the premise that the profession's defining mission is to help prevent and alleviate health problems (Kass, 1985). To the extent that physicians go beyond healing to attempt to improve on perfectly normal human traits, they are no longer providing health care, and our moral suspicions about what they are doing should increase for a number of reasons (Juengst, 1998). From this perspective, the cen- tral issue in evaluating the professional propriety of anti-aging medi- cine is to decide whether, and in what senses, human aging itself is either a pathological phenomenon, or a perfectly normal character- istic of our species, or both at once (Boorse, 1977; Caplan, 1982; Callahan 1993). If, as the A4M suggests, aging does conceptually amount to a collection of maladies, then attempts to combat it are at least philosophically bona fide medicine. On the other hand, if aging is not pathological, then, as biogerontologist Leonard Hayflick sug- gests, "the concept of seeking a cure for aging is tantamount to seek- ing a cure for embryogenesis or child or adult development" (Hayflick, 2001–2002, p. 21).

This issue has generated a fascinating literature on whether or not human aging should be considered a disease (Caplan, 1982, this volume; Murphy, 1986; Callahan, 1995), how best to distinguish the health problems associated with older ages from the underlying mechanisms of normal aging (Forbes and Thompson, 1990), and how to relate the concept of human aging to the concepts of growth and development, duration through time, and senescence and decay (Logothetis, 1993). Although there are controversies in each area, two claims seem to be accepted by all sides. First, the frequency of some diseases and disabilities—maladies that can be described without reference to aging, like diabetes, heart disease, and cancer—does increase as adult humans get older. Second, there are universal intrinsic biological processes that, in combination with variable environmental factors, induce progressive senescence in all adult humans, incidentally putting them at risk for the age-associated maladies (Kirkland, 2002).

Even those who are most concerned with resisting the medicalization of normal aging readily agree that the professional mandate of medicine includes combatting the maladies that plague old age (Callahan, 1993; Hayflick, 2001–2002). Since the 1980s, this effort has gone under the banner of the *compression of morbidity* in biogerontology, to single out the goal of providing people with more years of productive life by delaying the onset of serious age-associated maladies as long as possible (Fries, 1980, 1988). The critics appear not to have noticed, however, that allowing the debate to be framed in this way is fatal to their cause. As long as the underlying aging processes are understood as the major risk factors for the morbidities of aging, those processes become rational targets for preventive interventions aimed at forestalling the maladies in question. Just as it makes sense for public health officials to attempt to prevent the behaviors that put people at risk for human immunodeficiency virus infection whether or not they are considered healthy in themselves, it does not matter for medicine whether the underlying mechanisms of aging in humans are pathological in themselves. To the extent that the changes that constitute aging in humans increase the risk that people will experience disease and disability, it is proper, even imperative, that medicine attempt to mitigate them. From this point of view, one foreseeable side effect of intervening at that level is that people might begin to live beyond the historical human life span. But as long as the intervention is successful in forestalling the morbidities of aging, that extraordinary outcome is neither here nor there.

In fact, it is just this conceptual move that biogerontologists make to justify their interest in developing interventions into the mechanisms of human aging. While some biogerontologists evidently have even more ambitious goals—to either decelerate or arrest the aging process altogether—the forestalling of age-related morbidities creates a broad common ground between the aging research community and its potential critics. As one recent review article puts it:

> In the last few years, new findings have made preventing the onset of age-related diseases by delaying the process of senescence a tangible prospect. . . . The hope of basic research on senescence is to understand the fundamental aging mechanisms that underlie all of these diseases and, with this understanding, to forestall them as a group and increase the duration of disease-free, youthful vigor.
>
> (Kirkland, 2002, p. 383)

In part, appealing to the goal of compressing morbidity is clearly politically motivated as a way of distinguishing the work of mainstream biogerontologists from the anti-aging entrepreneurs on the margins (Binstock, 2003). Biogerontologists admit that

> [S]cientists and their patrons—even those who have legitimate research interests in interventional gerontology—do not wish to be seen hanging out with snake-oil vendors. Perhaps for these reasons, discussions of research on life-span extension are carefully skirted in political discourse at the NIH and among similar custodians of public funding. One can sometimes get away with cautious circumlocutions, but to be safe, it is clearly better to focus on how to "add life to years" and how to "learn the secrets contributing to a healthy old age."
>
> (Miller, 2002, p. 167)

Even the clinical entrepreneurs touting anti-aging medicine are careful to couch their official goals in this language. The stated mission of the A4M is "the advancement of technology to detect, prevent and treat age-related disease and to promote research into methods to retard and optimize the human aging process" (Binstock, 2003, p. 9).

But, of course, the compression of morbidity can serve as a useful political shield for researchers and entrepreneurs because it also forms a legitimate conceptual platform for the field. It is on that platform that medical research institutions base their support for anti-aging research. Thus, when the U.S. Institute of Aging includes "Unlocking the Secrets of Aging, Health and Longevity" as an important research goal in its Strategic Plan for 2001–2005, it declares that "The ultimate goal of this effort is to develop interventions to reduce or delay age-related degenerative processes in humans" (NIA, 2001, p. 16).

Given the ease with which anti-aging interventions can be wrapped in the flag of the compression of morbidity, it will not be enough to show that aging is not a disease if one wants to advance the position that responsible physicians should eschew such interventions. Are there other ways to set the boundaries of proper medical practice? While no one has yet developed them fully, there are the beginnings of at least three other arguments in the literature that might be worth exploring.

Three Critiques of Anti-Aging Medicine

The secular professional ethic of medicine operates in a relatively limited axiological universe. If an appeal to the values of health, normality, and vitality (and the correlative disvalues of disease, disability, and suffering) cannot help physicians steer their course, they have few other obvious stars to go by. One that has grown increasingly bright over the last century is the profession's commitment to respecting the personal autonomy of patients. Given the clear public interest in anti-aging medicine, that is not likely to help set a course away from those shoals. Pale within the penumbra of patient autonomy, however, may exist other medical values. The nascent alternative arguments against medical attempts to control aging are interesting in this respect, because they expose three neglected questions about the medical profession's moral commitments that will need to be addressed as anti-aging technologies emerge from the laboratory. Anti-aging medicine challenges both physicians and philosophers of medicine to ask: (*1*) How prescriptively should medicine take the contemporary biological parameters of human life? (*2*) How seriously should medicine take the relational character of human identity? and (*3*) How much responsibility does medicine have to expose and police its own value assumptions?

To Age Is Human

The first, and most common, alternative medical argument against anti-aging medicine is that aging is part of the life cycle that defines human beings, and that tampering with that cycle could literally be *dehumanizing*. It is usually offered as a generic ethical critique for personal or public policy purposes, but it can be framed as a professional ethical position as well, and it is in that frame work that it gains interest here.

This view is what Dan Callahan calls *life cycle traditionalism*:

> It is based on the biological rhythm of the life cycle as a way of providing a biological boundary to medical aspiration. This view looks to find a decent harmony between the present biological reality of the life cycle as an important characteristic of all living organisms and the feasible, affordable goals of medicine. . . .
>
> (Callahan, 1995, p. 23)

For proponents of this view, even if anti-aging interventions can help forestall some health problems, they cannot do so without sacrificing patients' essential identity as human beings (Kass, 2001).

Appealing to the natural life cycle as a normative guide has interesting analogs within professional medical ethics, where it plays an important role in the debates of forgoing life-sustaining treatment. There, one often hears that a natural death is the proper goal of care for the terminally ill and that, quite apart from considerations of personal autonomy, extraordinary attempts to prolong life artificially can sometimes be demeaning and dehumanizing for patients. This argument assumes that there is a normative natural order to life's events and their pacing in individual human lives. Critics of anti-aging medicine argue that the fact that we can see the importance of this developmental pacing in our maturation and in our dying suggests that it is just as important in middle life, and that it is only a lack of perspective that keeps us from seeing it.

To illustrate their point, the critics of anti-aging medicine recall our moral intuitions about interrupting the development of a child at prepubescence. Biologist Leonard Hayflick writes:

> The goal of slowing the aging process might be viewed in the same light in which we view slowing developmental processes. Slow physical or mental development in childhood is viewed universally as a serious pathology. If retarding the mental and physical development of someone from birth to age twenty years, for ten years in order to gain a decade of extra life is

unattractive, then slowing one's aging processes in later life will
not be attractive, and for the same reasons.

(Hayflick, 2001–2002, p. 25)

What is worrisome about that scenario is not simply the psychological harm such a developmental distortion might produce. Nor is
it just a matter of violating the child's right to self-determination:
that right is not yet in full flower, and it is the parents' role to protect,
and to some extent define, the child's best interests. But some form
of autonomy, as self-governance, does seem violated here. The
child's bodily development is no longer progressing on its own
schedule, nor being driven by the complex automatic interplay of
genes and their reactions to the environment. This disruption of the
child's *developmental autonomy*, in turn, alienates his or her life story
from the temporal narrative that characterizes our species.

Postponing the normal biological changes of aging, the critics
argue, constitutes a similar disruption. Whether or not the biological
changes of aging are beneficial or harmful, they are meaningful:
they and their natural timing constitute part of the normal life cycle
for human beings and thus part of what it means to be human (Kass,
2001). Intentionally distorting that cycle alienates the elderly from
the definitive human life story and dehumanizes them in the process. Adults should be taught to seek the meaning of the later stages
of human development, and biomedical research should focus on
making the experience of that part of life as healthy and pleasant as
possible without interfering in its essential rhythm (Callahan, 2000).
For those who see human life as a fixed natural cycle from the
dependence of childhood to the dependence of old age, or for
whom the discomforts of dying are as important as the discomforts of
birthing for full human experience, even delaying age-associated
morbidity beyond *premature aging* would produce an inappropriately
distorted life experience.

In light of Hayflick's analogy to delayed maturation, it is instruc-
tive to think about the circumstance in which we do humor people's
concerns about the harms of aging without taking them as serious
calls to action. When my daughter was 12, she once responded to my
description of her behavior as *adolescent* with hot denial, saying she
was not a teenager and did not want to become a teenager, because
teenagers were all "gross." She had already seen her sister suffer

the bodily indignities of puberty, the aches and awkwardness of accelerated growth, the loss of previously enjoyed mutual interests, the runaway emotions, the truncation of sociability, and the decrease in energy that seemed to her to characterize that stage of life, and she saw all those changes as distinct harms. If she could have compressed the morbidity of adolescence by postponing those changes, I am sure she would have. In fact, she probably was at her lifetime physical peak on most measures of human health and fitness; why not let her maximize the benefits and opportunities that level of health can provide?

Growing pains is what these outbursts of anxiety are called at our house, and they tend to be humored indulgently as understandable but childish. If the anxiety persisted, we might worry about the *Peter Pan syndrome,* and if it seemed driven by some social aspiration or pressure, such as excelling in gymnastics, we would bristle protectively and rethink her activities. But we would not try to manipulate her endocrine system to prevent or postpone her adolescence, and most people would accuse any parents or physicians who did so with committing a grave moral wrong. Why is that so, and what does it imply for the ethics of adult anti-aging interventions?

First, we believe that some of the changes she perceives as harms—the emergence of sexual maturity and the shifts in interests and activities—are not harms at all. We see them as just natural parts of growing up, which, on balance, offer more benefits than losses. Moreover, we expect most of the worst symptoms to be transient: complexions clear, emotions stabilize, and awkwardness dissipates as adolescents adapt to their new life phase, early adulthood. Postponing puberty would deny children the wider benefits of growing up, which are thought by most persons who enjoy them to be well worth the price of adolescence.

Critics of anti-aging medicine suggest that a similar argument might be made for the biological changes of late adulthood if our society were not so pervasively influenced by the perspective of those who have not yet undergone them (Callahan, 1993). That is, perhaps not all the changes that young adults count as the harmful losses of aging are harms at all when seen from the other side. One familiar example of this is menopause: a loss of reproductive capacity, fraught with physical and emotional turbulence, but one that many women come to celebrate as opening new opportunities and life pleasures (Martin, 1985; Logothetis, 1993). Similarly, in many societies, the loss of physical strength and endurance that comes with aging is what allows one to relinquish responsibility for the labor of survival and move into an even more important role as an elder for one's community (Moody, 1986). Traditionally, even the frank health challenges of aging—failing senses, vulnerability to disease and accident—have been seen as contributing to the life experiences of the elderly in a way that gives them a level of equanimity and insight difficult to achieve at earlier stages in life (Post, 2000). Among twentieth-century authors, psychologist Erik Erikson looked to old age as a crucial source of generativity in the human life cycle (Erikson, 1982), and philosophers Daniel Callahan and Leon Kass argue that growing old provides special opportunities for teaching, wisdom, and altruism (Kass, 1983, 1985, 2001; Callahan, 1993, 2000). This does not mean that we should be unconcerned about the major diseases that threaten human health in late adulthood, any more than we should become complacent about the increased risk of fatal traffic accidents in adolescence. But it does hint, critics argue, that attempting to intervene in the aging process itself, for all its attendant complaints, may be shortsighted and harmful, by denying adults the wider human experience of growing old.

Of course, arguing that the traditional human life cycle is normative for human beings requires a good bit of philosophical work if it is not to be accused of making a virtue of necessity. Just because human beings have always lived within a particular pattern of life experiences is not necessarily a reason to continue doing so. In fact, the social, technological, and biological dimensions of the typical human life story have been rewritten continuously over our species' history without diminishing the moral status of those people whose lives have been made possible by that evolution. Given our history of pushing back the natural limits of our lives through technology, the burden of proof in this case, the advocates argue, is on the naturalists to complete their philosophical project convincingly (Overall, 2003).

How prescriptively should medicine take the contemporary biological parameters of human life? After all, the physical burdens that accompany aging are more serious than those of adolescence and less transient. It is harder to adapt to life with fragile skin and brittle bones than to life with oily skin and lengthening bones. Moreover, we do not now live in a society designed to optimize the role of the elderly. Given the social realities of aging in our culture, many adults would consider the price of the late stages of human development high enough to warrant attempts to postpone and compress them as much as possible. Moreover, unlike preadolescents, middle-aged adults have seen enough of life to allow them to project themselves and their interests beyond their current age and appreciate the trade-offs involved in postponing aging. Advocates of anti-aging research can point out that respecting that human ability to project and pursue a life plan is at the heart of what it means to respect self-determination and personal autonomy. In the bright light of that star, how could responding to informed adult requests for anti-aging interventions with new research and (elective) clinical services be wrong?

It is popular today to promote the *preservation of the human species* by protecting humanity against *species-altering interventions* like reproductive cloning, genetic enhancement, and life span extension (Annas et al., 2002). From proponents of responsible genetics (Council for Responsible Genetics, 1993) to defenders of our *genetic patrimony* as the "common heritage of all humanity," (Knoppers, 1991) to the anti-post-humanist life cycle traditionalists (Kass, 1985, 2001), the prospect of further human evolution is provoking resistance. But much philosophical work remains to be done to justify that resistance. Until it is clear why, in the light of all its other intrinsic values, it is important for medicine to conserve the human species in its current form, a commitment to life cycle traditionalism in medicine can only count as an idiosyncratic ideology, which autonomous physicians (and their patients) in a free society should have the right to assess, adopt, or reject as they will. While the dehumanization argument bears more development, at this point it cannot provide a strong basis for discouraging physicians from the practice of anti-aging medicine under the banner of the compression of morbidity.

Aging and Family Health

A second argument that might be mounted against anti-aging interventions as a medical practice draws on psychosocial studies of aging to assert that, while anti-aging interventions may benefit individuals, the individual is not the proper unit of analysis to use in assessing their medical merits. Instead, anti-aging medicine is primarily an intervention into the web of relationships in which individual patients live, and is best assessed as *health care* at that level. This argument is grounded in a particular view of patients and their welfare:

the "long recognized proposition by students of the family" that "[t]he lives of family members are interdependent such that each person's family life continually interacts with the lives of significant relatives" (Riley, 1983, p. 447). Gerontologists who work within this tradition observe that "to individuals within ageing populations, the meaning of aging is in many ways mediated by smaller groups of interacting and interrrelated individuals, among the most important being kin groups" (Smith, 1990, p. 81). A corollary of this observation is that the meaning of any changes in an individual's aging process will also be mediated by his or her relationships with other people. As Matilda Riley of the National Institute on Aging points out:

> Though many facts of life extension are familiar, their mean-ings for the personal lives of family members are elusive. Just how is increasing longevity transforming the kinship structure? Most problematic of all, how is the impact of longevity affecting those sorely needed close relationships that provide emotional support and socialization for family members?
>
> (Riley, 1986, p. 453)

Traditionally, familial obligations have revolved around a cycle of vitality and vulnerability: I care for my vulnerable parents and my vulnerable children, and when my children grow and I weaken, they care for me (Post, 1999). My obligations to my grandparents and my grandchildren, while real, become forceful mainly when the inter-vening generation cannot fulfill its role and the cycle is disrupted. If senescence is postponed and foreshortened, however, the basis of the cycle itself is challenged. Older adults will not only be less vul-nerable, but may even continue propagating new cycles, as they peri-odically become interested in childrearing again. Of course, the institution of marriage may also change as we find the natural limits to psychologically healthy human pair bonding (Hackler, 2001–2002).

If anti-aging interventions can enable multiple generations of one family to occupy the same life stage (at least physiologically), what might this do to the allegiances of responsibility and reciprocity that animate this cycle? For example, once I, my children, and my parents all have the bodies and brains of young adults, are there any reasons why we should continue to take special responsibility for each other's welfare? We may find that, at best, we have the allegiances of siblings, bound by genetics and shared childhood experiences. At worst, we could find ourselves competing for the same opportunities and roles. If some of us are continuing to bear new children, our obligations to them will complicate the system even further. As Hayflick notes:

> We interact with each other to a substantial extent as a function of our perceptions of relative age. The destruction of that relationship would have enormous negative personal and societal consequences.
>
> (Hayflick, 2001–2002, p. 25)

For example, one fundamental tenet of family psychology is the importance of the development of *filial maturity* in multigenerational families. On this view, the "the essential psychological task associated with old age is coping with loss and fear while accepting dependency" (Golden and Saltz, 1997, p. 58). In that context, filial maturity is the ability of a family to adapt to the challenges of genuine caregiving for dependent older members without disrupting even further the elders' uncertain sense of self. On this view, "making room in the family system for the wisdom and experience of the old without taking over for them is essential" (Golden and Saltz, 1997, p. 59). Without the timely emergence of the stimulus for this trait—that is, increasingly dependent parents—this developmental stage could be retarded, to the detriment of all the family members, including the nominal elders.

How seriously should medicine take the relational character of human identity? Once again, this argument depends upon an increasingly popular intellectual proposition, but one that has hitherto had only a tenuous grip on the medical mind. Unlike the argument from dehumanization, however, there is at least a body of empirical evidence to support this argument's premise. The health outcomes and psychosocial family studies that suggest that there does seem to be reason to interpret the impact of anti-aging interventions at the level of family systems are provocative enough to warrant more consideration, even within a patient-centered medical ethos.

Unfortunately, even if aging is interpreted relationally, it is not yet clear what the consequences of anti-aging interventions would be for family systems. How do we know that the impact of such a change would be negative? For example, some argue that, far from destroying the traditional family, anti-aging interventions may make possible new forms of family that can take the traditional familial virtues to a new level of realization by destabilizing dysfunctional power hierarchies, bridging cultural generation gaps, and providing more opportunities for equitable sharing of childrearing roles (Bengston, 2001). Matilda Riley, after questioning the impact of increased longevity from the relational perspective, also comes to a positive conclusion. She argues that her research shows that with the gains in life expectancy we have already experienced.

> [t]he options for close family bonds have multiplied. Over the century, increased longevity has given flexibility to the kinship structure, relaxing both the temporal and spatial boundaries of optional relationships.
>
> (Riley, 1983, p. 445)

Thus, again, while the prospect of anti-aging medicine presses physicians to adopt a different philosophical understanding of their patients, it is not clear that taking that perspective will necessarily require medicine to abandon anti-aging interventions. If anything, it suggests that, given our empirical equipoise about the consequences of anti-aging interventions at the level of patients' relational identities, clinical research on such interventions would be justified as a means of determining those consequences

Anti-aging and Ageism

Finally, another argument against anti-aging medicine that bears scrutiny is the argument that, even if anti-aging interventions did forestall genuine health problems, even if they were not unduly dehumanizing, and even if they promoted the vitality of interpersonal relationships, they could do so only by involving medicine in exacerbating fundamental social injustices. Here the claim is that the anti-aging enterprise is complicitous with prejudicial social attitudes toward aging and the elderly and, like medical racism and sexism, should be eschewed as a professional perversion (Greene et al., 1986).

In considering biomedical enhancements generally, complicity with unjust social practices is one of the important moral issues involved in deciding whether to attempt to enhance oneself or one's children (Juengst, 1998). In practice, this confines the range of morally problematic enhancements to those that can be expected to exacerbate invidious social prejudices—in the way, for example, that homogenizing aesthetic enhancements like orthodenture reinforce prejudices against snaggle-toothed outliers in a high school class. Even then, as this example suggests, parents are usually excused for putting the social interests of their own children ahead of broader justice concerns, and claims of personal autonomy can protect most self-improvement attempts by individuals. Only where the unenhanced are clearly disadvantaged in unfair ways—as athletes can be in competitive sports—is strong moral censure warranted (Mehlman, 2000).

Would the widespread use of anti-aging interventions feed prejudice against or unfairly disadvantage those who do age normally? Answering this question will mean examining what we already know about the social context of aging in the United States today. First, despite efforts to valorize contemporary life expectancies and reform the medical model of aging, the aging process itself has become increasingly stigmatized as pathological (Greene et al., 1986). At the same time, the elderly portion of the population is growing quickly and will become an ever larger proportion of the voting public (Binstock, 2000). As the youthful old retain more interests in common with young adults than with the aging old, what is likely to happen to their political allegiances? If it remains strong, a larger population of youthful elderly might benefit the interests of the aging elderly. If other interests realign allegiances, however, the aging elderly could find themselves increasingly marginalized.

Again, this argument founders on the need for better clues to the likely consequences of anti-aging medicine. Further research may be able to triangulate more presciently from what we know today about the social status of aging to the justice issues of a long-lived society. However, whatever that research tells us, concern for the equality and social welfare of those who age normally in an era of anti-aging interventions does challenge medicine again to think about its underlying moral commitments. To what extent should physicians take the interests of nonpatients—the normal agers, in this case—into consideration?

In providing clinical medical care, physicians are usually enjoined not to put social policy concerns ahead of the best interests of their patients. On the other hand, in public health contexts, social policy concerns are given precedence over the welfare of specific patients.

Between those two contexts lie a range of medical practices, such as giving growth hormone to short children, *normalizing* cosmetic surgery for children with Down's syndrome, and providing skin-lightening treatments for African-Americans, that help people avoid socially stigmatizing characteristics. All of these, to varying degrees, advance the interests of individual patients at the risk of acknowledging and tacitly endorsing the unjust prejudices that make a problem of otherwise unproblematic physical traits.

When physicians conscientiously object to performing procedures in this socially volatile middle range, they do so on the grounds that their complicity with those prejudices would be undermining the interests of the class that displays the features being stigmatized (Little, 1998). But medicine as a profession has not accepted a special duty to police its professionals' complicity with biased social attitudes. Rather, it has generally tolerated a wide range of medically unnecessary medical practices of this sort out of respect for the clinical judgment of its members and the wishes and welfare of its patients. This means that, in practice, medicine is likely to police anti-aging interventions for reasons of justice only when it becomes clear that the social problems created by their availability as elective medical services are severe enough to be compared with public health emergencies. According to some critics, such crises are not unforeseeable in a long-lived society (Hayflick, 2001–2002). But until it is clearer that medicine should steer by social justice as well as patient welfare, the argument of complicity is not likely to stand in the way of anti-aging medicine.

Conclusion

Are there professional ethical grounds for physicians to decry the advent of an effective anti-aging medicine? Perhaps, but it will not be because of a commitment to the view that aging is not a disease. As long as anti-aging interventions serve to forestall the morbidities associated with the aging process, they have a legitimate place in the armamentarium of preventive medicine. Rather, the prospect of anti-aging medicine forces medicine to directly face three other philosophical limit questions: (*1*) How prescriptively should medicine take the contemporary biological parameters of human life? (*2*) How seriously should medicine take the relational character of human identity?

(3) How much responsibility does medicine have to expose and police its own complicity with invidious social biases? The state of our thinking on each of these questions is too preliminary to convincingly evict anti-aging interventions from the proper domain of medicine. But as biogerontological research advances, the importance of these questions will grow.

Acknowledgments

Support for this chapter came from a research grant (1R01AGHG20916-01) from the National Institute on Aging and the National Human Genome Research Institute. I am indebted to my collaborators on this research project—Robert H. Binstock, Maxwell J. Mehlman, Stephen G. Post, and Peter J. Whitehouse—and to the invaluable research assistance of Roselle S. Ponsaran.

References

Annas, G., Andrews, L., and Isasi, R. (2002). Protecting the endangered human: Toward an international treaty prohibiting cloning and inheritable alterations. *American Journal of Law and Medicine,* 28, 151–178.

Bengtson, V. (2001). Beyond the nuclear family: The increasing importance of multigenerational bonds. *Journal of Marriage and Family,* 63, 1–16.

Binstock, R. (2003). The war on "anti-aging medicine." *Gerontologist,* 43, 4–140.

Boorse, C. (1977). Health as a theoretical concept. *Philosophy of Science,* 44, 542–573.

Butler, R., Fossel, M., Harman, S., Heyward, C., Olshanshy, S., Perls, T., Rothman, D., Rothman, S., Warnes, H., West, M., and Wright, W. (2002). Is there an anti-aging medicine? *Journal of Gerontology: Biological Sciences,* 57A(9), B333–B338.

Callahan, D. (1993). *The Troubled Dream of Life: Living with Mortality.* New York: Simon & Schuster.

Callahan, D. (1995). Aging and the life cycle: A moral norm? In: Callahan, D., ter Meulen R.H.J., and Topinka, E., eds. *A World Growing Old: The Coming Health Care Challenges.* Washington, DC: Georgetown University Press, pp. 21–27.

Callahan, D. (2000). Death and the research imperative. *New England Journal of Medicine,* 342, 654–656.

Caplan, A. (1982). The unnaturalness of aging: A sickness unto death? In: Caplan, A., Engelhardt, H.T., and McCartney, J., eds. *Concepts of Health and Disease: Interdisciplinary Perspectives.* Reading, MA: Addison-Wesley, pp. 331–345.

Council for Responsible Genetics. (1993). Position statement on human germ-line manipulation. *Human Gene Therapy,* 4, 35–39.

Erikson, E. (1982). *The Life Cycle Completed: A Review.* New York: W.W. Norton.

Forbes, W.F. and Thompson, M.E. (1990). Age-related diseases and normal aging: The nature of the relationship. *Journal of Clinical Epidemiology,* 43(2), 191–193.

Fries, J.F. (1980). Aging, natural death, and the compression of morbidity. *New England Journal of Medicine,* 303, 130–136.

Fries, J.F. (1988). Aging, illness and health policy: Implications of the compression of morbidity. *Perspectives in Biology and Medicine,* 31(3), 407–428.

Golden, R. and Saltz, C. (1997). The aging family. *Journal of Gerontological Social Work,* 27, 55–64.

Greene, M., Adelman, R., Charon, R., and Hoffman, S. (1986). Ageism in the medical encounter. *Language and Communicaiton,* 6, 113–124.

Hackler, C. (2001–2002). Troubling implications of doubling the human life span. *Generations,* 24(4), 15–19.

Hayflick, L. (2001–2002). Anti-aging medicine: Hype, hope and reality. *Generations,* 24(4), 20–27.

Juengst, E. (1998). What does enhancement mean?" In Parens, E., ed. *Enhancing Human Traits: Ethical and Social Implications.* Washington, DC: Georgetown University Press, pp. 29–34.

Juengst, E., Binstock, R.H., Mehlman, M., and Post, S.G. (2003). Antiaging research and the need for public dialogue. *Science,* 299, 1323.

Kass, L. (1983). The case for mortality. *The American Scholar,* 52, 173–191.

Kass, L. (1985). *Toward a More Natural Science: Biology and Human Affairs.* New York: Free Press.

Kass, L. (2001). L'Chaim and its limits: Why not immortality? *First Things,* 113, 17–25.

Kirkland, J. (2002). The biology of senescence: Potential for prevention of disease. *Clinical Geriatric Medicine,* 18, 383–405.

Knoppers, B. (1991). *Human Dignity and Genetic Heritage.* Montreal: Law Reform Commission of Canada.

Little, M. (1998). Cosmetic surgery, suspect norms, and the ethics of complicity. In: Parens, E., ed. *Enhancing Human Traits: Ethical and Social Implications.* Washington, DC: Georgetown University Press, pp. 162–177.

Logothetis, M.L. (1993). Disease or development: Women's perceptions of menopause. In: Callahan, J., ed. *Menopause: A Midlife Passage.* Bloomington: Indiana University Press.

Martin, M. (1985). Malady and menopause. *Journal of Medicine and Philosophy,* 10, 329–339.

Miller, R. (2002). Extending life: Scientific prosopects and political obstacles. *The Milbank Quarterly,* 80, 155–174.

Moody, H. (1986). The meaning of life and the meaning of old age. In: Cole, T. and Gadow, S., eds. *What Does It Mean to Grow Old? Reflections from the Humanities.* Durham, NC: Duke University Press, pp. 9–41.

Murphy, T. (1986). A cure for aging? *Journal of Medicine and Philosophy,* 11, 237–257.

National Institute on Aging. (2001). *Action Plan for Aging Research: Strategic Plan for Fiscal Years 2001–2005.* Washington, DC: U.S. Department of Health and Human Services.

Olshansky, S.J., Hayflick, L., and Carnes, B. (2002). Position statement on human aging. *Journal of Gerontology: Biological Sciences,* 57A(8), B292–B297.

Overall, C. (2003). *Aging, Death and Human Longevity: A Philosophical Inquiry.* Berkeley: University of California Press.

Post, S. (1999) *Spheres of Love: Toward a New Ethic of the Family,* Dallas, TX: Southern Methodist University Press.

Post, S. (2000). The concept of Alzheimer disease in a hypercognitive society. In: Whitehouse, P., Maurer, P., and Ballinger, J., eds., *Concepts of Alzheimer Disease: Biological, Clinical and Cultural Perspectives.* Baltimore: Johns Hopkins University Press, pp. 245–247.

Riley, M.W. (1983). The family in an aging society: A matrix of latent relationships. *Journal of Family Issues,* 4, 439–454.

Shelton, D. (2000, December 4). Dipping into the fountain of youth. *AMA News,* p. 25.

Smith, J. (1990). Aging together, aging alone. In: Ludwig, F., ed. *Life Span Extension: Consequences and Open Questions.* New York: Springer, pp. 81–93.

16

The Social and Justice Implications of Extending the Human Life Span

Audrey R. Chapman

*T*ypically, our society proceeds in a *reactionary mode*, scrambling to deal with scientific developments after the announcement of new breakthroughs. But doing so has serious limitations. When a potential scientific development raises profound theological, ethical, and/or social issues, it seems far preferable to assess the implications in advance and to decide whether and how to proceed. The fundamental issue of whether we will determine or be determined by science and technology depends on our ability to discern the challenges and respond wisely. Moreover, it is far more feasible to undertake an informed and unemotional examination of the broader societal implications of a new technology before rather than after it becomes a reality. And when such an evaluation suggests that there are likely to be serious problems, either because of the nature of the technologies or because of their ethical and social consequences, it may be preferable to regulate or block their development.

Clearly, the prospect of prolonging the human life span through genetic or other types of biomedical interventions requires such a careful evaluation before proceeding. Any prospective biomedical or genetic technology that is likely to impinge on the understanding of what it is to be human and to have significant social, ethical, religious, and justice implications should be treated very cautiously. These concerns are even more warranted when the technology has significant long-term risks, especially if it is likely to affect the genes that are transmitted to future generations and the prospects of future societies. Extending the human life span by a considerable number of years, even if well short of efforts to achieve immortal life, would have profound consequences, not only for the individuals who were given the seeming gift of long or longer lives, but also for their societies and possibly for the rest of the world as well. If such efforts were to succeed and be available to a large number of people, they would likely bring about not only a medical but also a social revolution. Human societies are built around expectations of a life cycle of a limited duration. Increasing the life expectancy would challenge these arrangements and the web of social relationships based on them.

So that brings us to the question of how to go about making such an evaluation, especially when the desires of some individuals for longer life may be in conflict with the best interests of their society and/or the human community. How do we best anticipate the likely implications of a technology well in advance of its development? What kinds of questions should we ask? How do we make unprecedented choices to alter the biological basis of life? What kinds of ethical norms, theological concepts, social issues, and scientific factors should be taken into account? Is the decision best left to societies to regulate or to the individuals who may opt to take the risk of using the new technology? This chapter discusses the importance of using a social and justice framework for undertaking such an assessment.

A study of inheritable genetic modifications conducted by a working group of eminent scientists, ethicists, theologians, and policy analysts convened by the American Association for the Advancement of Science (AAAS), for which I served as the codirector, offers a potential model of how to proceed with such an evaluation (Frankel and Chapman, 2000). Rapid breakthroughs in genetic research, spurred by the Human Genome Project, advances in molecular biology, and new reproductive technologies have advanced our understanding of how we might approach genetic interventions as possible remedies for diseases caused by genetic disorders, particularly those caused by abnormalities in single genes. In theory, modifying the genes that are transmitted to future generations could offer the possibility of preventing the inheritance of some genetically based diseases and preventing irreversible damage attributable to defective genes before it occurs. However, these techniques could also confer the power to mold our children in a variety of novel ways and thereby offer extraordinary control over biological properties and personality traits that we currently consider essential to humanness. Therefore, the mandate to the working group was to assess whether inheritable genetic modifications offer a theologically, socially, and ethically acceptable alternative to other approaches under development to treat genetic diseases. The working group also considered whether current and prospective technologies could meet the high safety standards required for shaping the genetic future of multiple descendants across generations. The analysis here will build some of my work in conjunction with that project (Chapman and Frankel, 2003).

Using a Social and Justice-Oriented Framework

Doubtless many people will regard any decisions about extending the human life span as intensely personal and therefore inappropriate to assess and regulate from a social perspective. In a liberal and individualistic society such as ours, there is a presumption in favor of individual freedom of action, absent strong arguments about the need to protect others from harm. Many in our society believe they have an unlimited right of control over their own bodies. Others would likely argue that they should not be restricted from purchasing any treatment or enhancement that they can afford for themselves, for other members of their family, or perhaps even for their descendants. They might accept the appropriateness of the federal government's exercising some very limited regulatory oversight to prevent the introduction of unsafe technologies, but they would be reluctant to acknowledge a broader sphere of social control. Others might go so far as to claim that they even have the right to experiment with risky biomedical interventions should they desire to do so. Individuals who use illegal or untested performance enhancing drugs and hormone supplements despite scientific risks and social condemnation provide examples of this attitude.

In contrast, this chapter proceeds from the supposition that any new biomedical and genetic interventions that are likely to have profound consequences for human dignity, social relationships, and justice considerations should not be left solely to individuals to determine.

Instead, these technologies should be examined initially and perhaps primarily from an ethical, social, and justice perspective, and decisions regarding how to proceed should be made by an appropriate regulatory agency or political body after extensive public consultation. The need to apply a social and justice frame of reference is even greater when prospective technologies carry significant safety risks and have potential multi-generational implications.

Religious thinkers dealing with genetic issues have frequently stressed the need for a social and community framework for decision making (Chapman, 1999). In contrast with the radical individualism prevalent in our culture, most religious traditions have a vision of human beings as basically social and interdependent. The monotheistic religions with which I am most familiar—Judaism, Christianity, and Islam—and likely virtually all other faiths as well, conceptualize persons as moral and social beings created to live in communities linked by relationships of mutual caring and responsibility. As Sondra Wheeler comments, "The picture of the self possessed individual deciding his or her own fate in splendid isolation is one wholly alien to the Christian understanding of moral existence" (1996, p. 46). The same could be said of most faith communities. Religious perspectives generally recognize that the choices made by individuals affect other members of their families, their communities, and the wider society and therefore conclude that individuals bear a responsibility for their social impacts. The religious concept of covenant captures this sense of interconnectedness between humanity, God, and the creation. Classical interpretations of covenant stress the importance of the interrelationships among persons in a moral community in which the common good and the good of each member are sought as a dimension of faithfulness to God's mandates.

Many religious traditions translate this vision of human life into an ethic of responsibility for the way individuals and communities manage their lives, their social relationships, and the well-being of this fragile planet and its resources. The stewardship tradition, which is rooted in Scripture, characterizes the vocation of humanity as a servant who has been given the responsibility for the management and service of something belonging to another, in this case the Creator. Granted, the classical notion of stewardship predates modern science and assumes that we are living in a static, finished, and hierarchical universal in which stewardship implies respecting the natural order and not seeking to change it. This makes it very

difficult to apply to decision making regarding scientific developments (Chapman, 1999, pp. 42–44). But whether one draws on the
notion of stewardship or the more recent terminology of humanity
as the *created co-creator* (this term was first suggested by Philip Hefner
and has its most extended exposition in Hefner, 1993) or God's partner, there is a sense of limits, of the obligation to work for the long-
term good of the human race and for the flourishing of life on our
planet (Peters, 1997, pp. 177–178).

The wide web of relationships in which religious traditions typically conceptualize human life is very inclusive both in time and in
breadth. In many instances, these links and the moral obligations
they confer extend to future and sometimes past generations as well.
It is true that the topic of intergenerational ethics is controversial,
with philosophers and ethicists disagreeing on the nature and basis
of obligations to future generations. But most of these differences
relate to the nature of our responsibilities to specific *future contingent
persons* who may or may not be born, depending on the decisions
made by members of the current generation. That is not the issue
here. Instead, I am proposing a standard of intergenerational obligations that at the least requires us to desist from major undertakings
likely to make the world less equitable and sustainable for those who
follow us. As will be discussed below, extending the human life span
would have significant implications for intergenerational equity.

Similarly, extending the human life span would have justice
implications. Justice is a multifaceted and complex concept, with theorists differing in their approaches. The biblical conception is quite
broad and associates justice with *right relationship* or *righteousness*.
Most secular treatments are narrower, but generally concur that justice,
at a minimum, requires fair, equitable, and appropriate treatment in
light of what is due or owed to persons. Conversely, a wrongful act or
omission that denies an individual or a group the benefits to which
the person or group has a rightful claim, or alternatively fails to distribute burdens in a fair manner, constitutes a form of injustice. Justice
has social as well as individual dimensions. *Distributive justice,* the type
of justice most relevant to the issues raised in this chapter, refers to
the morally justifiable distributions of benefits and burdens in a society
as defined by the norms that structure the terms of social cooperation
(Beauchamp and Childress, 1994, p. 327).

This commitment to justice has a corollary to avoid injustice.
Indeed, one treatment of justice by a Christian ethicist conceptualizes

our task as nothing less than identifying the sources of injustice as the basis for restructuring political and social realities in the direction of greater equity and justice (Lebacqz, 1987). For people of faith, social inequalities violate the belief that the benefits of creation, including those that come from human effort, are to be widely shared. In keeping with this concern, many of the religious thinkers who were members of the AAAS working group on inheritable genetic modifications were particularly sensitive to the justice implications of this technology and recommended not proceeding unless these issues could be resolved. Other working group members were also concerned that this technology had the potential to enable us to enhance offspring in socially desirable and competitive ways, thereby further privileging the wealthy and powerful (Frankel and Chapman, 2000, esp. pp. 7–8, 31, 38–39, 40–43). For reasons that will be discussed below, I believe that extending the human life span also is likely to aggravate existing social inequalities within and across societies.

Scientific research and the development of technologies that have human applications may appropriately be considered to be a social enterprise and as such an activity about which society can justifiably make collective decisions. As a society, we have invested significant resources in the education and training of scientists, in research on important health issues, and in the infrastructure essential for sustaining scientific research. To date, much of our scientific research in the biomedical and genetic areas has proceeded with an important infusion of public funding. Such public funding, combined with increasing apprehension about the effects of science, particularly in the biomedical arena, has led to increasing social controls over science.

These considerations have forged a linkage between scientific freedom and responsibility. A policy statement of AAAS describes the relationship as follows: "scientific freedom . . . is an acquired right, generally approved by society as necessary for the advancement of knowledge from which society may benefit." But "scientific freedom and responsibility are basically inseparable" (1975, p. 5). This perspective clearly rules out pursuing potential scientific avenues of research and application with potentially harmful consequences just because it can be done.

It is also important to recognize that the determination of acceptable levels of safety related to a new technology is in itself a social decision. Safety is a relative, not an absolute, standard. For this reason, the AAAS working group emphasized the need to promote extensive public education and discussion to ascertain societal attitudes about proceeding with inheritable genetic modifications and to develop a meaningful process for making decisions about the future of the technology. It also recommended that before proceeding, there should be a method in place for assessing the short, and long-term risks and benefits of such interventions, and that society must decide how much evidence of safety, efficacy, and moral acceptance will be required before allowing human clinical trials (Frankel and Chapman, 2000, pp. 9–10). Any new technologies for purposes of extending the human life span should be treated in a similar manner.

Potential Technologies for Delaying Aging or Prolonging Life in a Social Context

It has been suggested that efforts to delay aging or extend human life might use one or a combination of three approaches. Each of these differs in feasibility and social implications. The first is using hormones and new protein-based drugs, some of which would have been developed for other purposes—for example, taking human growth hormone to stimulate physical vigor. At the time of writing none of these anti-aging remedies has proved effective (Olshansky et al., 2002), but in the future other products may be useful. Nevertheless, it seems more likely that these hormones, proteins, or drugs, if efficacious, would improve vigor and/or the quality of life and in that way help delay some of the effects of aging rather than extend the life span.

The second approach involves potential developments in the new field of regenerative medicine based on applications of human stem cells. If successful, stem cell research would provide medicine with a new, more effective, and less invasive way to repair tissue and organ damage and cure some diseases, but research is still at a very early stage. Moreover, it will be far more feasible to develop stem cell therapies for some organs and bodily systems than others. Most significantly, stem cell therapies are unlikely to be applicable to reversing the effects of mental as compared with certain forms of physical deterioration. Like the development of hormones to rejuvenate older bodies, stem cells therapies are therefore more likely to improve health in selective ways and contribute only indirectly to lengthening the life span by reducing the toll of some age-related infirmities. Even if science is successful in developing some significant stem cell therapies, aging will continue to occur and bodily systems will still be susceptible to catastrophic failure.

Scientists seeking to control the biological process of aging are more likely to attempt to do so through genetic manipulations. The relevance of genetic interventions for this purpose, however, is a subject of considerable controversy. Many scientists understand aging as the result of a complex series of processes and not as due to a single simple mechanism. A position paper written by a group of 51 of the leading scientists who study aging, published in conjunction with an article in *Scientific American*, defines aging as the accumulation of random damage in the building blocks of life that begins early in life and gradually impairs the functioning of cells, tissues organs, and organ systems, thereby giving rise to the characteristic manifestations of aging, including vulnerability to diseases like Alzheimer's disease, stroke, heart disease, and cancer (Olshansky et al., 2002, p. 93). Viewed in this manner, aging, though inevitable, is not a genetically programmed process (Olshansky et al., 2002).

Although scientists in this field have generally assumed that aging is a complex process in which many genes and proteins play a role, some scientists have hypothesized that there may be a master gene or genes for this purpose. Consistent with this perspective, they reason that to prolong the life span, they just have to identify the relevant genes and then modify them. A few experiments with laboratory animals, like the roundworm, the fruit fly, and the mouse, have enabled them to live far beyond their normal life spans. On the human side of the equation, studies show that patterns of longer than average life sometimes run in families, suggesting that genetics may play a role in the ability of some people to survive to unusually old ages. Currently, a few scientists are searching for human genes and regions of mitochondrial DNA that affect longevity (Kaiser, 2001).

Even if genetic factors are shown to contribute to aging, there is an obvious need for caution about the feasibility or desirability of reengineering the genetic constitution of people to attempt to extend their life span. On the grounds of feasibility, there are significant limitations in applying research and findings about simple animal models to human beings. What can be done with worms, fruit flies, or even mice is often of little relevance to far more complex human organisms. Moreover, a recent experiment suggests that efforts to modify relevant genes would likely have serious unforeseen consequences. A paper published in *Nature* found that the *p53* protein, which works to suppress cancer, most likely by affecting how cells respond to damage, also has effects on aging. Increases in *p53* activity reduced the incidence of cancer in mice but also accelerated the rate of aging. Conversely, decreases in *p53* may decrease the rate of aging but at the cost of an increased incidence of tumors. The authors of the paper hypothesize that the influence of *p53* on the life span may result from a delicate balance between its antitumor and pro-aging effects (Ferbeyre and Lowe, 2002). This relationship suggests that interventions to modify the genetic mechanisms of aging may have profound unanticipated negative consequences.

But there are even more fundamental grounds on which to question both the feasibility and the appropriateness of seeking to modify the human genome so as to try to alter any of the genes potentially influencing the human life span. In the early stages of its development, human gene therapy was heralded as "a symbol of hope in a vast sea of human suffering due to heredity" (Fletcher and Anderson, 1992, p. 31). Despite this hype, gene therapy has not fulfilled its promise. Thus far, the major contribution of genetic science has been to diagnose rather than to treat genetically based disorders. While some patients have been helped and a very few cured, the overwhelming majority of the several thousand patients who have enrolled in gene therapy trials have not received any benefit.

Moreover, the state of genetic science and technologies is inappropriate for sensitive genetic modifications, particularly when interventions are likely to affect multiple genes and have multigenerational effects. Current methods for somatic gene transfer are inefficient and unreliable because they involve addition of DNA to cells rather than correcting or replacing a mutated gene with a normal one. Scientists have not yet developed vectors that deliver genes to the intended locations within the cell or the means to assure proper gene expression over time. Because gene addition techniques introduce viruses and other foreign matter into cells, they also increase the risk of iatrogenic harms (Frankel and Chapman, 2000, pp. 23–25). Clearly, we do not have sufficient biological knowledge and understanding of the human genome to alter single defective genes, let alone multiple genes and their interaction effects. Given the state of our knowledge and technology, it is not surprising that the AAAS working group found that inheritable genetic modification cannot presently be carried out safely and responsibly on humans (Frankel and Chapman, 2000, pp. 8, 24).

The social consequences of any efforts to reduce the effects of aging and to prolong life will depend on many factors, including the relative success of any of these technologies, the cost and degree of access within and across societies, and the potential balance between innovations that improve the quality and length of life. Here it is important to note the trend toward population aging that began in the twentieth century. The twentieth century was marked by a dramatic decrease in mortality primarily through improvements in health conditions, sanitation, and nutrition and secondarily through the introduction of modern medicine. These trends have also fueled significant population growth, particularly in countries in the South. The demographic transition from high to low levels of fertility and lower mortality rates means that people are living longer while families are getting smaller, particularly in the industrialized countries of the North. Globally, the population of older persons is growing more rapidly than other age group. In the more developed regions, nearly one-fifth of the population was already aged 60 or older in the year 2000. Even without the introduction of any of the technologies discussed above, older people are expected to constitute one-third of the total population of these countries by 2050 (United Nations Department of Economic and Social Affairs, Population Division, 2002, p. xxviii). This will be an unprecedented development.

Given these trends, the impact of innovations affecting the aging process will depend in part on the balance between their improving the quality and length of life. Further life extensions that are not accompanied by a reduction in age-related morbidity and mental deterioration would result in a rapidly growing population of dependent, frail elderly. If there is any extension of the life span or if regenerative medicine enables a greater proportion of the population to live even longer without improving their physical and mental vitality, society may come to resemble something like a giant nursing home (Fukuyama, 2002, p. 67). The social and economic implications of the changing age composition of societies will be discussed in greater detail later in the chapter.

Distributive Justice:
The Issue of Societal Investments

Problems of distributive justice typically arise under conditions of scarcity and competition when resources are insufficient and/or trade-offs are required. The development and dissemination of prospective technologies to reduce the effects of aging or extend the life span would raise such justice issues. Development will likely require considerable resource investments, particularly if scientists are to develop new forms of genetic technology to make clinical applications safe and effective. There are three potential scenarios. If such efforts are financed with public funds to ensure proper regulatory oversight, the resources invested will most likely come at the expense of other social investments, including research to produce other types of medical innovations. Alternatively, if the technology for greater longevity is developed by the private sector, like other privately funded high-technology innovations such as somatic cell genetic therapy, it will probably be very expensive. This will raise significant access issues within and across societies. Finally, if this field emerges from a public–private partnership, it may not eliminate either set of disadvantages—the burdens of public investment or the limitations of access.

Would a major public investment in these efforts be wise, fair, or equitable from a societal perspective? Therapeutic needs should be the primary criterion for public investments. The human aging process is not a disease or a serious health problem that requires elimination. Efforts to engineer longer life cannot be justified as a potential contribution to improving health status or relieving suffering. Instead such initiatives would be akin to other types of prospective enhancements, that is, non-disease-related interventions intended to improve normal human characteristics. A stronger case can be made for efforts to reduce the incidence of diseases that accompany aging, particularly if the technologies would have wider applications. Stem cell therapies would be one such example, with potential broad health contributions benefiting all population groups. Initiatives to improve the vigor and productivity of older persons could also have broad societal benefits.

Efforts to develop new medical technologies also need to be viewed in the context of other types of investments that are far more likely to contribute to public health and welfare. Although the United

States has the highest per capita health expenditures in the world, health-care economists estimate that approximately 40 million persons, nearly one-sixth of the U.S. population, lack health insurance, and many other persons have insufficient coverage (Freudenheim, 2002). Lack of health insurance often leads to delayed diagnoses, life-threatening complications, and ultimately, premature deaths (Connolly, 2002). Access to health care is already unfairly distributed throughout our society. Blacks, Hispanics, and other minorities tend to receive lower-quality health care than whites. This disparity is generally attributed to lower incomes, inadequate health insurance, and the lack of doctors in their areas of residence. Minorities are far more likely than whites to be uninsured: minorities comprised 46% of the uninsured in 2000, although these groups represented only 24% of the U.S. population (Guy, 2000). Various studies have also shown that minorities with insurance are more likely to have only minimal or basic coverage (Guy, 2000, p. 71) and to suffer from various forms of *therapeutic discrimination* that limit their access to a wide variety of procedures and therapies. A disturbing report issued by the Institute of Medicine of the National Academies of Science in March 2002, based on a review of 100 studies conducted during the past decade, concludes that racial and ethnic minorities in the United States receive notably lower-quality health care, even when they have the same incomes, insurance coverage, and medical conditions as whites. The report attributed these disparities to biases, prejudices, and negative racial stereotyping (Stolberg, 2002). These disparities particularly affect high-technology interventions. It can therefore be assumed that current limitations on access to care for minorities will also likely operate with respect to technologies related to countering the effects of aging.

On a global level, it is relevant to keep in mind the gross inequality in the health status of people between developed and developing countries and particularly the devastating toll of the HIV/AIDS (human immunodeficiency virus/acquired immunodeficiency syndrome) pandemic and other infectious diseases on poor countries. A recent report prepared by the Commission on Macroeconomics and Health at the request of the World Health Organization shows that an investment of some $66 billion per year, with the costs shared between high-income donor countries and low-income countries, could save around 8 million lives per year. This proposal is based on focused well-targeted measures, using existing technologies, to counter HIV/AIDS as well as two other scourges, tuberculosis and malaria. Not only would this scaling up to respond to infectious diseases reduce misery and save millions of lives, it would also remove significant obstacles to economic development. With the disease burden lifted, many of those living in poverty would also be able to increase their capacity to improve their economic circumstances (World Health Organization, 2002).

My position is that our first priority for health-related investments should be to provide basic medical services to everyone in our own country and to ameliorate health needs elsewhere in the world. Pursuing efforts to extend the human life span seems like a frivolous investment in comparison with these imperatives. Research to reduce age-related diseases would have a somewhat higher priority, but it still cannot compare with the need to provide basic health services for those currently going without them.

Some people may counter that the above analysis is based on unlikely trade-offs in investments. By this they mean that funds saved by foregoing research and trials intended to reduce the effects of aging or to extend the human life span will not then be made available for the purposes proposed here of extending access to health care and scaling up to deal with the toll of major infectious diseases in poor countries. While they may agree that the failure to deal with these critical health problems is unfortunate, they would not consider this to be relevant. However, as the analysis in the final sections of this chapter indicates, increasing the number and proportion of people in a society who live longer lives would have major economic and social implications and costs, particularly on the health system. It is even questionable whether such an aging society would be economically and socially sustainable. So I think we are warranted in placing the issue in a wider social context.

More significantly, I think that a narrow approach fails to recognize the role of our central values and commitments in allocating scarce resources. Our priorities and acceptance of wider relationships of responsibility have a great deal to do with whether we choose to rectify serious health problems and needs. The failure of health care reform in our society, itself an ethical scandal, reflects a fundamental lack of concern for others who are less fortunate. Many national commissions and task forces have proposed measures to extend access to health care, but in the end, legislators and their constituents did not care enough to spend the funds or to counter the lobbying efforts of private interests. Investing in new and very expensive high technologies for enhancement interventions while people in our own country lack access to basic health care and millions of people die prematurely of preventable diseases in poor countries would be yet another step toward moral bankruptcy.

The Implications of the Aging of Society

Suppose that scientists do manage to identify and manipulate genes that affect the aging process at some point in the future and make this technology available to a sizable number of people. Or, alternatively, what if regenerative medicine were able to confer additional years of life on a significant proportion of the elderly by limiting the effects of some age-related diseases? What would the implications be for the web of social and economic relationships on which societies are based?

As noted, a significant trend toward population aging began in the twentieth century and is likely to accelerate in the twenty-first. Globally, the population of older persons is already growing more rapidly than any other age group. This is particularly the case in advanced industrialized societies, where increased life expectancy is accompanied by decreased fertility rates, which in some countries are now below population replacement levels. If these trends continue, the populations of these European countries will become both older and smaller. Even without the introduction of new geriatric-related technologies, demographers estimate that in 2050 the median age in several developed societies will be far older than in any other period in history. They project that the figures will be 58 years of age in Italy, 56 in Japan, and 54 in Germany. The United States, with a higher fertility rate and greater immigration, will be in a better situation, with a median age of 40 (Fukuyama, 2002, p. 61). The introduction of new technologies to extend the life span or to let more people live longer within the normal life span would, of course, raise the median age still further. As a result, increasing proportions of the population would not only be older, they would be the *oldest old*, those 80 and over. The very elderly, who currently have no clear social role, would then become a major social group.

There are likely to be serious economic problems because an aging society will not be economically viable. As the population ages, the relative proportion that is economically active and productive is reduced. Longer years of life also decrease the relative period in which persons are contributing economically during their lifetimes and increases the period of dependency. The potential support ratio (the number of persons aged 15–64 years per one person aged 65 or older) is already projected to fall globally from the 1950 level of 12 economically active people supporting each older person to 4 working-age persons for each older person by the mid-twenty-first century (United Nations Department of Economic and Social Affairs, Population Division, 2002, p. xxix). The figures are far more dramatic for many countries in the North, where the support ratio will be far lower. It is possible to anticipate situations in the not too distant future where there will be only one or two working persons for each retired person in these countries, which is certainly insufficient to support retirement systems. These demographic trends will also have significant implications for economic savings, investment, growth, and sustainable consumption patterns.

Of course, people who are living longer could postpone retirement. However, countries with high per capita incomes tend to have lower participation rates of older workers (United Nations Department of Economic and Social Affairs, Population Division, 2002, p. xxxi). Moreover, a delay in retirement would introduce other problems. Workers and professionals in several countries already face significant bottlenecks in advancement. Having people remain in the labor force until they are 75 or 80 years of age or even older would aggravate these problems. And having older workers in senior management positions for ever longer periods of time would likely have implications for the introduction of innovations.

In addition, the aging of society will place serious strains on the health sector and likely undermine the viability of the Medicare program in this country. The health of older persons typically deteriorates with increasing age. An aging population will increase demands on the health sector, particularly for the management of chronic health conditions. There will be increasing demand for various forms of long-term care. Even if hormone therapy and stem cell research become viable options, they will be very expensive and likely selective in their applications. Moreover, they are less likely to be effective in dealing with mental health declines and the incidence of dementia. There are already 4 million Americans suffering from Alzheimer's disease, which leads to memory loss and eventually dementia, with these figures projected to rise to 15 million by 2030 (Dewar, 2002). Since the incidence of Alzheimer's disease rises proportionately with age, prolonging life would significantly increase the number of persons suffering from this terrible affliction. Extending life expectancies would therefore likely mean that sizable numbers of people would be living well into senility, when they would require supervised or institutionalized living arrangements.

The challenges of an aging population are already looming for a few countries, including our own. Pressures are mounting on the health-care system, Social Security, and private pension plans. Many developed countries are already having serious problems meeting the financial, health, and housing needs of older people. Traditional support systems for the elderly are also deteriorating in many areas (Population Reference Bureau, 1999, p. 4). It is therefore questionable whether societies will be able to sustain their already aging populations, let alone increasing numbers of the aged, many of whom may live well beyond current life expectancies.

Clearly, a major age reconfiguration of society would have significant social and political consequences. Older retired persons will have different political interests than those who are still in the work force. Interest groups representing older persons, like AARP (formerly the American Association for Retired Persons), already wield considerable political power. As society ages, the political clout of these groups will continue to increase. Class, ideological, and interest politics may therefore be displaced or cross-cut by conflicts between age cohorts.

Moreover, these patterns will have global implications. Successful technologies will be far more readily available within affluent industrialized countries. Current fertility trends have already produced a situation in which there is a considerable age differential between an aging North and a youthful South. Dramatically falling birth rates in affluent countries, compared with lower reductions in poor countries, have also resulted in significant differences in their respective rates of population growth. Further increases in life expectancy in the developed part of the globe without a comparable change in poor countries would reinforce these trends. This would create a situation in which a tier of aging, affluent Northern nations are considerably outnumbered by the younger, poorer, and more populous countries of the South. Such a North–South divide would inevitably increase pressures for mass immigration. The Northern countries would probably agree to accept increasing numbers of guest workers, but given the anti-immigration backlash already noticeable in European politics, they may be reluctant to integrate these workers and grant them full citizenship. While it is difficult to predict what the nature of domestic or international politics would be in such a situation, it does not seem like a scenario likely to result in stability, peace, and equitable relationships.

Intragenerational Equity

Intragenerational equity refers to principles of justice to determine how societal resources should be allocated to different age groups living at the same time. *Intergenerational equity*, in contrast, refers to the relationship between current living and future generations. To date, the topic of intragenerational equity has not received much attention from philosophers and social thinkers. Norman Daniels' book *Am I My Parents' Keeper?: An Essay on Justice between the Young and the Old* (1988) stands out in the skimpy literature on this subject. But in an aging society, whether based on current trends or accelerated by new technologies to extend life, this will be a key issue. An aging of society will accelerate resource transfers from younger to older persons, with significant implications for intragenerational relationships. It is even possible that the implicit social covenant of interlocking social roles and mutual support could break down under the strain.

We are already seeing the emergence of problems. Because many federal budget items, like defense and repayment of the national debt, are basically fixed, greater expenditures on programs for elderly persons can only come at the expense of categories that are considered to be discretionary expenditures. Daniels foresaw that this would result in increasing competition among various age groups, particularly between the old and children. When Daniels wrote his book, he estimated that federal per capita expenditures for programs devoted to children like education, food stamps, child nutrition, Aid to Dependent Children (welfare), and health amounted to about one-sixth of the resources devoted to Social Security and Medicare for the elderly (1988, pp. 4–5). This differential reduces investment in the young, who, of course, constitute the future hope of society. This trend is likely to become even more pronounced in the years ahead as the government acts to protect the long-term solvency of the Social Security and Medicare systems. In such a situation, younger people may question whether their futures should be mortgaged to care for those who are not making productive contributions to society.

The situation has implications for family relationships as well as patterns of public expenditures. Despite rising public expenditures on long-term care, the majority of ill and partially disabled elderly are still cared for by other family members. As the population ages, there will be increasing numbers of noninstitutionalized elderly requiring home care. Daniels anticipated that adult children will increasingly have to spend resources saved for their own retirement, or for their children's or grandchildren's education on the care of their own parents. With age expectancies rising, it is conceivable that adults in their 70s and 80s might still have the burden of caring for their parents. Obviously this would place a strain on families and could intensify conflict among family members (Daniels, 1988, p. 7).

Daniels' goal in writing was to frame a principle of distributive justice to resolve disputes about how income, support, health care, and other societal resources should be allocated to different age groups in society. He proposed an approach he termed the Prudential Lifespan Account as the basis for designing institutions that distribute fair shares of basic social goods over the life span. The Prudential Lifespan Account is based on the premise that fully informed persons could determine a standard of welfare or budgeting of resources and health care for each person that would be just over a lifetime and then allocate the benefits to different stages of life. Viewed in this way, Daniels argued that treating the young and old differently does not necessarily mean violating principles of equality. He suggested that transfers from the young to the old might be conceptualized as transfers within lives, that is, subsidies from the young for the old considered a type of savings (1988, chap. 3).

Does the Prudential Lifespan Account offer a viable approach? I think not. As Daniels acknowledges, the Prudential Lifespan Account is an ideal or general-compliance moral theory (1988, p. 139). It is predicated on a kind of social covenant based on prudential reasoning among generations that cannot be formulated in a meaningful way. Also, to work, even in principle, it would require relative stability in the size of various age cohorts, and the real societal situation is problematic precisely because of the ballooning of the older age groups. In the real world, there are likely to be significant intercohort inequalities in prospects for support in old age. Thus, younger age cohorts will be asked to make sacrifices without the expectation that they can count on similar levels of support when they reach a comparable age. It is also probably unrealistic to assume that older cohorts will willingly ration their consumption of resources so as to live within the boundaries of the principles of fairness. Obviously, then, there is a great need for more thinking about this topic.

Global Sustainability

The past 30 years have been marked by increasing awareness of and heightened concern for the impact of human societies on our planet. There has been growing understanding that the Earth's natural systems, and human population are inherently interconnected. Accelerating population growth—from 2 billion people at the beginning of the twentieth century to 6 billion at the end—and increases in consumption have taken a major toll on the Earth's resources and ecological systems. The impact of population growth on the environment, on development, and on the quality of life is compounded by the fact that the greatest increase is taking place in poor countries that are less able to provide services and infrastructure for growing numbers of persons. The average number of children per couple has been slowly falling in less developed countries, but the total population is growing faster than ever because of the large number of young people entering their childbearing years. At least another 1 billion persons are likely to be added by 2020.

In assessing human pressure on the environment, it is important to note that high rates of natural resource consumption and pollution, primarily in affluent countries, have at least as much impact as demographic pressures. Members of consumer-oriented societies are responsible for a disproportionate share of the global environmental challenges now facing humanity. Each year the richest 20% to 25% of the world's population consumes approximately 75% to 80% of all resources and produces most of the planet's pollution and waste. It is estimated that each child born today in a Northern country is likely to consume and pollute 20 to 30 times as much as a child born in the South. Americans rank near the top in most categories of resource use and waste even when compared to other European countries and Japan (World Wildlife Fund, 1994, p. 7).

In looking at the implications of these trends, some analysts believe that the cumulative impact of human activity is pushing against the limit of the Earth's life-supporting or carrying capacity, perhaps even exceeding it (Chapman et al., 2000). Many scientists fear that humanity is threatening not only the web of life on Earth but also its own survival. According to these assessments, "We are exceeding the planet's 'metabolic' capacity to absorb, replenish, and restore" (McMichael, 1993, p. 1). As one theologian starkly comments, "If current trends continue, we will not. And that is qualitatively and epochally new" (Maguire, 1993, p. 13).

Obviously, prolonging human life would further accelerate these problems, especially if it involved significant numbers of people. With people living longer, the total size of the population would continue to increase. More significantly, the very people most likely to benefit from increases in longevity—affluent members of developed countries—already have disproportionately high consumption rates and would impose the greatest toll on the environment. Moreover, people in affluent societies, Americans in particular, have been very reluctant to deal meaningfully with the impact of their consumption patterns on the environment.

The above analysis clearly underscores that increasing the human life span is not sustainable for the planet. It would also likely undermine efforts to attain more equitable resource use patterns within and between societies. Enabling a minority of wealthy individuals to secure long life for themselves at the expense of further endangering the environment and depriving the poor of resources needed for development would therefore be a fundamental violation of justice norms.

Conclusion

As noted, it is difficult to make decisions about future technologies, especially ones that may offer some benefits, even if only to a small minority. The approach recommended here is to inquire whether the development of the technology offers the prospect of a more or less just future society or world. The analysis in this chapter underscores that even if efforts to develop interventions to increase average life expectancies or lengthen the human life span can overcome significant scientific hurdles, they would impose many negative societal and environmental consequences. In an essay dealing with the prospects of immortality, Leon Kass suggests that a result of the retardation of aging would be that many individuals would be worse off throughout most of their lives (2002, p. 323). He is considering the issue from the perspective of an individual's existential quality of life. Viewing the issue from a societal and justice perspective, I would agree with his assessment. Increasing numbers of persons living many years beyond the current life expectancy in an already aging society would pose economic, health, and care burdens that societies would be hard pressed to sustain. The required resource transfers would have a profound impact on intra- and intergenerational equity. Developing life span–extending technologies would be even more problematic. Thus, from a justice perspective, it seems preferable not to go forward with the development and application of interventions for this purpose.

References

AAAS Committee on Scientific Freedom and Responsibility. (1975). *Scientific Freedom and Responsibility.* Washington, DC: AAAS Committee on Scientific Freedom and Responsibility.

Beauchamp, T.L. and J.F. Childress. (1994). *Principles of Biomedical Ethics,* 4th ed. New York: Oxford University Press.

Chapman, A.R. (1999). *Unprecedented Choices: Religious Ethics at the Frontiers of Genetic Science.* Minneapolis: Fortress Press.

Chapman, A.R. and Frankel M.S., (Eds.). (2003). *Designing our Descendants: The Potential and Limitations of Inheritable Genetic Modifications.* Baltimore: Johns Hopkins University Press.

Chapman, A.R., Petersen, R.L., and Smith-Moran, B. (Eds.). (2000). *Consumption, Population, and Sustainability: Perspectives from Science and Religion.* Washington, DC: Island Press.

Connolly, C. (2002, May 22). Study: Uninsured don't get needed health care: Delayed diagnoses, premature deaths result. *The Washington Post,* sec. A, p. 3.

Daniels, N. (1988). *Am I My Parents' Keeper?: An Essay on Justice between the Young and the Old.* New York: Oxford University Press.

Dewar, H. (2002, April 1). Alzheimer's patients get Medicare break. *The Washington Post,* sec. A, p. 3.

Ferbeyre, G. and Lowe, S.W. (2002). The price of tumour suppression? *Nature,* 415(6867), 26–27.

Fletcher, J.C. and Anderson, W.F. (1992). Germ-line gene therapy: A new stage of debate. *Law Med Health Care,* 20(1–2), 26–39.

Frankel, M.S. and Chapman, A.R. (2000). *Human Inheritable Genetic Modifications: Assessing Scientific, Ethical, Religious, and Policy Issues.* Washington, DC: American Association for the Advancement of Science.

Freudenheim, M. (2002, February 9). Coalition forms to reverse trend of fast-rising ranks of uninsured Americans. *The New York Times,* sec. A, p. 18.

Fukuyama, F. (2002). *Our Posthuman Future: Consequences of the Biotechnology Revolution.* New York: Farrar, Straus & Giroux.

Guy, H.V. (2000). Uninsured minorities: Who goes without and why? Available at http://accounting.smartpros.com/x19733.xml

Hefner, P. (1993). *The Human Factor: Evolution, Culture, and Religion.* Minneapolis: Fortress Press.

Kaiser, J. (2001). Hints of a "master gene" for extreme old age. *Science,* 293, 1570–1571.

Kass, L.R. (2002). Why not immortality? In: Kirstol, W. and Cohen, E., eds. *The Future is Now.* Lanham, MD: Rowman & Littlefield, pp. 321–332.

Lebacqz, K. (1987). *Justice in an Unjust World: Foundations for a Christian Approach to Justice.* Minneapolis: Augsburg.

Maguire, D.C. (1993). *The Moral Core of Judaism and Christianity: Reclaiming the Revolution.* Minneapolis: Fortress Press.

McMichael, A.J. (1993). *Planetary Overload and Human Health: Global Environmental Change and the Health and Survival of the Human Species.* Cambridge and New York: Cambridge University Press.

Olshansky, S.J., Hayflick, L., and Carnes, B.A. (2002). No truth to the fountain of youth. *Scientific American,* 286(6), 92–95.

Peters, T. (1997). *Playing God?: Genetic Determinism and Human Freedom.* New York and London: Routledge.

Population Reference Bureau. (1999). *World Population: More Than Just Numbers.* Washington, DC: Population Reference Bureau.

Stolberg, S.G. (2002, March 21). Race gap seen in health care of equally insured patients. *The New York Times,* sec. A, pp. 1, 30.

United Nations Department of Economic and Social Affairs, Population Division. (2002). *Executive Summary: World Population Ageing, 1950–2050.* New York: United Nations.

Wheeler, S.E. (1996). *Stewards of Life: Bioethics and Pastoral Care.* Nashville: Abingdon Press.

World Health Organization. (2002). *Scaling Up the Response to Infectious Diseases: A Way out of Poverty.* Geneva: World Health Organization.

World Wildlife Fund. (1994). *World Wildlife Fund, Population and the Environment.* Gland, Switzerland: World Wildlife Fund.

17

The Prolonged Old, the Long-Lived Society, and the Politics of Age

Robert H. Binstock

For several decades gerontologists have been writing about the *aging society* (e.g., Neugarten, 1978/1996; Pifer and Bronte, 1986), well aware from demographic analyses that the numbers and proportions of older persons in industrialized societies would swell substantially in the early decades of the twenty-first century. In the United States, for example, it has long been clear that the aging of the baby boomers—an exceptionally large birth cohort of 76 million persons born between 1946 and 1964—would result in one in five Americans being aged 65 and older by the year 2030 (Hobbs, 1996).

The societal implications of the phenomenon of population aging have been the subject of much speculation by scholars from a variety of disciplines and professions, as well as other observers of public affairs. Many of them have come to ominous conclusions. In a book called *Gray Dawn*, for instance, Wall Street banker and former Secretary of Commerce Peter Peterson (1999) has sounded the alarm:

> [G]lobal aging . . . threatens to bankrupt the great powers. As the populations of the world's leading economies age and

362

shrink, we will face unprecedented political, economic, and moral challenges. But we are woefully unprepared.

(p. iii)

Similarly, biomedical ethicist Daniel Callahan (1987) has described the growing population of older Americans as a "social threat" and "a demographic, economic, and medical avalanche" that could do "great harm" (p. 23). One of his main concerns is that "programs benefiting the aged [are] one of the great fiscal black holes" (p. 216) imposing an enormous and perhaps unsustainable economic burden. Consequently, in his book *Setting Limits: Medical Goals in an Aging Society*, Callahan (1987) draws on both his philosophical and social analyses to urge that life-extending health care be categorically denied in the United States to anyone who has achieved an age of about 80 (which he posits as a proxy for the end of a natural life span).

If these are the types of concerns and proposals engendered by the aging of the baby boomers, a specific birth cohort population bulge that will eventually die off, more drastic implications of these and other issue areas may attend a society in which average life expectancy and the maximum human life span are radically increased. As noted in the Introduction and in Chapter 1 of this book, the pursuit of prolongevity—effective anti-aging interventions to achieve such radical increases—has become part of a mainstream research agenda of the National Institutes of Health (NIH).

The Prolonged Old and the Long-Lived Society

The achievement of prolongevity through any of several paradigms that biogerontologists are pursuing through their research—compressed morbidity, decelerated aging, or arrested aging (see the Introduction)—could add tens of millions of healthy, active, and exceptionally long-lived persons to the future populations of the United States and other nations in which effective anti-aging interventions would be available. Just how many additional persons would depend, of course, on such factors as whether the interventions were universally or selectively accessible and the increases achieved in life expectancy and maximum life span. A leading proponent of achieving decelerated aging through the development of pills that mimic the biochemical effects of a calorie-restricted diet states that "one can, with some confidence expect that an effective antiaging intervention might increase the mean and maximal human life span by about 40 percent" (Miller, 2002, p. 164). His prolongevity estimates are far from the most radical that have been published by biogerontologists (e.g., de Grey, 2000).

Although the achievement of prolongevity may seem improbable at present, many biomedical innovations that once seemed impossible have come to fruition (Bonnicksen, 2002; Henig, 2002). If not during the lifetimes of baby boomers, then perhaps during those of their children, we may see a new large stratum of elderly people added to the older age groups that are currently described by a trio of conventional labels: the *young old*, aged 65–74; the *old old*, aged 75–84; and the *oldest old*, aged 85 and older (Binstock, 1996). Effective anti-aging measures may produce the *prolonged old* as a descriptive term for persons aged 95 and older who may heavily populate what could fairly be called the *long-lived society*.

A long-lived society populated by numerous prolonged old persons would certainly witness considerable changes in virtually every social institution and pattern of societal norms. The nature and implications of such changes have begun to be discussed as biological research on the fundamental mechanisms of aging has made progress. Among biogerontologists, Leonard Hayflick, in his book *How and Why We Age* (1994), briefly expressed his concern that radical prolongevity could cause extreme worldwide overpopulation accompanied by disastrous ecological and human consequences. Some of the anthropological, economic, ethical, kinship, legal, psychological, sociological, and policy implications of major increases in life expectancy and life span have been explored in two compendia: *The Impact of Increased Life Expectancy: Beyond the Gray Horizon* (Seltzer, 1995) and *Life Span Extension: Consequences and Open Questions* (Ludwig, 1990). Bioethicist Chris Hackler (2001–2002) has posited a doubling of the human life span and has devoted a paragraph or two to considering what things might be like in each of a number of sectors—marriage, the family, work, careers, the penal system, and the consequences of overpopulation. And a futurist and a journalist have coauthored a book (Cetron and Davies, 1998) in which they briefly speculate on the characteristics of a *postmortal* world by applying the assumptions of substantially expanded life expectancy to a standard package of extrapolated trends within a number of economic and social arenas.

One of the key influences on the nature of these and other arenas will be whether or not government intervenes in them, the substance of such interventions, and their consequences. For example, in the long-lived society, would there be anything resembling the present Old-Age Welfare State in the United States, on which the federal government presently spends over one-third of its annual budget (Binstock, 2002)? Would it be possible for the United States or any other nation to maintain old-age entitlements for groups that include the prolonged old, who could greatly swell the ranks of those already eligible for old-age benefit programs? The absence of public income transfers to elderly people would have strong effects on the nature of family life, the labor market, access to health care, and myriad other behavioral patterns and social arrangements.

In his interesting exploration of likely government policies toward older people in a society with a mean life expectancy of 100 years, Robert Hudson (1995) recognized the complexity of any such predictions because of the many contextual variables that could have an impact. For purposes of a manageable discussion, he selected only three such variables—economic growth, biomedical advances, and population growth. By constructing the various possible combinations of positive and negative trends among these variables, he described eight different scenarios for the future. A major dimension that Hudson did not address, however, is the impact of politics on what government does—the political behavior of the electorate, organized interest groups and social movements, and governmental and nongovernmental political elites.

Although innumerable factors shape the nature of politics in any society and in every era, one of the major features of politics in the long-lived society, by definition, will be a very large increase in the number and proportion of citizens who are elderly. The prolonged old may be part of the voting electorate, could possibly be harnessed as participants in old-age-based mass membership political organizations and social movements, or might establish political parties of their own. In short, the politics of age may play a critical role in shaping government policy and, thereby, individual lives and social institutions.

The remainder of this chapter explores what the politics of age might be like if life expectancy and/or life span become radically increased. First, it reviews what is already known about the politics of old age. Then, building on this background, it speculatively explores what the politics of aging might be like in a society that includes the prolonged old. It concludes by briefly addressing the implications of this exploration for how anticipatory actions might shape the politics of age in a long-lived society.

Examining the Conventional Senior Power Model

For the past several decades a *senior power* model of the politics of age has been generally subscribed to by journalists, politicians, political advisors, political observers, and some academicians (Preston, 1984; Cook et al., 1994; Peterson and Somit, 1994; Binstock, 1995). This model is widely used to explain the contemporary politics of aging and to predict the future of politics in an aging society. In principle, it could be used to forecast the politics of age in the long-lived society.

The senior power model builds on the fact that older people constitute a numerically significant portion of the electorate, and then assumes that their political behavior is guided by their self-interests and that most of them perceive their interests to be the same. Applying these assumptions, one expects older people to be homogeneous in political attitudes and voting behavior and consequently, through sheer numbers, to be a powerful, perhaps dominating, electoral force. Moreover, the model also assumes that interest groups representing older people are very influential forces that can motivate and swing the votes of older persons and thereby intimidate politicians. Based on all these assumptions, one can believe that older voters and old-age interest groups function effectively as a powerful *gray lobby* (Pratt, 1976), able to exert substantial control over policies on aging and, indirectly, other allocational decisions. (For fuller discussions of the senior power model see Pratt, 1993, 1997; Binstock, 1997a; Rix, 1999; Street, 1999).

When these assumptions have been used (explicitly and implicitly) to predict the nature of politics in societies that will have sharply increased numbers and proportions of older people, the typical result has been a vision of intergenerational political conflict. For example, economist Lester Thurow's application of the senior power model to the phenomenon of population aging in the early decades of the twenty-first century produces this apocalyptic scenario:

[N]o one knows how the growth of entitlements can be held in check in democratic societies. . . . Will democratic governments be able to cut benefits when the elderly are approaching a voting majority? Universal suffrage . . . is going to meet the ultimate test in the elderly. If democratic governments cannot cut benefits that go to a majority of their voters, then they have no long-term future. . . . In the years ahead, class warfare is apt to be redefined as the young against the old, rather than the poor against the rich.

(Thurow, 1996, p. 47)

One could also apply the same assumptions to a long-lived society populated by the prolonged old, even envisioning a more extreme outcome than Thurow's picture of class warfare between the young and the old—perhaps a gerontocracy, a country ruled by the aged. Indeed, as early as 1974, the senior power model was used at a meeting of the American Association for the Advancement of Science to address seriously the issue of whether the United States would become a gerontocracy beginning in the 1990s (Binstock, 1974), a period when the anticipated size of the elderly population was relatively small compared to what it will be in 2030 (Hobbs, 1996) or in a long-lived society.

However, some of the assumptions in the senior power model are flawed, both logically and empirically. Consequently, it is advisable to briefly review the complexities of what is actually known about the politics of age (as opposed to assumptions in the model) before speculating about the possible impacts of a prolonged old population on the nature of politics.

Older People and Voting Participation

One respect in which the senior power model is sound is in its assertion that older people constitute a numerically important component of the electorate. Studies of voting participation over several decades have shown that voter turnout is lowest among young adults, increases rapidly up to ages 35–45, and then continues to increase (more slowly) during the life course, declining only slightly after the age of 70 or 80 in the United States, and at somewhat younger ages in Sweden and Germany (Glenn and Grimes, 1968; Hout and Knoke,

1975; Wolfinger and Rosenstone, 1980; Delli Carpini, 1986; Myers and Agree, 1993; Miller and Shanks, 1996). Consequently, the percentage of the total vote cast by older people in elections is greater than their proportion of the voting-age population. In the 2000 U.S. presidential election, for example, people aged 65 and older were 17% of the voting-age population but cast 20% of the vote (Jamieson et al., 2002).

Why do older people turn out to vote at higher rates than middle-aged and younger people? Although the connection between age and voting participation has been investigated a great deal, overall the reasons for this relationship remain a source of controversy. Various explanations for age group differences in turnout have helped to define the issues, but they have not resolved them.

Miller and Shanks (Miller, 1992; Miller and Shanks, 1996) are among those who hypothesize that the relatively high voting rate of older Americans during the past several decades can be attributed to birth cohort replacement. They focus on the contrasting participation rates of the New Deal cohort and subsequent cohorts whose political attitudes and behavior have been shaped by the effects of historical periods and specific political events that they have lived through (e.g., the Vietnam War and Watergate) at different ages in the life course. Supporting this view is the fact that during these decades the rates of age-group participation have been dynamic, not static, as the various cohorts have entered different stages of the life cycle. From the 1972 presidential election through the 1996 election, the participation rate of persons aged 65 and older increased by 6.5%, while the rates for all other age groups declined—by 9% in the 45–64 category, 21.5% in the 25–44 category, and 34.7% in the 18–24 category (Binstock, 2000).

But other analyses (e.g., Teixera, 1992; Rosenstone and Hansen, 1993) suggest that the contribution of cohort replacement to voting turnout rates may be overestimated. In fact, a study by Myers and Agree (1993) found age-group differences in voting turnout in Sweden and Germany over four decades to be similar to those in the United States, despite the fact that cohorts in these three nations experienced different political events distinctive to their respective countries. This suggests that life course effects may be more important than cohort replacement in determining age-group voting participation rates.

One factor contributing to the higher voting rate of older persons is age-group differences in voting registration, an essential precursor to voting. A two-stage study of voter registration and turnout in U.S. national elections (Timpone, 1998) found that increased age (from age 18 to 88) is monotonically related to being registered and that another aging-related factor, length of residence in one's home, also has a substantial influence.

Another contributing factor is that persons who are comparatively well informed about politics and public affairs are more likely to register and vote (Palfrey and Poole, 1987; Flanigan and Zingale, 1998); older people are more likely than younger people to pay attention to the news (McManus, 1996), are more generally knowledgeable about politics (Luskin, 1987; Delli Carpini and Keeter, 1993), and report having the highest level of interest in political campaigns and public affairs generally (Jennings and Markus, 1988).

Still another contributing factor is the well-established connection between the strength of political party identification and higher rates of voting (see, e.g., Caldeira et al., 1985; Rosentone and Hansen, 1993; Flanigan and Zingale, 1998). Older people identify with the major political parties more strongly than do younger persons (McManus, 1996). A long-standing hypothesis is that the longer individuals identify with a party, the stronger their partisanship is (Converse, 1976).

How Do Older People Vote?

Although older people vote at a high rate, they do *not* vote cohesively (even though the senior power model suggests that they do). Older people are as diverse in their voting decisions as any other age group; their votes divide along the same partisan, economic, social, gender, racial, ethnic, and other lines as those of the electorate at large. Accordingly, the various cohorts of older Americans during the past 50 years, for example, have tended to distribute their votes among presidential candidates in roughly the same proportions as other age groups do; exit polls show sharp divisions within each age group and very small differences between age groups (Campbell and Strate, 1981; Connelly, 2000). As Street (1999, p. 117) asserts, "[T]here is no credible evidence in the United States that age-based voting blocs are a feature of national election landscapes." The empirical evidence from European nations is similar. Naegele and Walker (1999, p. 202), summarizing the situation there, conclude that "empirically numerous pieces of evidence . . . [show that old age] . . . is no authoritative means of predicting political opinions and behavior."

The senior power model also mistakenly assumes that old-age policy issues play a major role in influencing the electoral choices of older voters because the elderly have a self-interested stake in government policies that provide old-age benefits. This assumption has its roots in neoclassical economics and statistical decision theory, which predict that each voter's decision among candidates is rationally calculated on the basis of complete and accurate information to optimize her or his self-interest. But there are intellectual flaws in this model of electoral behavior (e.g., Downs, 1957; Simon, 1985; Flanigan and Zingale, 1998) and substantial empirical evidence that policy issues have little impact on voters of all ages (e.g., Gelman and King, 1992; Miller and Shanks, 1996; Abramson et al., 1999). Moreover, the self-interests of older people in relation to old-age policy issues and the intensity of their interests may vary substantially. Consider, for example, the relative importance of Social Security as a source of income for U.S. aged persons who are in the lowest and highest income quintiles. Social Security provides about 80% of the income for those in the lowest two quintiles but only about 18% for those in the highest (Federal Interagency Forum on Aging-Related Statistics, 2000). Some older persons have much more at stake than others do in policy proposals that would reduce, maintain, or enhance Social Security benefit payments.

There is no evidence from exit polls that old-age policy issues critically influence older persons' votes for candidates, and there are many reasons to expect that they would not be so influenced. Old age is only one of many personal characteristics of aged people, and only one with which they may identify themselves and their self-interests. Even if some older voters identify themselves primarily in terms of their age status, this does not mean that their self-interests in old-age policies are the most important factors in their electoral decisions. Other policy issues, strong and long-standing partisan attachments, underlying political attitudes, and many other electoral stimuli in an electoral campaign can be of equal or greater importance. Even in local referenda, when issues (rather than candidates) are presented on the ballot, there is little evidence that older people are more likely than other voters to oppose taxes for services that do not directly benefit them (Chomitz, 1987; Button and Rosenbaum, 1989). Overall, the weight of the evidence indicates that older people's electoral choices have rarely, if ever, been based on age-group interests.

Organized Political Action

An element of the senior power model that has some empirical validity is the assumption that old-age-based interest groups (Van Tassel and Meyer, 1992; Morris, 1996; Binstock, 1997b; Price, 1997; Day, 1998), casting themselves as representatives of a large constituency of older voters, have some forms of power. Although they have not demonstrated a capacity to swing the votes of older persons, they do play a role in the policy process. In the classic pattern of American interest group politics (Lowi, 1969), public officials find it both useful and incumbent upon them to invite an organization such as AARP (formerly the American Association of Retired Persons), which has over 30 million members, to participate in policy activities. In this way, public officials are provided with a ready means of being in touch symbolically with tens of millions of older persons, thereby legitimizing subsequent policy actions and inactions. A brief meeting with the leaders of some of the more than 40 old-age organizations (which are politically diverse) can enable an official to claim that he or she has obtained the represented views of a mass constituency.

The symbolic legitimacy that old-age organizations have for participating in interest group politics gives them several types of power. First, they have easy informal access to public officials: members of Congress and their staffs; career bureaucrats; appointed officials; and occasionally the White House. Second, their legitimacy enables them to obtain public platforms in the national media, congressional hearings, and national conferences and commissions dealing with old age, health, and a variety of subjects relevant to policies affecting aging. Third, old-age interest groups can mobilize their members in large numbers to contact policymakers and register displeasure when changes are being contemplated in old-age programs.

Perhaps the most important form of power available to the old-age interest groups might be termed the *electoral bluff*. Although these organizations have not demonstrated a capacity to swing a decisive bloc of older voters, the perception of being powerful is in itself a source of political influence (Banfield, 1961). Incumbent members of Congress are hardly inclined to risk upsetting the existing distribution of votes that puts them and keeps them in office. Few politicians, of course, want to call the bluff of the aged or any other latent mass constituency if it is possible to avoid doing so. Hence, when congressional offices are flooded with letters, faxes, e-mail messages, and phone calls expressing the (not necessarily representative) views of older persons, members of Congress take heed.

Nonetheless, these forms of power have been quite limited in their impact. The old-age interest groups have had little to do with the enactment and amendment of major old-age policies such as Social Security and Medicare. Rather, such actions have been largely attributable to the initiatives of public officials in the White House, Congress, and the bureaucracy who were focused on their own agendas for social and economic policy (e.g., on Social Security, see Derthick, 1979; Light, 1985; on Medicare, see Cohen, 1985; Iglehart, 1989; Ball, 1995; cf. Pratt, 1976, Pratt, 1993). Nor have the old-age organizations been able to prevent significant policy reforms that have been perceived to be adverse to the interests of an artificially homogenized constituency of "the elderly" (see Binstock, 1994; Day, 1998). Indeed, the political legitimacy of old-age interest groups began eroding in the mid-1980s in the United States and has been decreasing since (Binstock, 1997b; Day, 1998; Street, 1999).

The Politics of Age in the Long-Lived Society

As this review of the politics of aging indicates, the accuracy of the senior power model has been mixed in its depiction of the political behavior of older persons to date. In harmony with the model, older people have been a disproportionately sizable component of the electorate because they vote at higher rates than the rest of the voting-age population. On the other hand, the political attitudes and attachments of older persons are diverse, and their ballots have not been cast in a cohesive fashion. Old-age-based interest groups do have some limited power, but they have shown no capacity to influence the votes of older people and have had virtually no impact on major old-age policy decisions.

These major elements of what is known about the politics of aging in the twentieth century and early in this century could very well undergo substantial change in the years and decades immediately ahead as the baby boom cohort becomes old and if the prolonged old are added as a component to the population. But at least these elements can serve as frameworks for speculating about the nature of politics in the long-lived society.

From the present vantage point, of course, there are too many imponderables involved to posit how many prolonged old persons may inhabit a long-lived society and what proportion of the population they might constitute. However, the exact quantities are not as important as the magnitude of the increases involved and some of the substantive developments that might accompany them. Hence, the aging of the baby boom cohort can serve as a reasonable proxy for considering some aspects of the political consequences of implementing prolongevity interventions. For one thing, it involves a massive increase in the number of older Americans, a doubling of the number of older people, in a space of just 30 years (Hobbs, 1996). In addition, it has already generated some thoughts regarding what may happen or ought to happen when there is a large increase in the number and proportion of older persons.

A Voting Majority or New Electoral Rules?

The U.S. Bureau of the Census (1998) projects that the percentage of voting-age citizens aged 65 and older will increase from 17% in 2000 to 27% in 2035, when all members of the baby boom cohort will have reached the age category of 65 years and older. An even higher proportion of those who actually vote will be in the old-age range because, as indicated above, older people vote at a higher rate than other age groups. Two models have been constructed to extrapolate the percentage of votes that will be cast by aged baby boomers. One forecasts that the proportion of votes cast by persons aged 65 and older will be as high as one-third of all votes in the mid-2030s, and the other projects that the votes of older people will constitute 41% of the total in 2044 (Binstock, 2000). Add in many millions of prolonged old persons and the proportions would be greater, approaching or reaching the "voting majority" comprising older persons that Thurow envisions.

But extrapolation, of course, is the poorest mode of prediction (Bell, 1964). Many factors can affect the future voting participation rates of age groups substantially—and probably will (Williamson, 1998; Binstock, 2000).

One of the most dramatic possibilities is that the rules of voting might be changed in response to fears that the votes of older people will dominate politics and policy decisions. Lest this notion seem entirely fanciful, it should be noted that some radical proposals have already been put forth to change electoral provisions in order to contain the political influence of older people. Over three decades ago, for instance, Douglas Stewart (1970), a humanist, proposed that all Americans be disfranchised at retirement or age 70, whichever is earlier, because he blamed older people for the election of conservative politicians. In 1981, a former Assistant Secretary of Health and Human Services, fearing that the old-age lobby would win a pitched battle against the children's lobby in a competition for shrinking social welfare resources, proposed that parents with children under the voting age of 18 be enfranchised with an extra vote for each of their dependent children (Carballo, 1981). Apparently, this phenomenon of suggesting changes in electoral rule is not confined to the United States. In 1999, Peter Peterson (1999, p. 210) reported that a senior minister in Singapore's government proposed that "each taxpaying worker be given two votes" to balance the political power of retirees.

To be sure, most modifications of electoral rules in modern democracies have been for the purposes of expanding the principle of one person/one vote. Until the Fourteenth Amendment to the U.S. Constitution was passed, for instance, an African American was weighted as three-fifths of a person for purposes of apportioning the number of congressmen that a state would have in the U.S. House of Representatives. Women were not allowed to vote until the Nineteenth Amendment was ratified in 1920. And it was not until 1971 that the Twenty-Sixth Amendment guaranteed the right of suffrage to 18-year-olds throughout the nation, even though they had long been subject to military conscription (Woll and Binstock, 1991).

Yet, the senior power model has already generated suggestions for limiting the impact of voting by older people even though the baby boomers have still not begun entering the ranks of old age. If effective anti-aging measures begin to be developed and implemented, measures to curb or offset the voting participation of the prolonged old might readily gain popularity and be instituted preemptively.

Would Age-Group Consciousness Trump Other Social Identities?

Although all age groups have been heterogeneous in their political attachments and behavior for as long as modern political scientists have observed them, would this pattern change in the long-lived society? Would age-group identity become more important than socio-economic status, gender, race, ethnicity, and other characteristics in shaping political preferences? The rhetoric and actions of politicians would play an important role in answering these questions.

Despite the fact that older persons are diverse in their voting behavior, contemporary politicians have persistently courted their votes through campaign promises regarding old-age benefit programs and through sympathetic portrayals of their actions in the governing process. Incumbents and challengers in electoral campaigns are eager to capitalize on (and are wary of) what they erroneously perceive to be "a huge, monolithic, senior citizen army of voters" (Peterson and Somit, 1994, p. 178). As indicated above, however, these courtships have not had a demonstrable impact on the votes of older people, while the impact of gender, race, and other identities on voting behavior is very clear (Connelly, 2000).

Perhaps one of the reasons that age has had little if any impact on the distribution of votes is that in the perceptions of most voters there is little to choose between candidates regarding their stances on age-related issues. For example, in the 1996 presidential election campaign both candidates, President Bill Clinton and Senator Robert Dole, labored hard to convey the impression that they had been trying to "save" Medicare, even though their approaches were very different (*New York Times*, 1996a,b). Similarly, in the 2000 campaign, both Vice-President Al Gore and Governor George W. Bush promised to add a prescription drug benefit to Medicare (*New York Times*, 2000; Sack and Dao, 2000).

However, this pattern through which the candidates convey similar stances to the electorate regarding old-age issues might not persist in the long-lived society or even in the aging society of the 2020s or 2030s. The difficult economic challenges of maintaining old-age programs for an aged baby boom cohort have already been depicted by numerous policy analysts (see, e.g., Altman and Schactman, 2002). Adding an additional layer of benefit-eligible prolonged old persons would sharply exacerbate the fiscal burdens involved in maintaining the Old Age Welfare State. Given that there are already a number of skeptics regarding the long-run viability of old-age programs (e.g., Peterson, 1999), one can readily imagine a twenty-first-century election in which two presidential candidates take starkly different positions regarding the future of Social Security and/or Medicare. One candidate might propose sharply curtailing or eliminating these programs, and the other might vow to defend them. Except for the wealthy aged, the identity of old age (i.e., being eligible for old-age benefits) could well become more important than any other and lead to strong support for the candidate who promises to protect the programs. At the same time, younger age groups, who by then may anticipate a crushing burden of taxes to support old-age benefits, might flock to support the candidate who wants to curtail the programs.

Would There Be Class Warfare
Between the Young and the Old?

The possibility that age-group consciousness could become relevant to politics—particularly in the form of a clash between the young and the old—is hardly a new notion. As early as the late 1970s, various writers and organizations attempted to frame a political conflict between age groups. At that time, journalists (e.g., Samuelson, 1978) and academicians (e.g., Hudson, 1978) discovered the "graying of the budget," a tremendous growth in the proportion of federal dollars expended on benefits to aging citizens. Subsequently, an artificially homogenized group, *the aged,* began to be blamed for a variety of societal problems such as the plight of youngsters who had inadequate nutrition, health care, and education and insufficiently supportive family environments (e.g., Preston, 1984). The epithet *greedy geezers* was coined to characterize older people (Fairlie, 1988) and subsequently became a familiar adjective in journalistic accounts of federal budget politics (Salhoz, 1990). A writer in *Fortune* magazine declaimed that "The Tyranny of America's Old" is "one of the most crucial issues facing U.S. society" (Smith, 1992).

In the mid-1980s, a variety of concerns for which the aged had become a scapegoat (Binstock, 1983) were thematically unified as issues of *intergenerational equity*—really, intergenerational inequity—through the efforts of Americans for Generational Equity (AGE). Formed in 1985, and led by several congressman, this organization obtained most of its funding from insurance companies, health-care corporations, banks, and other private sector businesses and organizations that are in competition with Medicare and Social Security (Quadagno, 1989) and therefore would benefit from their curtailment or elimination. Central to AGE's credo was the proposition that older people were locked in an intergenerational conflict with younger age cohorts regarding the distribution of public resources. The organization disseminated this viewpoint effectively from its Washington office through press releases, media interviews, and a quarterly publication, *The Generational Journal*, as well as through conferences with such titles as "Children at Risk: Who Will Support an Aging Society?" Although AGE faded from the scene in the early 1990s, its themes of intergenerational equity and conflict were carried forward prominently by the Concord Coalition, which favored scaling back Social Security benefits (Concord Coalition, 1993).

The theme of a war between the generations was adopted by the media, academics, and a variety of commentators on public affairs as a routine perspective for describing many social policy issues (Cook et al., 1994). It also gained currency in elite sectors of American society. The president of the prestigious American Association of Universities, for instance, asserted: "[T]he shape of the domestic federal budget inescapably pits programs for the retired against every other social purpose dependent on federal funds, in the present and the future" (Rosenzweig, 1990, p. 6). And at the end of the twentieth century, Peter Peterson (1999) warned that population aging in developed countries could "enthrone organized elders as an invincible political titan" and that "'intergenerational war' . . . should not be ruled out anywhere in the developed world" (p. 209).

Although age-group consciousness has not been manifested seriously in voting behavior to date, the growing costs of the Old-Age Welfare State and the continuing reiteration of the message that intergenerational warfare is inevitable undoubtedly increase somewhat the probability of eventual political conflict between age groups as the baby boom cohort ages. The addition of a prolonged old population to the mix would certainly increase that probability sharply. Yet, the alignments in age-group political conflict might be more complex than simply the *class warfare* between young and old which commentators such as Peterson and Thurow envision.

Would Older Age Groups Make Common Cause?

Despite the fact that U.S. old-age-based organizations are politically diverse today, in principle one can imagine that a political party based on the mutual interests of older people might be formed in the long-lived society. In the Netherlands, for example, controversial national policies relevant to older people led to the establishment of two national parties, the General Senior Citizens' Union and Union 55+, which together won 7 of the 150 seats in parliament in 1994 (Schuyt et al., 1999).

More likely, however, is that various age groups within the broad category that might be sweepingly labeled as elderly—which for many years has commonly been age 65 and older—would develop a sense of age-group consciousness that would be rather different politically. Even as individuals within age groups have diverse characteristics, the young old, the old old, the oldest old, and the prolonged old might have varied political tendencies. A major factor shaping these differences could be the details of age-related public policies.

The contemporary senior power model that tends to lump older persons together as if they were a politically monolithic group is in large measure a product of public policies on aging. The very existence of public programs that distribute benefits on the basis of old age creates a latent political constituency that has a stake in the maintenance and enhancement of those programs. Similarly, old-age policies shape the concerns and aims of those who scapegoat older people and envision intergenerational warfare; they are concerned about the growing costs of old-age benefits and how those costs may harm their interests.

But old-age policies in the long-lived society might very well make important distinctions among the young old, the old old, the oldest old, and the prolonged old, thereby creating separate old-age constituencies and defusing concerns about intergenerational warfare. For instance, the ages of eligibility for old-age benefits could be substantially raised—say, excluding the young old and the old old. Or, as Callahan (1987) has proposed, government financing of life-saving care might be denied for anyone aged 80 or older. Or the prolonged old, as a condition of their receiving anti-aging interventions, might be declared ineligible for old-age benefits.

In addition to such possible distinctions *between* older age groups, it is very likely that policy distinctions *within* old-age groups would be in effect in a long-lived society. Since the mid-1970s, a number of reforms have differentiated among older people with respect to their economic status in determining benefits and burdens in U.S. policies toward older persons (Binstock, in press). For instance, the Social Security Reform Act of 1983 rendered the old-age retirement benefits of wealthier older persons subject to taxation for the first time. The Tax Reform Act of 1986, even as it eliminated the extra personal exemption that had been available to all persons aged 65 and older when filing their federal income tax returns, provided new tax credits to low-income older persons on a sliding scale. The Older Americans Act programs of supportive and nutrition services, for which all persons aged 60 and older (and their spouses) are eligible, was gradually targeted to low-income older persons through a series of congressional amendments over the years. This sensitivity to the economic status of older persons was also applied to the health arena beginning in 1988 through a provision of the Medicare Catastrophic Coverage Act that made special health-care financing benefits available to older people with low incomes and minimal assets. This approach was amplified in the Balanced Budget Act of 1997.

Although there are still a number of respects in which old-age programs treat almost all older persons the same, these various policy reforms have established the principle that it is politically feasible for nonwelfare policies on aging to treat older people differently based on their economic status. Consequently, a workable framework has been established for maintaining governmental benefits to those older persons who truly need help through public programs (and not to those who do not), both in the near term and in the years when baby boomers will be elderly. There is no reason why this principle could not be applied to the prolonged old as well as the young old, old old, and oldest old.

In short, any of a number of imaginable policy distinctions regarding the elderly population could fractionate the political stakes that older people have in public policy. Accordingly, even though they might develop some dimensions of age-group consciousness, the various older age groups may not have a common ground of political behavior, attachments, and causes between them or within them.

A Concluding Note: Demography Is Not Destiny

As the preceding discussions surely illustrate, any attempt to speculate about the societal implications of prolongevity is fraught with uncertainties. This chapter has explored only one aspect of societal activity, the political arena, and within that arena the exploration has been confined to just the politics of age in a long-lived society. Any number of developments could take place in this arena in the next few decades and later in the century, even without the emergence of the prolonged old. Only a few selected possibilities have been offered for consideration, and each of these could shape and be shaped by developments in other societal arenas. Moreover, the discussions could have been even further complicated by postulating that the anti-aging interventions producing the prolonged old would not be universally available but distributed in response to economic status, social and political status, ascribed merit or lack thereof, nationality, or some other distinguishing criteria. The endeavor in this chapter has been simply to provide some basic tools for thinking about various political implications of prolongevity and illustrating their use.

Nonetheless, the various scenarios discussed regarding the politics of age in a long-lived society should convey one central message: *Demography is not destiny!* The political consequences of effective anti-aging interventions cannot be simply extrapolated from present behavioral patterns, social institutions, and public policies. In addition, a society that anticipates the emergence of the prolonged old can take deliberate steps to shape the ensuing political consequences. Electoral rules could be changed, as has already been suggested, to curb the voting power of older people. Alternatively, in an effort to safeguard the principle of one person/one vote, bulwarks against electoral rule changes could be erected. Similarly, the general tendency to provide public benefits on the basis of old age could be continued, providing a basis for age-group consciousness among older people. Or the relatively recent tendency to distinguish among older people in policies on aging could be nurtured, thereby reducing the likelihood that older people—even various age-group categories of older people— would have a collective political identity in a long-lived society.

Whatever might happen, however, it is certainly safe to make at least one assertion: the politics of age in a long-lived society would be very, very different from the politics of age today.

Acknowledgments

Support for the preparation of this chapter was provided by the John F. Templeton Foundation (JTF) and by Grant No. 1R01AGHG20916-01 from the National Institute on Aging (NIA) and the National Human Genome Research Institute (NHGRI), Eric T. Juengst, Ph.D., Principal Investigator. The opinions expressed are solely those of the author and do not reflect those of JTF, NIA, or NHGRI.

References

Abramson, P.R., Aldrich, J.H., and Rohde, D.W. (1999). *Change and Continuity in the 1996 and 1998 Elections.* Washington, DC: CQ Press.

Altman, S.H. and Shactman, D.I. (Eds.). (2002). *Policies for an Aging Society.* Baltimore: Johns Hopkins University Press.

Ball, R.M. (1995). What Medicare's architects had in mind. *Health Affairs,* 14(4), 62–72.

Banfield, E.C. (1961). *Political Influence: A New Theory of Urban Politics.* New York: Free Press.

Bell, D. (1964). Twelve modes of prediction—a preliminary sorting of approaches in the social sciences. *Daedalus,* 93, 845–880.

Binstock, R.H. (1974). Aging and the future of American politics. *Annals of the American Academy of Political and Social Science,* 415, 199–212.

Binstock, R.H. (1983). The aged as scapegoat. *The Gerontologist,* 23, 136–143.

Binstock, R.H. (1994). Changing criteria in old-age programs: The introduction of economic status and need for services. *Gerontologist,* 34, 726–730.

Binstock, R.H. (1995). Policies on aging in the post–cold war era. In: Crotty, W., ed. *Post–Cold War Policy: The Social and Domestic Context.* Chicago: Nelson-Hall, pp. 55–90.

Binstock, R.H. (1996). Continuities and discontinuities in public policy and aging. In: Bengtson, V.L., ed. *Adulthood and Aging: Research on Continuities and Discontinuities.* New York: Springer, pp. 308–324.

Binstock, R.H. (1997a). Do the elderly really have political clout? In: Scharlach, A.E., and Kaye, L.W., eds. *Controversial Issues in Aging.* Boston: Allyn & Bacon, pp. 87–91.

Binstock, R.H. (1997b). The old-age lobby in a new political era. In: Hudson, R.B., ed. *The Future of Age-Based Public Policy.* Baltimore: Johns Hopkins University Press, pp. 56–74.

Binstock, R.H. (2000). Older people and voting participation: Past and future. *Gerontologist,* 40, 18–31.

Binstock, R.H. (2002). The politics of enacting reform. In: Altman, S.H. and Shactman, D.I., eds. *Policies for an Aging Society.* Baltimore: Johns Hopkins University Press, pp. 346–377.

Binstock, R.H. (in press). Old-age provisions and economic status. In: Vitt, L.A. and Siegenthaler, J.K., eds. *Encyclopedia of Financial Gerontology,* 2nd ed. Westport CT: Greenwood Press.

Bonnicksen, A.L. (2002). *Crafting a Cloning Policy: From Dolly to Stem Cells.* Washington, DC: Georgetown University Press.

Button, J.W. and Rosenbaum, W.A. (1989). Seeing gray: School bond issues and the aging in Florida. *Research on Aging,* 11, 158–173.

Caldeira, G.A., Patterson, S.C., and Markko, G.A. (1985). The mobilization of voters in congressional elections. *Journal of Politics,* 47, 490–509.

Callahan, D. (1987). *Setting Limits: Medical Goals in an Aging Society.* New York: Simon & Schuster.

Campbell, J.C. and Strate, J. (1981). Are older people conservative? *Gerontologist*, 21, 580–591.

Carballo, M. (1981, December 21). Extra votes for parents? *The Boston Globe*, p. 35.

Cetron, M. and Davies, O. (1998). *Cheating Death: The Promise and Future Impact of Trying to Live Together.* New York: St. Martin's Press.

Chomitz, K.M. (1987). Demographic influences on local public education expenditures: A review of econometric evidence. In: Committee on Population, Commission on Behavioral and Social Sciences and Education, National Research Council, ed. *Demographic Change and the Well-Being of Children and the Elderly.* Washington, DC: National Academy Press, pp. 45–53.

Cohen, W.J. (1985). Reflections on the enactment of Medicare and Medicaid. *Health Care Financing Review, Annual Supplement*, 3–11.

Concord Coalition. (1993). *The Zero Deficit Plan: A Plan for Eliminating the Federal Budget Deficit by the Year 2000.* Washington, DC: The Concord Coalition.

Connelly, M. (2000, November 12). Who voted: A portrait of American politics, 1976–2000. *New York Times,* as indicated, the wk section, p. 4. (News of the week in Review).

Converse, P.E. (1976). *The Dynamics of Party Support: Cohort-Analyzing Party Identification.* Beverly Hills, CA: Sage.

Cook, F.L., Marshall, V.M., Marshall, J.E., and Kaufman, J.E. (1994). The salience of intergenerational equity in Canada and the United States. In: Marmor, T.R., Smeeding, T.M., and Greene, V.L., eds. *Economic Security and International Justice: A Look at North America.* Washington, DC: Urban Institute Press, pp. 91–129.

Day, C.L. (1998). Old-age interest groups in the 1990s: Coalition, competition, strategy. In: Steckenrider, J.S. and Parrott, T.M., eds. *New Directions in Old-age Policies.* Albany: State University of New York Press, pp. 131–150.

de Grey, A.D.N.J. (2000). Gerontologists and the media: The dangers of over-pessimism. *Biogerontology*, 1, 369.

Delli Carpini, M.X. (1986). *Stability and Change in American Politics: The Coming of Age of the Generation of the 1960s.* New York: New York University Press.

Delli Carpini, M.X. and Keeter, S. (1993). Measuring political knowledge: Putting first things first. *American Journal of Political Science*, 37, 1179–1206.

Derthick, M. (1979). *Policymaking for Social Security.* Washington, DC: Brookings Institution.

Downs, A. (1957). *An Economic Theory of Democracy.* New York: Harper and Brothers.

Fairlie, H. (1988). Talkin' bout my generation. *New Republic*, 198(13), 19–22.

Federal Interagency Forum on Aging-Related Statistics (2000). *Older Americans 2000: Key Indicators of Well-Being.* Washington, DC: U.S. Government Printing Office.

Flanigan, W.H. and Zingale, N.H. (1998). *Political Behavior of the American Electorate,* 9th ed. Washington, DC: CQ Press.

Gelman, A. and King, G. (1992). *Why Do Presidential Election Campaign Polls Vary So Much When the Vote Is So Predictable?* Cambridge, MA: Littauer Center, Harvard University.

Glenn, N.D. and Grimes, M. (1968). Aging, voting, and political interest. *American Sociological Review,* 33, 563–575.

Hackler, C. (2001–2002). Troubling implications of doubling the lifespan. *Generations,* XXV(4), 15–19.

Hayflick, L. (1994). *How and Why We Age.* New York: Ballantine Books.

Henig, R.M. (2002, December 17). Adapting to our own engineering. *New York Times,* p. A35.

Hobbs, F.B. (1996). *65+ in the United States.* U.S. Bureau of the Census, Current Population Reports, Special Studies, P23-190. Washington, DC: U.S. Government Printing Office.

Hout, M. and Knoke, D. (1975). Change in voting turnout, 1952–1972. *Public Opinion Quarterly,* 39, 52–68.

Hudson, R.B. (1978). The "graying" of the federal budget and its consequences for old age policy. *The Gerontologist,* 18, 428–440.

Hudson, R.B. (1995). Political implications of an extended life span. In: Seltzer, M.M., ed. *The Impact of Increased Life Expectancy: Beyond the Gray Horizon.* New York: Springer, pp. 109–126.

Iglehart, J.K. (1989). Medicare's new benefits: Catastrophic health insurance. *New England Journal of Medicine,* 320, 329–336.

Jamieson, A., Shin, H.B., and Day, J. (2002). *Voting and Registration in the Election of November 2000.* Current population reports, series p20-542. Washington, DC: U.S. Census Bureau, Economics and Statistics Administration, U.S. Department of Commerce.

Jennings, M.K. and Markus, G.B. (1988). Political involvement in the later years: A longitudinal survey. *American Journal of Political Science,* 32, 302–316.

Light, P.C. (1985). *Artful Work: The Politics of Social Security Reform.* New York: Random House.

Lowi, T.J. (1969). *The End of Liberalism.* New York: W.W. Norton.

Ludwig, F.C. (Ed.). (1990). *Life Span Extension: Consequences and Open Questions.* New York: Springer.

Luskin, R.C. (1987). Measuring political sophistication. *American Journal of Political Science,* 31, 856–899.

McManus, S.A. (1996). *Young v. Old: Generational Combat in the 21st Century.* Boulder, CO: Westview Press.

Miller, R.A. (2002). Extending life: Scientific prospects and political obstacles. *The Milbank Quarterly,* 80, 155–174.

Miller, W.E. (1992.) The puzzle transformed: Explaining declining turnout. *Political Behavior*, 14(1), 1–43.

Miller, W.E. and Shanks, J.M. (1996). *The New American Voter.* Cambridge, MA: Harvard University Press.

Morris, C.R. (1996). *The AARP: America's Most Powerful Lobby and the Clash of Generations.* New York: Times Books.

Myers, G.C. and Agree, E.M. (1993). Social and political implications of population aging: Aging of the electorate. In: *Proceedings of the International Population Conference, Montreal 1993*, vol. 3. Liege, Belgium: International Union for the Scientific Study of Population, pp. 37–49.

Naegele, G. and Walker, A. (1999). Conclusion. In: Walker A. and Naegele, G., eds. *The Politics of Old Age in Europe.* Buckingham, PA: Open University Press, pp. 197–209.

National Institute on Aging. (2001). *Action Plan for Aging Research: Strategic Plan for Fiscal Years 2001–2005.* Washington, DC: U.S. Department of Health and Human Services.

Neugarten, B.L. (1978/1996). Social implications of life extension. Presented at a symposium entitled "Extending the Human Lifespan," 11th International Congress of Gerontology, Tokyo, Japan, August 1978). Reprinted in D.A. Neugarten (Ed.), *The Meanings of Age: Selected Papers of Bernice L. Neugarten.* Chicago: University of Chicago Press, pp. 339–345.

New York Times. (1996a, October 8). A transcript of the first televised debated between Clinton and Dole, pp. A14–A17.

New York Times. (1996b, October 18). Excerpts from the second televised debate between Clinton and Dole, pp. C22–C23.

New York Times. (2000, May 16). Excerpts from prepared remarks by Bush and Gore, p. A18.

Palfrey, T.R. and Poole, K.T. (1987). The relationship between information, ideology, and voting behavior. *American Journal of Political Science*, 31, 511–530.

Peterson, P.G. (1999). *Gray Dawn: How the Coming Age Wave Will Transform America—and the World.* New York: Times Books.

Peterson, S.A. and Somit, A. (1994). *Political Behavior of Older Americans.* New York: Garland.

Pifer, A. and Bronte, E. (Eds.). (1986). *Our Aging Society: Paradox and Promise.* New York: W.W. Norton.

Pratt, H.J. (1976). *The Gray Lobby.* Chicago: University of Chicago Press.

Pratt, H.J. (1993). *Gray Agendas: Interest Groups and Public Pensions in Canada, Britain, and the United States.* Ann Arbor: University of Michigan Press.

Pratt, H.J. (1997). Do the elderly really have political clout? In: Scharlach, A.E. and Kaye, L.W., eds. *Controversial Issues in Aging.* Boston: Allyn & Bacon, pp. 82–85.

Preston, S.H. (1984). Children and the elderly in the U.S. *Scientific American*, 251(6), 44–49.

Price, M.C. (1997). *Justice between Generations: The Growing Power of the Elderly in America.* Westport, CT: Praeger.

Quadagno, J. (1989). Generational equity and the politics of the welfare state. *Politics and Society,* 17(3), 353–376.

Rix, S.E. (1999). The politics of old age in the United States. In: Walker, A. and Naegele, G., eds. *The Politics of Old Age in Europe.* Buckingham, PA: Open University Press, pp. 178–196.

Rosenstone, S.J. and Hansen, J.M. (1993). *Mobilization, Participation, and Democracy.* New York: Macmillan.

Rozensweig, R.M. (1990). Address to the President's Opening Session, 43rd Annual Scientific Meeting, Gerontological Society of America, Boston, November 16.

Sack, K. and Dao, J. (2000, August 31). Gore and Bush battling for control of the policy agenda. *New York Times,* p. A16.

Salhoz, E. (1990, October 29). Blaming the voters: Hapless budgeteers single out "greedy geezers." *Newsweek,* p. 36.

Samuelson, R.J. (1978). Aging America: Who will shoulder the growing burden? *National Journal,* 10, 1712–1717.

Schuyt, T., García, L.L., and Knipscheer, K. (1999). The politics of old age in the Netherlands. In: Walker, A. and Naegele, G., eds. *The Politics of Old Age in Europe.* Buckingham, PA: Open University Press, pp. 123–134.

Seltzer, M.M. (Ed.). (1995). *The Impact of Increased Life Expectancy: Beyond the Gray Horizon.* New York: Springer Publishing Company.

Simon, H.A. (1985). Human nature in politics: The dialogue of psychology with political science. *American Political Science Review,* 79, 293–304.

Smith, L. (1992). The tyranny of America's old. *Fortune,* 125(1), 68–72.

Stewart, D.J. (1970). Disfranchise the old: The lesson of California. *The New Republic,* 163(8–9), 20–22.

Street, D. (1999). Special interests or citizens' rights? "Senior power," Social Security, and Medicare. In: Minkler, M. and Estes, C.L., eds. *Critical Gerontology: Perspectives from Political and Moral Economy.* Amityville, NY: Baywood, pp. 109–130.

Teixera, R.A. (1992). *The Disappearing American Voter.* Washington, DC: The Brookings Institution.

Thurow, L.C. (1996, May 19). The birth of a revolutionary class. *New York Times Magazine,* pp. 46–47.

Timpone, R.J. (1998). Structure, behavior, and voter turnout in the United States. *American Political Science Review,* 92, 145–158.

U.S. Bureau of the Census. (1998). *Current Population Reports, Series P25.* Washington, DC: U.S. Government Printing Office.

Van Tassel, D.D. and Meyer, J.E.W. (1992). *U.S. Aging Policy Interest Groups: Institutional Profiles.* New York: Greenwood.

Williamson, J.B. (1998). Political activism and the aging of the baby boom. *Generations,* XXII(1), 55–59.

Wolfinger, R.E. and Rosenstone, S.J. (1980). *Who votes?* New Haven, CT: Yale University Press.

Woll, P. and Binstock, R.H. (1991). *America's Political System: A Text with Cases,* 5th ed. New York: McGraw-Hill.

Epilogue
Extended life, Eternal Life:
A Christian Perspective

....

Diogenes Allen

t is very easy to become confused in discussing the relationship of
the scientific prospect of extending our life indefinitely and the
Christian teaching on eternal life. Both deal with life and its
longevity, but Christianity is primarily concerned with the kind of life
we have. This can be seen perhaps in the contrast between a physician
and a moralist. A physician is concerned with the health of a person,
regardless of the kind of person that is being treated. It does not matter whether the person is kindly, helpful, and honest or vicious, selfish,
and a criminal. A moralist, however, makes evaluations: some ways of
living are more praiseworthy, more worthwhile, and more to be aspired
to and encouraged than others. Christianity is very concerned with
the kind of life we lead. So to prevent confusion in our examination
of the relation of extended life and eternal life, we must at the outset
distinguish between life itself and the kind of life that is spoken of in
the Christian understanding of eternal life.

As far as life itself is concerned, Christianity believes and teaches
that it is good. (In fact, being itself, not just life and human life, is
good. Traditionally, Christianity has opposed cruelty to animals and
has prohibited abortion, suicide, and euthanasia. From their earliest

days the Christian churches have been very active in providing hospitals and health care, especially through their religious orders, offering care to people regardless of their moral and spiritual conditions. As far as the issue of the extension of life is concerned, it has been argued that "there is no reason from the Christian point of view to be especially critical of the idea so long as health and cognition are reasonably intact." And, I might add, as long as we recognize the large number of major social and political implications of the immensely increased longevity that is now envisioned by some scientists. Indeed, we are already experiencing some of these implications with the modest increase in longevity achieved in recent decades. A great extension to the length of life also does not affect our need to repent of evil and to seek to obey God.

Eternal life in Christian teaching is a very different kind of life than the life whose great extension is being sought by some scientists. If we do not have this distinction clear, confusions arise. At least one participant at the March 2000 conference thought that science and religion are rivals. He mistakenly assumed that belief in eternal life arose in Christianity from the human quest for immortality. Now that a scientific alternative for extending life is possibly available, the attraction of Christianity and other religions that promise life beyond death has diminished. He did not realize that eternal life is not the infinite extension of life as we know it, but a different kind of life, which we can experience and have to a degree in this life, but can have fully only after death.

Because eternal life is so superior to the life we presently live, it may appear that Christianity devalues this life. But, life is good and death is an enemy. According to St. Paul, death is the "last enemy" to be abolished by Christ's redemptive death. The fact that life is good and death is an enemy does not warrant unqualified praise of this life or a failure to recognize that death has some moral and religious benefits. However good this life is and may become, it is still far less good than eternal life. On the surface of the sun there are places that look black. These so-called sunspots are actually very bright, but they are less bright than the rest of the surrounding sun and so appear black against its surface. So too with this life. However good it is, and however much we are to protect and support life and encourage attempts to prolong it, it is significantly less good than eternal life. In addition, it is because we are made to receive eternal life that we find the kind of life we now have, even if prolonged indefinitely, incapable of satisfying our aspiration for eternal life that is awakened by Christ.

In Christian teaching the concern is not primarily to keep the lives we now have going forever. Rather, it is to transform our present lives. Christian teaching is not that, after a temporary interruption by death, this life continues forever. This is clear from the very basis of belief in eternal life, namely, the resurrection from the dead of Jesus. His resurrection is not a resuscitation after death, as was the case with Lazareth. Jesus' own return from the dead was a transformation. For example, his disciples did not immediately recognize him. Although it was Jesus, he looked different. This is why St. Paul points out that a plant and a seed look very different. There is continuity with the present but also discontinuity.

The transformation is not merely reflected in the difference between the resurrected body and our present bodies. It is also reflected in the kind of life we receive. We do not create the never-ending life. Eternal life is a relationship with God, a relationship in which God seeks to share God's life with us. It must also be emphasized that since it is God's life in which we share, what God is specifies what eternal life consists of. To know what eternal life is, then, we need some understanding of what God is.

The aspect of God's nature that is relevant to our concern is that God is perfect love. Jesus said, "Love your enemies and pray for those who persecute you, so that you may be children of your Father in heaven; for he makes his sun rise on the evil and on the good, and sends rain on the righteous and on the unrighteous. . . . Be perfect, therefore, as your heavenly Father is perfect" (Matthew 5:44–45, 48). Let us examine the nature of perfect love and show its relevance to the extended-life, eternal-life discussion.

The Experience of Perfect Love

All of us rightly believe that we know what love is; we have exercised and experienced it in one form or another. But most of us have exercised and experienced it only to a limited degree or in less than a perfect form. Perfect love is rare. So my procedure here will be to present an example of perfect love.

W. H. Auden, in his introduction to *Protestant Mystics*, gives this masterful description of it.

One fine summer night in June 1933 I was sitting on a lawn after dinner with three colleagues, two women and one man. We liked each other well enough but we were certainly not intimate friends, nor had any one of us a sexual interest in another. Incidentally, we had not drunk any alcohol. We were talking casually about everyday matters when quite suddenly and unexpectedly, something happened. I felt myself invaded by a power which, though I consented to it, was irresistible and certainly not mine. For the first time in my life I knew exactly—because, thanks to the power, I was doing it—what it means to love one's neighbor as oneself. I was also certain, though the conversation continued to be perfectly ordinary, that my three colleagues were having the same experience. (In the case of one of them, I was able later to confirm this.) My personal feelings towards them were unchanged—they were still colleagues, not intimate friends—but I felt their existence as themselves to be of infinite value and rejoiced in it.

I recalled with shame the many occasions on which I had been spiteful, snobbish, selfish, but the immediate joy was greater than the shame, for I knew that, so long as I was possessed by this spirit, it would be literally impossible for me deliberately to injure another human being. I also knew that the power would, of course, be withdrawn sooner or later and that, when it did, my greed and self-regard would return. The experience lasted at its full intensity for about two hours when we said good-night to each other and went to bed. When I awoke the next morning, it was still present, though weaker, and it did not vanish completely for two days or so. The memory of the experience has not prevented me from making use of others, grossly and often, but it has made it much more difficult for me to deceive myself about what I am up to when I do. And among the various factors which several years late brought me back to the Christian faith in which I had been brought up, the memory of this experience and asking myself what it could mean was one of the most crucial, though, at the time it occurred, I thought I had done with Christianity for good.

(1964, pp. 13–18)

The rarity of the exercise and experience of perfect love suggests that it is to be regarded as a *goal* to be attained. It is an extraordinarily difficult goal. The difficulty is well worth emphasizing by giving another example of an occurrence of perfect love. Laurens van der Post recounts the experience in a prisoner-of-war camp of men who, in the closing months of World War II, fully expected to be slaughtered by their captors.

> It was amazing how often and how many of my men would confess to me, after some Japanese excess worse than usual, that for the first time in their lives they had realized the truth, and the dynamic liberating power of the first of the Crucifixion utterances: "Forgive them for they know not what they do."
>
> I found the moment they grasped this fundamental fact of our prison situation, forgiveness became a product not of an act of will or of personal virtue even, but an automatic and all-compelling consequence of a law of understanding: as real and indestructible as Newton's law of gravity. The tables of the spirit would be strangely and promptly turned and we would find ourselves without self-pity of any kind, feeling deeply sorry for the Japanese as if we were the free men and they the prisoners.
>
> (1963)

We need not fully experience perfect love ourselves to recognize it. Some degree of recognition of the independence of other things of our wishes, needs, and ambitions allows us to exercise and experience perfect love to an extent, as when, for example, we recognize in an argument the validity of another point of view, or we do not misuse scholars' data, or we become absorbed in our attention to a child or in the beauty of the natural world. These partial exercises of perfect love enable one to extend the line of vision toward the ideal case, the perfect recognition of other things, independent of whether they are useful to us or not, and undeflected by the moral or immoral behavior of people. But the way we usually experience things is not the way they are but the way they interest, enhance, repel, or threaten us.

There is a considerable body of empirical data that shows that our perception is affected by such things as expectations, emotional conflicts, and stress, and there are experiments that seek to measure the effects of these with precision. There are also theories, such as Freud's, that put great emphasis on unconscious desires over which we do not have much control, attempts to gratify them in a physical and social environment that is not always amenable to their gratification, and the role of fantasy as a major means of controlling and satisfying them.

My own claim about distortion in our perception of other things does not rest on either empirical studies of perception or Freudian-type views. It hinges on the fact that each of us is a conscious center, aware of how his or her body feels, and with an unreflective concern for himself or herself that is enormous. We usually perceive everything from the perspective of ourselves in terms of how it affects us.

We have, in addition, the power to occupy a position that is a type of solipsism; that is, when we have a *unique* concern for ourselves, we see things from our selves as the center and estimate the value and significance of all things in terms of their worth for us. Their value is conditional; our own is not. We are an unconditional end, and nothing else is so perceived or regarded. We are not only ontologically primary, since our concern is for ourselves and for other things only as they relate to ourselves, but we are ontologically unique, since usually there is no experience of other centers as centers (in the case of people, animals, or plants) and little regard for nonliving things as existing independently of their relation to us and of their value and significance to us. We can occupy the position of this type of solipsism and, while occupying it, truly say that there are other minds, that other things feel, and that things exist independently of us, and yet be *experiential* solipsists.

But this position is a distortion, for each of us is but one item among many; each of us is not the center of the universe but only one focus. Other items exist independently of us, and so their significance and value are not to be measured solely in terms of their relation to ourselves. But we have the capacity to resist recognizing other centers as centers and to resist valuing any item independently of ourselves. We can keep things in orbit around ourselves and not release them. Such a position is unrealistic since they in fact are not in orbit around us.

This view of our power to prevent ourselves from recognizing the reality of other things allows us to draw a distinction between two kinds of self: what I call a de facto person and a *moral* person. To be a de facto person is to have a unique self-regard, and thereby to judge all things only as they relate to oneself. One does not actually experience oneself as standing in the relationship of but one being among others, one item among many. We do not as de facto persons experience or have ontological humility.

A moral person is aware that he or she is but one reality among other realities. Rousseau made a similar distinction. For him a moral person was one who has moved from a private interest to a public interest, from private will to the general will or good. This view is related to my distinction and is quite a demanding goal. It moves in the right direction, but it does not go as far as to call for perfect love. Moreover, it is not at all clear to me that anyone is able to occupy the position of perfect love all the time, that is, to perceive others as independent and valuable in their own right and to remain in that relation to them all the time, or even for very long or very often. Nonetheless, one can be aware of the idea of what becoming a moral person is. To grasp even the idea of what a moral person is is to move toward becoming a moral person; it is to move toward a more realistic relation to others. It is more realistic because some of the distortion of the original position has been removed.

The commandment "Love your neighbor as yourself" means that one is to have the same unreflective concern for others as one *already* has for oneself. No one has to be taught to have self-concern; no one has to develop it. It is there and is all-encompassing, even when one feels miserable and full of self-deprecation and self-hatred, since one is very much the center. What must take place is for one to shed that unique self-concern so that one may recognize the reality of others with that immediate, unreflective, untaught concern that one now has only for oneself.

The Meaning of Death

This understanding of one aspect of eternal life, namely, perfect love, gives us a new perspective on death. Death that is overcome by a resurrection of the dead is not a continuation of a de facto life, but the realization and consummation of a life of perfect love, begun in this life but only partly and fitfully realized in this life.

This view has several implications for the present situation in which human life is of limited duration. First, it is a blessing that this life is limited in duration, not because it is not good but because this kind of life cannot satisfy. Were life to go on as it now is on this Earth, with what we are and with what is available to us, it would never satisfy our aspirations and potential. Once we have tasted perfect love, we desire to be always as we are only fitfully and at best only for a short time, as we saw in the case of W.H. Auden. We find this explicit in the experience that drove and inspired Dante's entire life. Dante tells us that he once saw a young girl of 16 who was so lovely that he was filled with love. He said that for several days, if anyone had done him an injury, he would have been unable not to forgive him. This in itself is not unusual. When one falls in love, one often feels as if one is walking on air, and indeed finds it easy to pass over things that would otherwise make one angry. What is unusual in Dante's case is that he took as his standard and goal to become always the way he was for a few days, that is, to be a person so possessed by love that he would always be able to forgive injuries automatically. This aspiration to perfection is also what inspired and drove the poet T.S. Eliot. Many of us waste these high moments of perfect love rather than seeing them as intimations of what we may and should become.

Second, this life as it now is, were it to continue indefinitely, would become a dreary business. Consider, for example, how in Hinduism and Buddhism escape from this life, not its prolongation, is the goal. This life, when viewed as continuing indefinitely in successive reincarnations, is thought to be a bondage. Or consider the Faust legend, in which Faust is given the power by Satan to explore and experience the entire range of human life without any dire consequences, with only one condition. The moment he becomes bored, he forfeits his soul to the Devil. In time, Faust grows weary and loses his zest.

Many people in fact do not live long enough to become weary of this life; indeed, many who do live a long life do not feel that this life cannot satisfy their aspirations. But this may well be because our life is in fact of limited duration. Because there is only a limited time, what we do have remains sweet, fascinating, and engaging. Nonetheless, it should be clear that Christianity does not offer an afterlife to meet the fear of *this* life's coming to an end. This life is not sufficient to satisfy our aspirations, at least once we are aware of perfect love.

Third, death is a blessing because it can also be an occasion for a more realistic assessment of oneself. We are not particularly anxious about the fact that we once did not exist. When we look, however, toward the opposite direction, to the fact that one day we will not be, for many there is a touch of dread, anxiety, and unease. This may not be only because of our inordinate self-concern but also because we have during our lifetime accumulated guilt, regrets, and failures. For an unjustified life, death has a sting. One dreads to meet one's end when one's life is unjustified. So a time limit forces one to examine oneself and to consider what to do with an unjustified life. Clearly, the fact of death does not impose a great burden on one who feels that one can justify one's life; the end poses no more problem for such a person than the fact that one begins. But the higher one's conception of one's obligations, and the less one condones one's failures, the more difficult it is to justify one's life. Death's sting is proportionate to one's yardstick. A major part of Christianity's view of our life is that God justifies it and thereby removes the sting of death. So the sting of death can lead one to look to God for relief.

But apart from any anxiety that results from an unjustified life, the very shortness of the life span calls for self-examination of one's life. Since life is of limited duration, it is wise to ask (whether or not one does so): What should I do with what I have? What is important? What is the truth of the reality about us so that I can judge rightly what to do with my life? Death is a blessing in that it calls us to examine the reality about us and ourselves in relation to it.

Fourth, death is a blessing because it threatens a de facto position and a de facto worth. It logically means that one is but one item among other realities, without unique ontological status. It logically means that our experiential solipsism is a distortion of reality. Death can thus be a spur to get one to ask: What do I amount to?

In brief, then, the Christian belief in an afterlife does not tells us not to worry about death, or that death is not real, or if real, not permanent. Death is indeed an enemy to be both resisted and accepted. Death is to be resisted because this life is good. It is to be accepted because this life cannot satisfy us and an allotted time helps makes this time precious. Christianity teaches us that death cannot keep us from attaining a justified life, and it drives us to seek one. It teaches us that an allotted time means that we should investigate the reality around us and ourselves in relation to it to determine how we are to use limited time wisely. But an afterlife is not intended to rid us of that part of the fear of death that arises from a de facto estimate of ourselves; it does not save one's de facto person from extinction. It promises the consummation of the erratic but persistent movement toward perfect love.

Death is a judgment of this life and our lives. Our lives are judged to be invalid because we cannot fully escape from the unreality of a de facto position and the outrage we thereby commit on other realities. A human life is a life of death, that is, a life of isolation from a true relation with others, and so it is to end. We have this time to seek to give up our de facto stance, that is, willingly to desire that our life of isolation come to an end. If we do not, when it ends, the loss is complete ("from him who has not, even what he has will be taken away": Mark 4:25).

Conclusion

It should be clear that life after death in Christianity under the interpretation I have given is not a doctrine entertained because of a self-centered fear of the loss of life. The entranceway to God's presence is by the death of the unreality of our present perception; the reward is the perception of the reality that God is and the reality God has conferred on others. The motivation to seek eternal life is not to escape death, but to escape the unreality of one's present position for that which is true. That this involves a never-ending life is indeed a reason for great joy. It is a joy that comes to those who seek to be moral ("to him who has will more be given": Mark 4:25). The more fully, clearly, and deeply we have perceived the presence of God through the presence of God's perfect love in our lives, the greater is our confidence in the completion of the life that is now being hectically, sporadically, and fitfully received from a reality that is not of this world but the source of this world.

References

Auden, W.H. (1964). Introduction. In: Freemantle, A. ed. *The Protestant Mystics*: An Anthology of Boston: Little, Brown and Co., pp.13–180.
van der Post, L. (1963). *The Seed and the Sower.* London: Penguin Books, 1983.

Annotated Bibliography

....

Roselle S. Ponsaran

Science

Allolio, B. and Arlt, W. (2002). DHEA treatment: Myth or reality? *Trends in Endocrinology and Metabolism*, 13(7), 288–294.

Dehydroepiandrosterone (DHEA), a product of the adrenal cortex that significantly decreases with age, has been touted as an anti-aging drug. However, studies demonstrating anti-aging, anticancer, and immune-enhancing properties have used extremely high doses of DHEA in mice, which have very little DHEA compared to humans. Studies of DHEA supplementation for the elderly indicate that although it may improve well-being, mood, and sexuality and may result in better body composition, it is unlikely to enhance already normal performance. In addition, there may be a risk of neoplasia. As a result, there is not enough evidence to recommend DHEA for the elderly.

Austad, S.N. (1997). *Why We Age: What Science Is Discovering About the Body's Journey Through Life*. New York: Wiley.

Austad, a zoologist and evolutionary biologist who specializes in aging, clearly summarizes the theories on why we age, the biological mechanisms of aging, and what might be done to ameliorate the process. Drawing from a wide range of disciplines, including evolutionary biology, anthropology, medicine, and particularly comparative zoology, he provides a comprehensive overview of aging research and longevity issues for both the scientific and general audiences.

He describes the theories of aging and death as an evolutionary mechanism, the link between menopause and aging, and the roles of hormones, oxidative damage, and genetic self-repair errors. In documenting the responses of science to the questions of aging, he paints illuminating portraits of such key scientists as J.B.S. Haldane and Peter Medawar. Austad disputes current proposed methods of postponing aging, including caloric restriction, exercise, and melatonin supplementation, as well as several notorious examples of age inflation, such as reports of extreme longevity in Pakistan, the Caucasus, and Ecuador. Generally, the anti-aging techniques currently available may only prevent premature death. However, while skeptical of anti-aging claims, he is also optimistic that further research will result in actual extension of the life span. Because aging is fundamentally determined by genetics and chance, genetic engineering will be the key to this future achievement.

Banks, D.A. and Fossel, M. (1997). Telomeres, cancer, and aging: Altering the human life span. *Journal of the American Medical Association*, 278(16), 1345–1348.

A shift in the conceptualization of aging now acknowledges the possibility of extending the maximum human life span. Recent research on cloning, cancer, and aging cells indicates that the aging process may be altered, at least on the cellular level. Aging is now viewed as the result of altered gene expression and cell metabolism due to a complex cascade of processes in cell division and telomere effects, rather than the passive accumulation of damage in the cell. Cell aging seems to be mutable, suggesting that projections of aging in developed countries, and their social and economic consequences, may need to be revised. The possibility of aging intervention will place fiscal and social pressures on the ability to care for the elderly, based on the level of functional impairment, health-care needs of developing countries, changes in work and retirement, and demand for long-term care on governments and individuals.

Bernarducci, M.P. and Owens, N.J. (1996). Is there a fountain of youth? A review of current life extension strategies. *Pharmacotherapy*, 16(2), 183–200.

This article reviews the scientific and medical research on various proposed life extension strategies, including nonpharmacological strategies such as caloric restriction, specific nutrient restriction (tryptophan-restricted), and exercise and pharmacological strategies such as the use of antioxidants, DHEA, and melatonin. The studies surveyed were limited by several factors: most were done in rodent strains that had a predisposition to disease or lived in a controlled experimental environment that could have modified specific disorders or environmental influences rather than aging itself, or with human subjects with specific diseases. These strategies require further study. Studies on life extension intervention should be done in samples that have a life span approximating that of the larger group.

de Grey, A.D.N.J., Ames, B.N., Andersen, J.K., Bartke, A., Campisi, J., Heward, C.B., McCarter, R.J.M., and Stock, G. (2002). Time to talk SENS: Critiquing the immutability of human aging. *Annals of the New York Academy of Science*, 959(1), 452–462.

Aging is a three-stage process: metabolism, damage, and pathology. The biochemical processes that sustain life generate toxins as an intrinsic side effect. These toxins cause damage that accumulates, driving age-related degeneration. Interventions can be designed at all three stages. However, intervention in metabolism can only modestly postpone pathology, and intervention in pathology is a losing battle if the damage that drives it is accumulating unabated. By contrast, intervention to remove the accumulating damage would sever the link between metabolism and pathology, and so has the potential to postpone aging indefinitely. The authors survey the categories of such damage and the ways in which, with current or foreseeable biotechnology, they could be reversed, suggesting that that indefinite postponement of aging—"engineered negligible senescence"—may be possible. With the demographic consequences it would entail, this possibility warrants immediate consideration and debate.

de Grey, A.D.N.J., Gavrilov, L., Olshansky, S.J., Coles, L.S., Cutler, R.G., Fossel, M., and Harman, S.M. (2002). Anti-aging technology and pseudoscience. *Science*, 296(5568), 656a.

In a response to Holden's (2002) article, the authors argue that not everyone who uses the term *anti-aging* is a quack; in fact, the term has been used by reputable scientists doing valid research on modifying aging. The public should be aware of both the scientific and nonscientific uses of the term *anti-aging medicine*. Misuse of the term has led some legitimate scientists to avoid using it at all.

Fries, J.F. (1980). Aging, natural death, and the compression of morbidity. *New England Journal of Medicine*, 303, 130–136.

This is a frequently cited article that first proposed the compression of morbidity model of aging. Based on the assumptions that the life span is fixed (natural death occurs even without disease) but that the chronic diseases and markers of age can be postponed, Fries predicts continued decline in premature death and the emergence of a pattern of natural death at the end of the natural life span. By promoting health and personal autonomy, the phenomena associated with aging may be postponed, resulting in the rectangularization of the survival curve and of the morbidity curve. Life can be vigorous until shortly before death.

Frolkis, V.V. (Ed.). (1982). *Aging and Life-Prolonging Processes*, trans. Nicholas Bobrov. New York: Springer-Verlag Wien.

This book reviews the research on aging and potential life extension techniques for a scientific audience. Frolkis focuses on the concept of the vitauct mechanism, the stabilizing of an organism's viability, its relationship with aging, the role of neuro-humoral mechanisms, and the possible ways to increase the life span. The main mechanisms of vitauct include DNA repair, while the main mechanism of aging is genome alteration; the relationship between the two determines the rate and extent of changes with age. The chapters address a range of topics from aging of the brain, thyroid regulation, and metabolism to cellular aging. The final chapter deals with experimental life prolongation antioxidants and other chemical agents, low-calorie or low-protein diets, exercise, hormones, energy metabolism, and genetic factors.

Frolkis, V.V. and Muradian, K.K. (1991). *Life Span Prolongation*. Boca Raton, FL; Ann Arbo, MI; Boston, and London: CRC Press.

This is an extensive and comprehensive review of the scientific research on the biology of aging and life span extension by two Russian gerontologists. It is highly technical, with little discussion or mention of social implications, ethical concerns, or historical or cultural context. Each chapter is well referenced, some with over 100 works cited. Aging is not a one-step or a genetically programmed state, but a genetically determined, probabilistic process connected to genome regulation, protein biosynthesis, and nervous and hormonal influences. The correlations between certain parameters and species life span suggest that some parameters might be modified for life extension. The question of life prolongation should not be approached with either complete denial or belief in extreme possibilities in the near future; both mislead the public and harm the scientific work. Present knowledge of aging offers grounds for a theoretical search for life prolongation. There are a variety of experimental approaches contributing to life span increase, and most geroprotectors studied can positively influence the adaptive potentialities of an organism, its biological age, and its quality of life.

Glannon, W. (2002). Extending the human life span. *Journal of Medicine and Philosophy*, 27(3), 339–354.

Research into the mechanisms of aging has suggested the possibility of extending the human life span. But there may be evolutionary biological reasons for senescence and the limits of the cell cycle that result in the infirmities of aging and the eventual demise of all human organisms. Genetic manipulations of the aging mechanisms over many generations could alter the course of natural selection and shift the majority of deleterious mutations in humans from later to earlier stages in life. This could harm people in the distant future by making them more susceptible to premature disease and mortality. Thus, there are biological and moral reasons to consider carefully the implications of exploiting this technology on a broad scale to extend the lives of people in the present and near future.

Gosden, R. (1996). *Cheating Time: Science, Sex, and Aging*. New York: W.H. Freeman.

Gosden, a biologist specializing in reproductive technology, reviews the science and theories that link aging with the decline in sexual health and function, with particular emphasis on the role of sex hormones. Understanding the aging process, and then knowing how to slow it down, would preserve youth and prolong fertility. It is not well referenced since it is intended for a general audience, but there is a list of further readings.

By comparing the life spans across species (plants and animals), Gosden concludes that the life span is not permanently fixed but flexible. Women's longer life expectancy may be due to lifestyle differences, but it is more likely due to the evolutionary argument that men are more expendable. Aging itself is not necessarily a disease, and disability can be prevented. Health promoters should not focus on the secondary conditions of aging but on slowing the aging process itself. Fertility triumphs over longevity when the two are set against one another in evolution; aging may exist because some genes have both good and bad effects at different parts of the life span. Aging is more complex than the decline of sex hormones, although in Gosden's view hormone replacement therapy does more good than harm, particularly for women. Humans are comparatively infertile as a result of choice, disease, miscarriage, and the quality of the germ cells, which are susceptible to diet, lifestyle, other environmental factors, and age. There does not appear to be an upper age limit to having a child, and with reproductive technology, later pregnancy may become more common.

Guarente, L. and Kenyon, C. (2000). Genetic pathways that regulate ageing in model organisms. *Nature,* 408, 255–262.

This is a review of the research on genes in the aging process in two model organisms, the yeast and the nematode worm *Caenorhabditis elegans.* Reviewing the studies of single-gene mutations in these and other organisms such as *Drosophila* and mice, these genetic studies establish that aging is regulated by specific genes, and reveal simple and complex mechanisms governing the pace of aging and the life span. These studies may indicate that the mutation may also impact regulatory systems that control aging in higher organisms.

Harman, D., Holliday, R. and Meydani, M. (Eds.). (1998). *Towards Prolongations of the Healthy Life Span: Practical Approaches to Intervention,* vol. 854. Annals of the New York Academy of Sciences. New York: New York Academy of Sciences.

The volume (a reprint of the Annals of the New York Academy of Sciences issue) contains 40 papers from the 1997 conference of the International Association of Biomedical Gerontology. Scientific and technical, the papers cover a range of theories regarding the causes (and potential means of life extension) of aging: molecular and cellular changes, exercise, mitochondria, pharmacological interventions such as oxyradical therapy, nutritional interventions, and antioxidants. The editors argue that it is reasonable to expect that the biogerontological research will promote compression of morbidity, focusing more on extending functional life expectancy than on extending the maximum possible life span.

Hayflick, L. (1994). *How and Why We Age.* New York: Ballantine Books.

Hayflick, a biologist considered by many to be one of the fathers of biogerontology, provides lay readers with a comprehensive overview of the research and theories of aging and longevity—what is known, why aging changes occur, and what may be possible in the future. Writing in a clear and understandable style (he does not provide references but includes an extensive list of additional and recommended readings), he focuses primarily on the biology, rather than on the social issues and consequences, in order to provide accurate information in view of increasing public interest in aging.

Hayflick defines aging by explaining the difference between chronological and biological age and how longevity is measured, as well as the differences in aging in other animals and plants, and strongly challenges the idea that aging is a disease. Going beyond the individual experience of aging, he considers the demographics of aging, including the *graying* of the United States, the rectangularization of the survival curve, and various issues concerning life expectancy. He also reviews what is known about the process of human aging, including Hayflick's limit, the inherently limited number of times that normal cells divide in laboratory conditions. The Baltimore Longitudinal Study of Aging is used to discuss the specific changes that occur in aging, including those affecting appearance, metabolism, cognition, strength, and various organs and systems.

While he discounts reports of superlongevity, centenarians are presented as models for healthy aging and as examples of the potential and limit (determined weight, metabolic rate, and particularly evolution) of the human life span. There are two groups of theories of aging: programmed theories (based on purposeful events) and damage theories (based on random events). Reviewed in detail, programmed theories include the neuroendocrine theory, while the random event theories include the wear and tear, free radical, cross-linking, immune system, and error and repair theories. Finally, he considers attempts to slow aging and increase the life span, including exercise, diet and nutrition, temperature manipulation, cryonics, and internal clocks. While these practices may prevent premature death, he concludes, it is unlikely that any intervention could truly increase the maximum life span.

Hayflick, L. (2001–2002). Anti-aging medicine: Hype, hope, and reality. *Generations*, 25(4), 20–26.

Anti-aging will not work for scientific reasons. Aging is not a disease because it occurs in every animal that reaches a fixed size, crosses all species barriers, occurs only after sexual maturation, and occurs even after animals are removed from the wild. Understanding geriatric diseases will not increase our understanding of aging. We must address the question "Why are old cells more vulnerable to pathology than new cells?" We should examine the social consequences of anti-aging technology, such as who would have access to it and at what age aging should be arrested. Slowing aging would not appeal to the poor, oppressed, or sick.

Holden, C. (2002). The quest to reverse time's toll. *Science*, 295, 1032–1033.

Aging research and the anti-aging industry are becoming increasingly popular. Recent work on the genetics of aging, particularly caloric restriction mimetics (drugs that produce the anti-aging effects of caloric restriction), has spawned several companies aimed at anti-aging, with many scientists affiliated with them. Some scientists suggest that some of these mechanisms may have problematic side effects or consequences. The association that some scientists have with anti-aging companies, because of the legitimacy of their own research or product claims, may also be problematic. The author concludes that anti-aging medicine in general is still considered quackery.

Johnson, T.E. (1997). Genetic influences on aging. *Experimental Gerontology*, 32(1–2), 11–22.

Genetic approaches have been used repeatedly to understand diverse biological phenomena but have only recently been applied to the analysis of aging and senescence. Areas where genetics has been successfully applied to the study of the aging processes include neurological diseases of the elderly, the limited life span of human cells in tissue culture (Hayflick's limit), studies on the mouse life span, and genetic analysis of the life span in shorter-lived organisms, such as *Drosophila melanogaster, Caenorhabditis elegans,* and the yeast *Saccharomyces cerevisiae.*

Kirkwood, T. (1999). *Time of Our Lives: The science of human aging.* Oxford and New York: Oxford University Press.

British gerontologist Kirkwood provides an overview of the evolution of aging and its mechanisms for lay as well as scientific readers. In a personal and informal style he focuses on the development of and evidence for the disposable soma theory. In contrast to other evolutionary theorists of aging, he argues that aging has nothing to do with population control or other deterministic mechanism, but is the result of genes essentially making the best of limited energy resources. Soma cells (body cells, in contrast to germline cells) are constantly being replicated, accumulating errors over time. This accumulation meant little when conditions of life meant that reaching old age was rare, but in modern industrialized nations the effects have become obvious. The variations in life span among species demonstrate that aging is a consequence of a kind of trade-off with reproductive needs.

Lane, M.A., Ingram, D.K., and Roth, G.S. (2002). The serious search for an anti-aging pill. *Scientific American*, 287(2), 36–41.

In this wide-reaching cover article, three scientists review their experiences and research in seeking a caloric restriction mimetic, a chemical compound that could replicate the anti-aging effects of caloric restriction. Although the compound they were working with, 2DG, has too narrow a safety zone, they believe that a more viable caloric restriction mimetic may be available in the future.

Lane, M.A., Mattison, J., Ingram, D.K., and Roth, G.S. (2002). Caloric restriction and aging in primates: Relevance to humans and possible CR mimetics. *Microscopy Research and Technique*, 59, 335–338.

According to data from ongoing primate studies, the effects of caloric restriction on aging and the life span may be universal and may have benefits for human aging and longevity. To have widespread application, however, caloric restriction will have to be mimicked rather than actually practiced. Initial studies of potential mimetics suggest that it may be possible to achieve some metabolic effects by metabolic inhibition at the cellular level.

Masoro, E.J. (2000). Caloric restriction and aging: An update. *Experimental Gerontology*, 35, 299–305.

Three hypotheses concerning the mechanisms underlying the anti-aging actions of caloric restriction are reviewed and combined into a single unifying scenario. There is evidence that caloric restriction protects against age-associated accumulation of molecular damage (attenuation of oxidative damage), but its significance is unclear. The hypothesis that caloric restriction modifies glucose and insulin levels has not yet been adequately tested. Another theory, that the anti-aging effects result from a response to low-intensity stressors, is supported by the nonmammalian studies and likely operates through stress response genes. The anti-aging effects of caloric restriction may have evolved in response to periods of scant food availability in nature when energy was diverted to maintenance. Each of the three hypotheses encompasses components of anti-aging action.

Moore, T.J. (1993). *Life Span: Who Lives Longer—and Why*. New York: Simon & Schuster.

Moore, a health policy analyst who specializes in prescription drug safety, examines the factors that impact average life expectancy as well as maximum life span, arguing that longevity is observed among those who adapt most successfully. Because his focus is on the population rather than on the individual, the discussion concentrates on epidemiology and public health aspects of longevity.

Despite differences in culture, diet, gene pools, and disease rates, mortality rates are similar: long-lived nations are stable, prosperous democracies that generally protect children from disease, violence, and malnutrition. Throughout history, life expectancy has been regulated by dynamic and shifting relationships with disease-causing bacterial/viral life forms, a battle that humans have not often won. The development of the germ theory, vaccines, and epidemiology led to greater understanding of these relationships and ways to adjust them, but these do not fully explain gains in life expectancy. The swine flu incident and the Ebola virus demonstrate that there is a certain amount of randomness in infectious disease epidemics; increased virulence could occur spontaneously in strains of influenza or other diseases to potentially wipe out gains in life expectancy.

Popular beliefs that modifying commonly identified risk factors (obesity, high blood pressure, and high cholesterol) increases longevity are misplaced in that such modifications likely have minimal impact and are often propelled by commercial interests rather than scientific evidence. Factors that seem to promote longevity, such as marriage, do not necessarily imply direct causation but should be understood as part of a complex interaction. Research on cells and animals has begun to address the basic process of aging and points to some potential anti-aging products techniques, such as human growth hormone, DHEA, caloric restriction, and antioxidants. Longevity is a product of a community, not the achievement of an individual, and the greatest threat to longevity (relationship with bacteria/viruses) must be managed on the levels of the community, nation, and world.

Olshansky, S.J. and Carnes, B.A. (2001). *The Quest for Immortality: Science at the Frontiers of Aging.* New York: W.W. Norton.

The explicit goal of this book is to educate the public about how and why aging occurs in order to prevent exploitation by the anti-aging industry and the claims made about its products. While scientists are optimistic about prevention of aging in the future, current products exaggerate and deceive the public about what is possible now. Aimed at the general public, the book is written in a casual, nonacademic style without references, often using personal experiences to illustrate points.

Through improved public health measures and medical technology, longevity has been increased. Changes in life expectancy indicate only that many more people have the opportunity to grow old; additional gains will be more difficult to obtain since there are limits to the life span that can only be addressed by genetic manipulation. The reason prolongevists have not been able to detect a limit to life expectancy is that this limit has already been passed in some populations; medical technology has "manufactured time" for many people who otherwise would have died. Although medical interventions can extend life by producing manufactured time, neither medicine nor lifestyle changes are likely to impact life expectancy the way public health did in the twentieth century.

However, while claims of an *elixir vitae* and antioxidants are false or greatly exaggerated, there may be pharmaceuticals in the future that can slow the aging process. The authors review possible scientific approaches, especially genetic manipulation, although the latter may be problematic since the gene for aging may also affect other critical processes, as well as raising ethical questions. This technology will be used, but it could lead to harm. Adding more years will not improve the quality of life; the better approach is to guard one's health during the years now available.

Olshansky, J.S., Hayflick, L., and Carnes, B.A. Position statement on human aging. Retrieved June 2, 2002 at http://www.scienceonline.org

In response to the growing anti-aging industry and its unproven products and techniques, 51 scientists who conduct research on aging issued a position statement condemning claims that suggest that contemporary interventions can slow, stop, or reverse human aging. While they are optimistic that such interventions may be available in the future, promotions of current anti-aging products are generally false and misleading. The statement includes a comprehensive summary of what is known about aging and potential anti-aging techniques.

Olshansky, S.J., Hayflick, L., and Carnes, B.A. (2002). No truth to the fountain of youth. *Scientific American,* 286(6), 92–95.

In light of the increasing number of entrepreneurs hawking unproven anti-aging products, three scientists explain the need and rationale for organizing a consensus position statement from an international group of 51 scientists against unproven anti-aging products. While they are optimistic that a technology to slow aging may be available in the future, current products and their claims are false and misleading. Due to the lack of a specific genetic program and the complexity of the human organism, there are no quick fixes for aging and death, and the lack of aging measurements makes it difficult to assess the rate of aging. In addition, anti-aging products, such as antioxidants and hormone replacement therapy, without the rigorous testing required for medications, may have dangerous side effects.

Perls, T., Kunkel, L.M., and Puca, A.A. (2002). The genetics of exceptional human longevity. *Journal of the American Geriatrics Society*, 50, 359–368.

As a result of demographic selection, centenarians delay and even escape age-associated diseases and may be the model for disease-delayed aging or compressed morbidity. Family studies indicate that there is a substantial familial component (genetic or shared environment) to extreme longevity. Selection for genes that actively promote aging seems unlikely, but there is evidence, based on the link between reproduction and life span, for genes that combat the aging process. In evolution, increased life span may be associated with longer periods of reproductive fitness. The disposable soma theory predicts a trade-off between fertility and longevity. These genetic factors are likely to influence basic mechanisms of aging that broadly influence susceptibility to age-related diseases. Lacking genetic variations that predispose to disease and having longevity-enabling genes are likely both important to survival advantage.

Perls, T., Levenson, R., Regan, M., and Puca, A. (2002). What does it take to live to 100? *Mechanisms of Ageing and Development*, 123, 231–242.

Centenarians are the model for aging because of their compressed morbidity—slow aging and lack of age-related illness until late in life. The evidence indicates genetic rather than environmental influence on extreme longevity. The authors argue for the existence of longevity-enabling genes, using several studies of late female fecundity to support the theory that the development of longevity-enabling is a result of the pressure to increase the age at which a woman can bear children and so have more of them. Two approaches to determining the significance of candidate longevity genes have been used in lower organisms: screening for polymorphisms or allelic frequencies in human homologues and association studies of centenarian subgroups. Claims that people will someday live to 150 or beyond are "outrageous and impossible." The authors' own findings however, may bring the population closer to being centenarian-like (age slowly and delay/escape age-related disease).

Schneider, E.L. and Reed, J.D. (1985). Life extension. *New England Journal of Medicine*, 312(18), 1159–1168.

In light of the increasing interest in life extension in the media, this article reviews the research on several proposed interventions to increase longevity, including caloric restriction, exercise, dietary antioxidants, immunological interventions, and DHEA. The data on these interventions are generally inconclusive and require further research. Interventions should be studied in strains that have life spans close to the maximum and in higher primates, rather than in rodent strains that may have diminished longevity. It is unlikely that a single intervention could reverse or arrest all aging processes, but segmental interventions may have important effects on specific aging processes. Potential problems include increased risks of autoimmune diseases and ethical issues, such as an increased period of disability. However, interventions could also increase the period of health and vigor, remove ageist biases, and place greater emphasis on basic aging research.

Vance, M.L. (2003). Can growth hormone prevent aging? *New England Journal of Medicine*, 348(9), 779–780.

The initial studies indicating the potential anti-aging properties of human growth hormone were limited and should not be considered conclusive. More recent and more extensive studies indicate that although human growth hormone improves body composition, it does not improve function and is very expensive. Resistance training is much more beneficial.

Walford, R.L. (1983). *Maximum Life Span*. New York and London: W.W. Norton.

Walford, a biologist, reviews several potential interventions (such as genetic therapy) but concludes that caloric restriction is the only "relatively sure" way to extend the maximum life span at this point (he himself has practiced a strict regimen for many years). Maximum survival is genetically determined, and currently the maximum life span probably stands between 110 and 120 years. But some time in the near future, the maximum life span will be 140 years. The diseases of aging, such as cancer, are secondary to the decline in resistance and adaptability that comes with the aging process, so the onset of these diseases will be delayed. Thus, interventions that retard aging should be considered more effective and more research-worthy methods than treating the individual diseases of aging.

Warner, H.R. and Hodes, R.J. (2000). Hype, hope, and reality: Telomere length, telomerase, and aging. *Generations*, 24(4), 6–8.

In light of recent hype surrounding telomeres as a fundamental key to aging and aging intervention, the authors examine the reality by summarizing the research on telomere length in aging and cancer. Telomeres, which shorten with successive cell division, determine replicative senescence (the Hayflick limit) and are maintained or rebuilt by telomerase, which is present in germline and cancer cells. Research on the telomerase genes and protein components indicates that there may be some potential ability to use telomere manipulation therapeutically for cancer and tissue-specific repairs (as in Alzheimer's disease), but many uncertainties and challenges remain; its use to extend the life span is even more speculative at this point.

Wick, G. (2002). "Anti-aging" medicine: Does it exist? A critical discussion of "anti-aging health products." *Experimental Gerontology*, 37, 1137–1140.

In this short opinion piece based on a U.S. General Accounting Office report on anti-aging health products, Wick argues that many of the so-called anti-aging medicines have no scientifically proven effect on the aging process and have the potential to inflict physical and economic harm on elderly consumers. Recommending treatments based on anti-aging effects (even those based on successful interventions in animals) is unethical and will damage the credibility of experimental gerontology.

Yamaza, H., Chiba, T., Higami, Y., and Shimokawa, I. (2002). Life span extension by caloric restriction: An aspect of energy metabolism. *Microscopy Research and Technique*, 59, 325–330.

This article reviews the data on aging and caloric restriction alterations of metabolism in rodents and discusses the data obtained from lower organisms. Genes related to metabolism are associated with longevity in lower animals and may also be a factor in mammals. The authors illustrate a hypothetical model unifying longevity-related pathways in lower and higher organisms, although there may be some discrepancies.

Yu, B.P. (Ed.). (1994). *Modulation of Aging Processes by Dietary Restriction*. Boca Raton, FL: CRC Press.

This edited volume reviews the research on caloric restriction for a scientific audience. After reviewing current and discredited theories of aging, the book evaluates the proposed molecular mechanisms of caloric restriction. Topics include the effect on neuroendocrine signaling, modulation of the cardiovascular system, and the deleterious effects of age-related pathologies such as hypertension, stroke, and heart failure. Also addressed is the role of endocrine systems and their ability to mediate the aging process through metabolism and the decline of protein turnover with age.

Ethics

Benecke, M. (Ed.). (1998). *The Dream of Eternal Life: Biomedicine, Aging and Immortality*, trans. Rachel Rubenstein. New York: Columbia University Press.

Benecke, a German forensic entomologist and philosopher-scientist, investigates the biological meaning of life and death and the prospects for human life extension and immortality for a general audience. He discusses the biological fundamentals of why death exists and what modern biology, especially genetics, knows about aging and death, based on cell death, cancer cell immortality and *immortal* species, evolution, and sexual reproduction. Humans cope with and resist a finite life span and the certainty of death in a variety of ways, including afterlife beliefs, myths of the undead, and life extension methods (gene therapy, cloning, organ and brain transplants, and cryonics). Despite numerous ethical considerations, the desire for immortality is inevitable, although it is uncertain whether immortality is possible. However, humans as a species can stay healthy only if the Earth is healthy; environmental problems such as climate change, overpopulation, and migration need to be addressed. Eternal life would involve biological and psychological problems such as issues of changed identity. In addition, it may prevent regeneration, reproduction, and adaptation to the environment and, thus, evolution.

Bonita, R. (1997). Added years, onus or bonus? *The Lancet*, 350, 1167–1168.

Increased longevity has been a bonus for developed countries: active life expectancy has increased and chronic age-related disability has fallen. However, in poorer countries, longevity is burdened with poverty and illness. To challenge this problem, the life expectancy gaps among and within countries must be reduced by focusing on the social determinants of ill health, recognizing the roles of poverty, socioeconomic disadvantage, and gender discrimination and emphasizing collective action rather than individualism.

Butler, R.N. (2001–2002). Is there an anti-aging medicine? *Generations*, 25(4), 63–65.

Complementary and alternative remedies are not regulated by the Food and Drug Administration and are often unsafe. Because there are no valid aging biomarkers, making it impossible to determine if a substance is actually slowing the aging process, it is difficult to test the efficacy of anti-aging medicine. In addition, artificially inducing human growth hormone has been shown to shorten rather than lengthen the life span of some laboratory animals, and an excess of human growth hormone can cause the disease acromegaly. Anti-aging medicine pictures normal aging as a disease and puts a negative connotation on the natural occurrence of growing old.

Butler, R.N., Fossel, M., Pan, C.X., Rothman, D., and Rothman, S.M. (2000) Anti-aging medicine: What makes it different from geriatrics? *Geriatrics*, 55(6), 36, 39–43.

The growth in popularity of so-called anti-aging medicine challenges physicians to examine their attitudes about aging. Does one define aging as a predisposition to pathology or as part of the life cycle? Is longevity without the chronic diseases associated with aging a realistic goal? Anti-aging treatments being prescribed by some practitioners include hormone replacement therapies, vitamin and mineral supplements, diet, and exercise. Although diet, exercise, and some vitamin and mineral supplements are recognized as preventive measures, hormone, megavitamin, and herbal therapies are controversial and unproven. Both the patient and the physician bring biases and values to the discussion of anti-aging medicine, and that combination will influence the treatment decisions.

Callahan, D. (1995). Aging and the life cycle: A moral norm? In: Callahan, D., ter Meulen, R.H.J., and Topinkova, E., eds. *A World Growing Old: The Coming Health Care Challenges*. Washington, DC: Georgetown University Press, pp. 20–27.

There must be a reciprocal relationship between medicine and aging. Callahan presents two models of the goals of medicine and the response to aging. In the first model, progressive incrementalism, there are no intrinsic biological limits in the progress toward extension of life expectancy and compression of morbidity. Culture should focus on the possibilities of individual development in the elderly rather than seeing older persons as a discrete group with shared characteristics and boundaries. Without a goal, this model is meaningless: it does not help us make sense of the place of aging in human life. In the second goal, life cycle traditionalism, medicine helps people remain in good health "within the boundaries of a finite life span and to help them cope well with the poor health they may have" (p. 23). Aging is not a disease but a condition to ameliorate. It is valid to think of the elderly as a group for policy purposes, since one could make valid generalizations to help them and to limit entitlements. This model critiques the ambivalence of what old age means in today's society, which has resulted in the aged person's loss of status in today's society. Life cycle traditionalism is the most promising way of making medical and human sense of aging because it is compatible with the results of efforts to overcome age-related disability. It does not see aging as a disease and recognizes age as a pertinent social category, allowing for the development of more equitable health policy. The goal of medicine should be to alleviate those conditions that rob old age of human meaning and social significance. Three values must be maintained as medical and social shifts occur: intergenerational reciprocity, the centrality of meaning in devising our ideals of old age, and moderate, clear medical goals for the care of the elderly.

Cetron, M. and Davies, O. (1998). *Cheating Death: The Promise and the Future Impact of Trying to Live Forever.* New York: St. Martin's Press.

Cetron is a well-known futurist and technological forecaster; Davies is a science writer. Assuming that anti-aging techniques will be available in the near future, they speculate on the impact that increased longevity will have on society. Although the projections are fairly specific, there are no references; the book is intended for a general audience. The projections are placed in the immediate rather than the remote future (mostly concerning 2000–2030) and focus primarily on economics and labor. In particular, they suggest that the fiscal difficulties of Social Security and the size of the baby boom generation will result in a *post-mortal revolution* that will include significant changes in our ideas of retirement. Tensions will be exacerbated in ethnic politics, between generations, in the labor market, and in relations with poorer nations. Compression of morbidity will result in the decline of the health-care industry. Five challenges of the *peri-mortal* world are adequate incomes for all people, modernization of "backward" nations, environmental reform, population control, and the search for new meaning when immortality becomes possible. The book contains two appendices: 74 trends for a post-mortal America and 50 trends for a post-mortal world covering education, labor, values, family, and institutions. Several of these predictions have already proven untrue, and some contradict each other, but other ideas are still interesting, such as reduced class disparities, greater value on cooperation, community, and the family, and greater risks of terrorism.

Cole, T.R. and Thompson, B. (2001–2002). Introduction: Anti-aging: Are you for it or against it? *Generations*, 24(4), 6–8.

Aging is "an offense to the reign of biotechnology and to postmodern dreams." Extended aging offers opportunities to become more fulfilled as human beings. The term *anti-aging* is antagonistic and forces people to choose whether they are for or against their "very existence as biological and temporal beings."

de Grey, A.D.N.J., Baynes, J.W., Berd, D., Heward, C.B., Pawelec, G., and Stock, G. (2002). Is human aging still mysterious enough to be left only to scientists? *Bioessays*, 24(7), 667–676.

Given recent research that indicates that reversing (not just retarding) the key components of mammalian aging may be possible in mice in the next decade, challenging the traditional consensus among biogerontologists dismissing such a scenario, serious public debate on the possibility of human anti-aging is now warranted. Reversing aging may have fewer side effects than retarding aging, although some aspects of aging may be more difficult to reverse. Extrapolation from the past indicates a continuing trend of postponing the age of death. Among biogerontologists there is resistance to predictions of life extension because of fears that it will increase periods of age-related morbidity, wariness of raising false hopes, and the association of such claims with anti-aging quackery. In addition, there is apprehension regarding overpopulation, the quality of extended life, and political and distributive justice. However, these arguments are inconclusive, and the moral and social issues and questions need to be considered and debated more fully by the public in preparation for the possibility that such technology will become widely available.

Fins, J.J. (1999). Death and dying in the 1990s: Intimations of reality and immortality. *Generations*, 23(1), 81–87.

This article focuses on the issues of assisted suicide, the right-to-die movement, and efforts to improve end-of-life care in the 1990s through research, legislation, and education. The conflict over the alternative view to the acceptance of human finitude (controlling one's death as a personal prerogative) will become even more contentious with scientific progress. This tension is a healthy one, however, which will help reconcile the desire for good health and for a good death.

Fukuyama, F. (2002). *Our Posthuman Future: Consequences of the Biotechnology Revolution*. New York: Farrar, Straus & Giroux.

This book by Fukuyama, a prominent and controversial scholar who has written extensively on international political economy and social capital in modern economic life, is an influential work that critiques the potential of biotechnology to fundamentally change human nature and society. Comparing visions of the future in Orwell's *1984* and Huxley's *Brave New World*, Fukuyama argues that the most significant threat of biotechnology is its potential to alter human nature and thus move us into a *posthuman* stage of history. Despite debate, human nature exists, is meaningful, and provides stability and continuity to our experience as a species. Because human nature shapes and constrains the possible kinds of political regimes, reshaping it through technology may have consequences for politics. Medical technologies may offer a devil's bargain: providing long life at the cost of some measure of humanity.

The first part of the book looks at what may potentially occur in medical science and the immediate consequences. Increasing knowledge of the brain and the sources of human behavior, even in the absence of technology to use it, will have important political implications, as it already has with intelligence, crime, and sexuality in the nature–nurture debates. Neuropharmocology and the manipulation of emotions and behavior, through drugs such as Prozac and Ritalin, demonstrate the ethical ambivalence regarding the use and criminalization of drugs that artificially enhance normal behavior or simply help one feel good. Political implications include increased disparity between wealthy and poor nations, the feminization of the voting population, the breakup of age-graded hierarchies, and the lengthening of power regimes. Political, social, and intellectual changes will occur much more slowly. Increasing life expectancies will also prolong disease and a national nursing home scenario will emerge, characterized by increasing loneliness, fewer family ties, and the view of death as an evil. Genetic engineering will follow genetic screening and human cloning, leading to designer babies and, consequently, skewed sex ratios, eugenics programs, and population-level changes. Objections to human genetic engineering, aside from fears of state-sponsored eugenics programs, are based on religion, utilitarian considerations, and philosophical principles.

Human nature is central to our understanding of right and wrong. Human rights rest on a concept of nature based on species-typical (genetic rather than environmental) behavior. The traditional concept of human nature has been critiqued in terms of there being no significant true human universals. Human physical appearance and behavior are shaped more by environment than by genetics, and humans are cultural creatures who have different natures, depending on their circumstances. In contrast to the tabula rasa model, there are innate human emotional responses that guide the formation of moral ideas. Finally, departing from the free-market capitalism Fukuyma endorsed in his previous work, he argues that a regulatory framework is needed to separate legitimate and illegitimate uses of biotechnology (as decided by democratically elected politicians, as well as scientists). There needs to be an international consensus on the control of biotechnology.

Hackler, C. (2001–2002). Troubling implications of doubling the human life span. *Generations*, 25(4), 15–19.

Hackler reviews the potential social issues and consequences of an increased life span, such as access to the anti-aging treatment, impact on the increasing divorce rate, and impact on family and work. New careers would be required, and power may be consolidated. There will also be an impact on the penal system and the right-to-die movement. Any human intervention should be strictly incremental (i.e., a 20-year extension) for the first several generations to allow social and political adaptations to take place at a gradual pace.

Haigh, R. and Bagaric, M. (2002). Immortality and sentencing law. *Journal of Philosophy, Science, and Law, 2.* Retrieved October 8, 2002 at http://www. pslijournal.com/archives/papers/immortality.html

The purpose of this article is to inform lawyers of the inevitable prospect of immortality and the consequent need to develop and refine legal principles to deal with this possibility. The authors focus in particular on the potential impact of immortality on criminal sentencing. Although there are some potential ethical and moral objections to immortality (e.g., it is inherently objectionable or will have undesirable social consequences), the desire for it will be so strong that people will aggressively seek anti-aging technology. Sentencing law and practice will need to change to account for greater longevity to maintain proportionality; for example, longer imprisonment will be needed to account for a longer life span. The severity of crimes may also change: an injury or property offence may be less significant but a homicide may be more so, given the changed nature and availability of time.

Harris, J. (2000). Intimations of immortality. *Science,* 288(5463), 59.

Harris, a bioethicist, discusses the prospect of scientifically achieved immortality and challenges the reasons critics of such a scenario propose. Because such technology would be available only to a few, the new *immortals* would be a small minority living among *mortals,* but criticisms based on justice, morality, and intergenerational conflicts are not completely convincing. Since it is unlikely that the progression to life extension or immortality can be stopped, and the ethical objections do not hold up, society should rather think about how to live with such a prospect.

Harris, J. and Holm, S. (2002). Extending human life span and the precautionary paradox. *Journal of Medicine and Philosophy,* 27(3), 355–368.

A precautionary approach to scientific progress of the sort advanced by Walter Glannon with respect to life-extending therapies involves both incoherence and irresolvable paradox. The authors demonstrate the incoherence of the precautionary approach in many circumstances and argue that, with respect to life-extending therapies, we have at present no persuasive reasons for a moratorium on such research.

Hayflick, L. (2000). The future of aging. *Nature,* 408, 267–269.

Because aging is not a disease, understanding the major causes of death in old age will not tell us much about the fundamental biology of changes with age, distinguishing between gerontology and geriatrics. Aging is not a programmed process governed directly by genes. Increasing the life span with a pill would bring up questions of the ideal age and the nature of interpersonal relationships. Arresting aging should be seen in the same light as arresting development in childhood—as serious pathology. It will also not be an attractive option to the poor, sick, or oppressed. A natural increase in the life span is occurring slowly. We must learn that aging and youth should be valued equally so that youth in the developed countries can experience that which they hold in low esteem. Thus, the anti-aging movement will be shown to be a superficial coverup for an irreversible process and a waste of money. Biogerontologists need to emphasize that the goal is to increase active longevity rather than increase longevity regardless of consequences.

Holstein, M.B. (2001–2002). A feminist perspective on anti-aging medicine. *Generations*, 25(4), 38–43.

Anti-aging will lead to further cultural devaluation of women's bodies and reinforce the idea that a woman's worth should be judged by her appearance and caretaking. Older women will experience negative effects of anti-aging more forcefully than will men, but will be judged or blamed if they choose not to accept the intervention. Marketing will target middle-aged women because they experience more discontent with their bodies. Like childbirth and menopause, aging of women will be medicalized. Continued living will not be desirable for women if they work in low-wage, physically taxing, and boring positions.

Juniper, D. F. (1974). *Man Against Mortality, or Seven Essays on the Engineering of Man's Divinity.* New York: Charles Scribner's Sons.

Juniper, an educational psychologist, speculates on how human immortality might be achieved and what that might mean. Contemporary attitudes toward the choice to live longer or forever are examined through a questionnaire: most would refuse an existence without a body, fearing loss of identity and lack of free will, in addition to fearing eugenics, boredom, and intergenerational conflict. Despite this, he concludes, after reviewing the technology and models for aging, that technologies that *upload* the brain may be the best approach to personal immortality. Societal implications include the need for a long-term contraceptive or mass medication, a legal framework to prevent exploitation of natural people by immortals with huge accumulations of wealth, an ambivalent relationship between mortals and immortals, and a shift in the meaning of marriage. Immortality might mean emancipation from uniqueness, death, cults, and religion. Possible sources of anxiety are the sense of self as unlimited and endless, increased dependence on technology, and a greater tendency toward recriminations and regrets due to greater responsibility for the future. However, immortals would have greater pleasure of future participation (being able to see the consequences of their work), may be more creative, and have a stronger commitment to the Earth and a greater degree of self-knowledge.

Kass, L. (1983). The case for mortality. *The American Scholar*, 52(2), 173–191.

Kass argues for mortality in light of scientific potential to achieve immortality or extend the life span. Such interventions would impact the entire population, and while they may be positive on the individual level, they will be disruptive and undesirable on higher levels. Intergenerational conflict and employment changes will result in people being worse off during most of their lives. Even a modest prolongation of life with vigor or preservation of youth with no increase in longevity would make death even less acceptable and would increase the desire to keep pushing it away. Individual dangers include boredom and tedium, lack of meaning/seriousness, loss of beauty, and loss of nobility. Mortality makes life matter: recognition of beauty requires the recognition of its fleetingness, and moral courage and virtue are possible only though detachment from the needs of survival. The interest in immortality is based not so much on longing for deathlessness as for wholeness and wisdom. The longing cannot be satisfied by prolonging human life; no amount of more of the same will satisfy our aspirations. Once we accept mortality, we can concern ourselves with living well rather than longer. To covet a longer life is both a sign and a cause of our failure to open ourselves up to a higher purpose.

Kass, L. (2003). Ageless bodies, happy souls: Biotechnology and the pursuit of perfection. *The New Atlantis: A Journal of Technology and Society, 1.* Retrieved May 6, 2003 from http://www.thenewatlantis.com/archive/1/kassprint.html

Kass methodologically critiques the attempts of biotechnology to prevent aging and mortality in a number of ways. The semantic device of making a distinction between *therapy* and *enhancement* does not solve the moral question, since human beings are by nature frail and finite. Three obvious objections include fears of its implications for health and safety, social inequity, and freedom. However, Kass objects to the essence of the activity rather than its consequences: the goodness of the ends, the fitness of the means, and the meaning of science's desire to *master* aging or death. There can be no such thing as full escape from our own (human and mortal) nature; to attempt to do so may be hubristic. While social and personal attempts to enhance oneself demonstrate one's own work, biomedical means prevent the subject from understanding the meaning of the effects in human terms: the subject has no role at all. Human experience then is mediated by unintelligible forces and vehicles separated from broader human significance. What is impeded is the human-being-in-the-world experience. Finally, there are many human goods that are inseparable from aging, mortality, and the natural human cycle: engagement, beauty, virtue. With regard to pharmacological drugs, he suggests that there is something misguided about the pursuit of psychic tranquility: guilt, shame, and painful memories may be appropriate and real. Furthermore, happy feelings are not the essence of human flourishing; the possibility of unhappiness is what makes genuine happiness possible.

Katz, S. (2001–2002). Growing older without aging? Positive aging, anti-ageism, and anti-aging. *Generations,* 25(4), 27–32.

Most chronological and generational boundaries that characterize the different stages of life have become blurred. The modern life course of industrial standardization and age-specific institutions that characterized the nineteenth century has changed into a postmodern life course organized around the priorities of a consumer culture. Positive aging outlooks tend to overlook the overwhelming poverty, illness, loneliness, and marginalization that characterize the lives of most elderly persons. So-called positive agendas based on activity devalue traditionally important values such as wisdom and disengagement by turning them into problems of inactivity and dependency.

Ludwig, F.C. (Ed.). (1990). *Life Span Extension—Consequences and Open Questions*. New York: Springer.

This collection of essays approaches the consequences of life span extension on three levels: (*1*) what current gerontology has accomplished and what can be realistically accomplished in the foreseeable future; (*2*) what the societal implications are, including ethical dilemmas for health-care providers, economic implications, and impact on law and on the form and function of kin groups; and (*3*) what the philosophical implications are, including who will benefit (current people, future people, or the human species). Using a model of decelerated aging, the essays supplement the biological approach and provide guidance in research, policy, and care. Although aging can treated as a disease, it is not.

Several essays examine the societal implications of life extension, specifically in the kinship group as care providers (aging alone will be more prevalent), in economics (the health and capacity to work of the aged must be improved, and limits that reduce their income must be removed), in the law (the distribution of assets to members of society who no longer contribute), and in policy. Ultimately, the book recommends against the development of an anti-aging drug, because one must be guided by the concern for the greater good over time, and thus it takes into account the interests of future generations. The period of old age is a time for the "discovery of an interior life" (p. 150) and the potential for transcendence. It is better to face old age and death with dignity than to continue to surround it with fear.

Moody, H.R. (1995). The meaning of old age: Scenarios for the future. In: Callahan, D., ter Meulen, R.H.J., and Topinková, E, eds. *A World Growing Old: The Coming Health Care Challenges*. Washington, DC: Georgetown University Press, pp. 9–19.

In this brief chapter, Moody presents four scenarios that define different approaches to the meaning of old age and the policy and resource allocation implications of these alternatives. Old age no longer has a fixed meaning, and public policy must take seriously a variety of ideas about what constitutes *good* old age. The author breaks down these scenarios neatly in a comparative table summarizing the key idea, origin, current impact, and policy.

(*1*) Prolongation of morbidity: the meaning of old age is defined by quality of life, so allocation policies favor determining treatment on the basis of quality (i.e., euthanasia). Heroically (though pessimistically) returning death to individual responsibility by self-imposed limits, this scenario has been advocated by Stoics and existentialists. (*2*) Compression of morbidity: there is a fixed limit to life, but old age can be made *successful*, so research and health promotion that delay morbidity are favored. Optimistic about old age, it finds hope within limits. (*3*) Prolongevity: aging is a disease that can be revised, and resources should be directed to basic aging research.

Life extension, however, would exacerbate all social inequalities. (*4*) Recovery of the life world: the meaning of old age is found in the finitude of life, to be accepted through collective action (not individual choice) and intergenerational concern. Resource allocation would favor research defined as appropriate insofar as it supports the values of the life world. Inequity would also be intensified, as some individuals would have access to available life extension. The *natural life course* argument is inadequate because what is considered natural in aging is constructed, contested, and problematic.

Moody, H.R. (2001–2002). Who's afraid of life extension? *Generations*, 25, 33–37.

Moody outlines common arguments on both sides of the anti-aging debate, including futility, quackery, side effects, diversion of scarce resources, prolonged disability, ecological balances, boredom, and the virtues of aging. Referring to the fictional Makropoulous Case (where the bored heroine turns down further life extension after 300 years) and to the Struldbruggs (*Gulliver's Travels'* life-prolonged but disability-plagued elderly), he suggests that whether we endorse life extension technology or not, we need to begin thinking about its consequences, since the science will probably expand whether we want it to or not.

Murphy, T. (1986). A cure for aging? *Journal of Medicine and Philosophy*, 11(3), 237–255.

Aging does not have to be classified as a disease in order for biomedicine to attend to it; medicine concerns itself with many other areas and issues that are not considered pathological states. The better approach to addressing aging in medicine is to ask whether there is good reason to want to eliminate or prevent aging. Broad interest in the person's well-being (i.e., a normative vision of medicine) might be enough to justify efforts to limit or eliminate aging. The question of its desirability rests on moral and metaphysical questions and guidelines. Aging and death have been interpreted as conditions for meaningful human life; therefore, it is not death or aging that is objectionable, but how one lives one's life. One must ask if longer or eternal life would ameliorate the human condition.

Overall, C. (2003). *Aging, Death, and Human Longevity: A Philosophical Inquiry*. Berkeley: University of California Press.

Overall dissects the arguments against prolongevity and concludes that they do not hold up. Systematic and clear, this is an excellent review of the philosophical questions and arguments regarding life extension. Ultimately, because many people do not have the opportunity to live their lives fully (particularly women), more life can be a good thing, and life extension may be an opportunity that should not be broadly rejected. The proponents of apologism failed to make an adequate case for accepting the life span as it is and for rejecting extension efforts. Such critics are mistaken when they insist that human life should not be broadly prolonged: their generalizations about aging and the value of extended life are unjustified. None of the arguments for a duty to die are successful: dying is not a duty even if we may be a burden to others, although there are situations in which there is a duty to die. Overall advocates prolongevitism because most people want to live longer, many have been deprived of life's goods, this life is the only one we have, and more life offers the prospect of more experience and action. The potential for boredom is neither unavoidable nor inevitable.

Rosenfeld, A. (1976). *Prolongevity*. New York: Alfred A. Knopf.

Rosenfeld, a science journalist, reviews the science and potential of anti-aging techniques. Aimed a lay audience, the book explores the scientific theories to explain why aging occurs and the evidence for potential techniques to eventually extend the life span and eliminate aging, which seems likely to be possible in the future.

Consequences of eternal life include immortality as a curse, loss of a sense of adventure and risk, stagnation, boredom, overpopulation, and state control of eugenics or population control programs. Profound changes are likely to occur at the personal, community, and national levels; even modest life extension would likely affect retirement. Intergenerational conflicts would increase, and death may be feared even more. Questions arise about access to life extension, how to end extended life, the relationship between the long- and short-lived, redefinitions of life and death, and human relationships. Nevertheless, gerontological research should be supported because it is probably inevitable and certainly desirable. Benefits of life extension include motivation to care about the future, the likelihood that today's values of right and wrong will still be honored in the future, and more time for greater achievements.

Stock, G. (2002). *Redesigning Humans: Our Inevitable Genetic Future.* Boston and New York: Houghton Mifflin.

Stock, a biophysicist who has written extensively on genetic engineering, examines the emerging reproductive technologies for selecting and altering human embryos, which culminate in germline engineering. Their advent will change evolution by transforming reproduction into a highly selective social process, ultimately leading to something that is posthuman and offering therapeutic enhancement, including arresting aging. Their increasing prevalence will result in difficult personal decisions about what is best for children and what risks are acceptable. The rapid technology-driven processes will result in transforming the range of what is human by expanding our diversity, although it is uncertain whether this will separate and isolate us. The impact of this transformation will hinge on who has access to these processes. A free market environment with real individual choice, modest oversight, and robust mechanisms to allow us to learn quickly from mistakes will protect society from potential abuses and channel resources to the proper goals.

Chapter 5 is of particular interest because it posits anti-aging technology as a potential example of the first human enhancement with widespread appeal; thus, the course of these procedures may shape more general attitudes toward biological enhancement and genetic modification. The social implications could include class conflict and intergenerational differences, greater inequity and unequal access, and the need to reorient biological drives to the elongated arc at the life span. Human growth hormone supplementation is an example of how people will eagerly take up anti-aging drugs. Because traditional testing would require long periods of time, the best route, given its probable popularity, would be to provide existing users with information on potential risks and involve them in voluntary trials, taking advantage of the massive self-experimentation. Such a procedure is not necessarily morally problematic; it may enrich society by preventing death and pain and by retaining wisdom and education.

van Tongeren, P. (1995). Life extension and the meaning of life. In: Callahan, D., ter Meulen, R.H.J., and Topinková, E., eds. *A World Growing Old: The Coming Health Care Challenges*. Washington, DC: Georgetown University Press, pp. 28–38.

The author, a philosopher, argues that the questions of life extension are not just about whether it is desirable, but why. The desire for life extension is universal, rather than a recent phenomenon, suggesting that we desire something about life itself. Stock critiques Callahan's *natural life span* because his criterion is subjective, and to normalize the definition is problematic and ahistorical. This construct is useful to determine the conditions for meaningful lives, but it does not answer the question of a natural end to life or to the meaning of life. The desire for life extension may in fact be an effort to escape death. For some philosophers, the meaning of life is the meaning of a finite and mortal existence: life must be oriented in mortality. Others view death as proof of the meaninglessness of life, which may bring a kind of relief. For example, Epicurius taught that fear of death was based on the mistaken idea that life and death were somehow connected, while Stoics taught indifference to that which is beyond our power. Part of our resources should be used to reflect on the meaning of life, rather than on the question of aging and prolongation of life. Rather than avoiding death, we should think of it in order to understand more about what life is.

Veatch, R. (Ed.). (1979). *Life Span: Values and Life-Extending Technologies*. San Francisco: Harper & Row.

This edited volume provides a comprehensive overview of the ethical and policy issues that accompany scientific efforts towards life extension. The contributors examine and propose guidelines for such research and the values that they promote. The questions of a *natural* death and of aging as a disease are debated. Issues of justice, freedom and uncertainty, and suicide and euthanasia are also examined.

Literature and Mythology (Secondary Analyses)

Bransom, S. (1994). The "curse of immortality": Some of the philosophical implications of Bram Stoker's *Dracula* and Anne Rice's *Interview with the Vampire*. *Popular Culture Review*, 5(2), 33–41.

The vampires of Bram Stoker and particularly of Anne Rice offer a different perspective on the nature of undeath and a new secular attitude toward immortality: even without a belief in an afterlife, everlasting life on earth is undesirable. Rice's Louis tells his story of becoming a vampire in order to discourage others from doing the same. While vampire life is the same as human life, with the same emotions, vampires mostly feel lonely: although they could live forever, they do not want to, often committing suicide because they are afraid of change. Immortality is a curse: vampires long for close relationships that are rarely realized, and experience sexual pleasure that does not result in happiness. Like human existence, vampire life is a state of confusion and longing in which individuals don't wish to die but don't want to live forever either. The secret to happiness is not in longevity but in self-forgiveness and self-love.

Bronstein, C. (2002). Borges, immortality and the circular ruins. *International Journal of Psychoanalysis*, 83(3), 647–660.

Drawing on two short stories by Jorge Borges and a case study based on 5 years of psychoanalysis, the author suggests that the compulsive search for immortality is rooted in the inability to handle the mental pain of ordinary human vulnerability and loss (death). Immortality is here pursued symbolically and metaphorically rather than literally, through daydreams of invulnerability instead of actual interest in life extension. These represent fantasies of ridding the self of emotional pain and fear, and a denial of the significance of time, separation, and difference from others. The individual's dissociation from feeling triumphs over awareness of pain, resulting in guilt, fear of death, and further withdrawal. Individuals become trapped in these "circular ruins" by a death drive that compels them to avoid the psychic pain of time, change and difference (individuality), and the "unconscious choice of narcissistic omnipotence as against awareness of psychic reality." Becoming a mere ghost of a person is a relief but also a humiliation and terror, as this state is self-destructive and static. Borges' characters eventually realize that this latter state may be worse than physical death, giving up the search for immortality to recover their specific, particular destiny (identity) and write, achieving literary immortality: "awareness of transience . . . increases the value of life."

Clark, S.R.L. (1995). *How to Live Forever*. London and New York: Routledge.

A philosopher examines the ways in which science fiction writers have imagined immortality. Recent philosophical work has dealt with issues of personal identity in resurrection or disembodied survival, the moral meanings of hopes or fears for immortality, theories that computers could imitate the mind, and the prospect of genetic engineering, transplants, anti-aging drugs, and other devices for prolonging life. The objections against wanting to live forever—inability to do so, possibility of prolonged senescence, threat of loss, boredom, inability to mature, and the (unnecessary) wish for more—are shown to be at least partly answerable, and are countered by positive reasons such as love of life and the desire to transcend set limits. Eternal life, however, requires a transformation of this life, not just continuance.

Clark presents several models for immortality, and their potential consequences and philosophical implications. Continued corporeal life brings up questions of bodily continuity and identity when immortality involves many different bodies, either cloned or duplicated. In the model of uploaded life, the elimination of the body could result in more control (although these worlds often move out of our control) and progression to a more evolved (godlike) noncorporeal state. But is a set of programs, even with memories and personalities, true continuity? The vampire model suggests that (corporeal) immortal societies would work through transformation and a greater understanding of humans' dual nature. The Byzantium model (immortality via permanent achievement) imagines immortal life as productive and worthwhile through pleasure, beauty, and creativity.

The later chapters are increasingly philosophical, reflecting on such topics as identity, time travel, and resurrection. Immortal life comes from increasing identification with a ruling passion and decreasing need to linger in the mundane world. The possibility of an *overmind*, in which the immortal one incorporates everyone into segments of its own being (analogous to beehives), again demonstrates the concern for shifting the boundaries of identity. Clark concludes that goal of immortality is "an unpleasant mirage" (p. 184).

Fortunati, V. (1998). Aging and utopia through the centuries. *Aging Clinical and Experimental Research*, 10, 77–82.

In this brief survey of literary utopias, old age—closely associated with death and illness—has always been problematic for utopians. Fortunati identifies three issues: (*1*) Utopians have always found old age, illness, and death problematic since they represent the failure to simplify anthropological complexity. (*2*) The tension in utopia between the desire to return to Edenic purity and an obsession with planning and control results in an ambivalent attitude toward the old as both wise and a problematic element of deterioration and disorder. (*3*) Utopia reflects the ambivalent attitude toward the elderly, positioning them as double figures. The author focuses on works of three periods: classic antiquity (More's *Utopia*), modernity (Swift's *Gulliver's Travels*), and Morris' *News from Nowhere*, as well as a comparative approach from LeGuin.

In More, the role of old people is to moderate the ardor and insolence of the young by making them profit from their experience, but when the old are not self-sufficient, common good must prevail over the individual, so they either commit suicide or are convinced to do so by priests. Swift's Struldbruggs demonstrate cultural aging, the difficulty of finding one's way in a system of unknown signs, posing a central question of the twentieth century: what is the role of the elderly when they are no longer the repository of knowledge in a society dominated by the idea of progress? In Morris, old age is not a biological fact but a cultural event whose quality depends on the collectivity's way of living, age being relative. Thus, in culturally and morally healthy societies (noncapitalistic), the old age more slowly. In LeGuin's work, old people are creative and dynamic, have well-integrated roles, and dialogue and interchange with young people. Old people can make important contributions, initiate change, and establish new meaning even in their final stages of life. Old age must be prevented in its negative aspects and actively lived. It should also be approached from a transcultural perspective.

Graham, E. (2002). *Representations of the Post/Human*. New Brunswick, NJ: Rutgers University Press.

This book does not deal with anti-aging or immortality per se, but with one of the central issues of anti-aging technology: the potential loss of humanity as digital, cybernetic, and biomedical technologies play increasing roles in one's bodily experience. The most definitive representations of human identity are in Western biotechnoscience and science fiction. New technologies have complicated the question of what it means to be human in several ways: the technologization of nature (cloning), the blurring of species boundaries, technologization of human bodies and minds, creation of new personal and social worlds, and redrawn boundaries between tools, bodies, and environments. However, technology is also seen as enhancing lives, relieving suffering, and facilitating human evolution. Responses fall along a continuum, from disenchantment to transhumanism and reenchantment. In particular, the author critiques the ideology of transcendence invoked in the representations of the post/human.

Technoscience and the genres of science fiction, myth, and literature provide narratives of what it means to be human. In the tradition of teratology, monsters delineate the faultlines of exemplary and normative humanity. Elements of Mary Shelley's *Frankenstein* and the Golem myth remain vital images for current debates about the nature of scientific inquiry, the potential and limits of powerful and creative personalities, and the gendered nature of technological endeavors. As marginal figures they demonstrate the hopes, fears, and anxieties surrounding humanity's engagement with its technologies.

The biotechnological, cybernetic, and digital age has prompted a recognition that humanity has always coevolved with its environment, tools, and technologies, suggesting a model of post/humanity that is bound up in relationality, affinity, and contingency. We need a reflexive model rather than the polarized responses to technology; ideological or reductionist representations reify assumptions about normative humanity at the expense of excluding others.

Lenker, L.T. (1999). Why? versus Why not?: Potentialities of ageing in Shaw's *Back to Methuselah*. In: Deats, S.M. and Lenker, L.T., eds. *Aging and Identity: A Humanities Perspective*. Westport, CN: Praeger, pp. 47–59.

George Bernard Shaw's play *Back to Methuselah* questions the accepted norms of the aging process. Written as a social commentary on the late Victorian controversies concerning the role and needs of the aging population, such as old-age pensions, the play critiques the ingrained idea that aging is inevitable and negative. The "Why not" of the article's title refers to the idea that experiences of old age are socially constructed, not biologically determined, and thus can be changed. The central theme is the human life span. For example, Adam arbitrarily sets the life span at 1000 years in order to resolve the paradox of mortal existence (the desire for immortality along with the tediousness of eternal life), while Eve contemplates the question of how much time is enough in life in order to accomplish things. In a following discussion, a group of experts suggest that humanity has devolved, and that an average life span of 300 years would be a more adequate maturation period for humans. The intergenerational conflicts that may result when people do live to such great ages include discouragement for the short-livers, especially when they interact with long-livers, which should be guarded against, since while years can be voluntarily added, one needs stamina to prevail. While long life will introduce difficulties and detriments such as lack of mutual appreciation for those at different stages of life, long-livers also embrace the emancipatory possibilities of old age. Human existence will evolve toward pure thought and reason, effectively eliminating the ravages of age on the body.

Mangum, T. (2002). Longing for life extension: Science fiction and late life. *Journal of Aging and Identity*, 7(2), 69–82.

Most science fiction treatments of immortality assume the consequences of suffering, loneliness, and boredom (the Tithonus myth). The author looks at science fiction rejuvenescence stories (regression to and prolongation of youth) which teasing out the consequences for reversing the aging process. These novels question the fundamental nature of loss. It involves adjustment of expectations, but this is a condition for living well through life stages rather than incarcerating oneself in anger, denial, or oblivion. In other words, attachment to youth is a trap, while acceptance of aging is a release. Rejuvenescence narratives, popular at the end of the nineteenth century, had two main plots, the *bildungsroman* (which traces a character from childhood to the advent of adulthood, like *Oliver Twist*) and the marriage plot (which marked early adulthood as the most interesting time in life). The origins of science fiction include anxiety about technological interventions in the human life span, as in *Frankenstein*. Bruce Sterling's novel *Holy Fire*, in which good citizens are rewarded with life extension while rebels are condemned to natural aging, is explored closely. The youth achieved by the gerontocrats, however, is a paradox because they have lost their humanity in the process. Joy is mistaken for youth but, like dressing young, the chemical simulation of youth cannot animate the essence of youth. All is that is left of youth is style rather than substance. The novel challenges the definition of old as simply not young. Rejuvenescence proves the bane of old age, since it is never a return to an earlier version of oneself. These narratives can also be seen as a mask for impatience with the elderly and their costs. Finally, the author argues that we employ these rejuvenscence fantasies even less self-consciously than the late Victorians or Sterling's gerontocrats in our use and popularity of anti-aging techniques.

Masing-Delic, I. (1992). *Abolishing Death: A Salvation Myth of Russian Twentieth-Century Literature.* Stanford, CA: Stanford University Press.

Early-twentieth-century Russian literature is reviewed for its representations of the immortalization myth, a vision of an earthly paradise where death has been conquered by science, art, and the fusion of multiple wills into One will. These works are not science fictions or utopias, but are set in contemporary Russian reality. Immortality is possible as a logical and natural outcome of a *war with death* by science, art, collective labor, and communal effort, not a fantastic dream that comes with divine grace. The immortal societies envisioned are analyzed primarily for their relation to religion and the ideologies of the Russian Revolution and Stalin, focusing on the philosophical justification of immortality. An overall salvation plan is identified, with negative parameters pointing to existing flaws that ensure the continued existence of death in the world (such as denigration of a False Deity for using death as a weapon) and positive parameters (such as the vision of the New World as a workshop where nature obeys human will) that indicate those conditions under which earthly immortality becomes reality. The immortality myth centers on the refusal to wait passively for death and humanity's readiness to shoulder the responsibility of its own salvation. The Soviet realist literature propagandized and popularized the myth of human immortality in the midst of Stalinist policies.

Roberts, M.M. (1993). "A physic against death": Eternal life and the Enlightenment—gender and gerontology. In: Roberts, M.M. and Porter, R., eds. *Literature and Medicine During the Eighteenth Century.* London and New York: Routledge, pp. 151–67.

The author looks at how eighteenth-century novelists portray gendered attitudes toward rejuvenation. The possibility of life extension became increasingly popular during the Enlightenment as a secular alternative to the more remote promise of spiritual immortality and a barometer of progress. The pursuit of longevity became an extensive commercial industry with the commoditization of various interventions, including elixirs and electroshock therapy. For some, extreme longevity was an appalling prospect that would interrupt the evolutionary path. Rejuvenation for men was often synonymous with increased sexual potency, possibly because it displaced fears of mortality, but for women, immortality was not linked to continued fertility. Although women tended to outlive men, aging was experienced as more negative due to the declining social value of women. Wollstonecraft in particular critiques men's valorization of female youth over female maturity. The *tyranny of the youth cult* may be interpreted as a means of undermining the power of mature women, whose sexual capacities are increasing at an age when men's are decreasing; the "lure of an elixir of youth serves to perpetuate the masculinist myth that women are disempowered by visible signs of aging" (p. 162).

Slusser, G., Westfahl, G., and Rabkin, E.S. (Eds.). (1996). *Immortal Engines: Life Extension and Immortality in Science Fiction and Fantasy.* Athens and London: The University of Georgia Press.

This collection of essays examines the use and meanings of immortality in science fiction and fantasy literature. Most of the essays, rather than focusing on individual works, look at the broad range of literary works and their use of a particular theme. There is a tension between immortality as negative (the Tithonus syndrome) and its attractiveness in future life. The first of the book part addresses approaches to immortality, including philosophical models. Myths about resurrection have interacted with the growth of medical technology to influence science fiction. Shaw's *Back to Methuselah* is set as a starting point for a hermeneutic study of writing about immortality as a reflection of an underlying class struggle. The next part examines aspects of science in immortality, such as the potential of cryonics and the possibility of living forever in a machine. The final, and longest, part of the book is a thematic examination of immortality in the literature, focusing not on the implications for eternal life, but on the process of writing and the context of the literature (the necessity of death in storytelling, feminist approaches, and children's literature).

Wagner, J. (1999). Intimations of immortality: Death/life mediations in *Star Trek*. In: Porter, J.E. and McLaren, D.L., eds. *Star Trek and Sacred Ground: Explorations of Star Trek, Religion, and American Culture*. New York: State University of New York Press, pp. 119–138.

This chapter looks at the way in which *Star Trek* uses secular narratives in a hypothetical future to blur and destabilize the boundaries and emotional valences of life/death. In contrast to traditional mythology, *Star Trek* uses the realm of science and natural law to pose various strategies for mediating between life and death, stressing the provisional nature of our metaphysical knowledge, proposing death as a contingent rather than a necessary part of life, and using the theme of resurrection to transform mortality into an elusive fact of life rather than an essential one. The ideas of multiple or parallel existences and the preservation of the human mind in technology question the finitude and reality of individual selves. The stories of androids, however, also normalize death as a potentially energizing aspect of life.

Yoke, C.B. and Hassler, D.M. (Eds.). (1985). *Death and the Serpent: Immortality in Science Fiction and Fantasy*. Westport, CT: Greenwood Press.

This book is a collection of essays on the treatment of physical immortality in science fiction and fantasy literature. Most chapters are specific treatments of one or two authors or works, rather than a general treatment of immortality in the genres a whole, including such contemporary and classic science fiction or fantasy authors as Heinlein, Tolkien, and Herbert. The last chapter is a compendium of works on immortality in science fiction. The essays map the "real existences in speculative fiction concerning the dystopias that result from extended longevity, the schemes for immortality, and the variations in the struggle against death" (p. 6). They explore the potential mechanisms for achieving longevity (drugs, transplants, fantasy) and the different forms life extension might take (radically increased life span to immortality), but seem to focus more on the implications of such possibilities for individuals, societies, and the human species. Most of the contributors observe ambivalence in writers' treatment of immortality or extreme longevity: it is an age-old human desire that comes with some price, most often one's humanity (exemplified alternately as empathy, morality, emotion, or sexuality). In fact, only one of the writers reviewed here envisions immortal life as distinctly positive. Many of the pieces can be read as explorations of the role or necessity of death and mortality, as demonstrated by the (imagined) failure of immortality; there is much less emphasis on the attitude toward youth or the aging process.

History

Achenbaum, W.A. (1995). *Crossing Frontiers: Gerontology Emerges as a Science.* New York: Cambridge University Press.

Achenbaum, a historian and gerontologist, argues in this well-researched history that gerontology did not emerge as an interdisciplinary scientific field of inquiry in the United States until the twentieth century. Tracing the origins of modern American gerontology from the colonial era to the early decades of the twentieth century, he describes the contributions of early pioneers such as Metchnikoff (who coined the term *gerontology* in 1908) and the diverse roots of modern American gerontology that led to methodological debates between the natural science and humanist perspectives.

Achenbaum highlights particular intellectual orientations and organizations within gerontology that emerged from the 1940s on, revealing the extent to which those early pioneers with a particular interest in aging were committed to empirical research, including longitudinal research, and how some academic traditions were used to develop a broader gerontological mission. Four case studies of institutional centers of academic research and writing illustrate how researchers from a range of disciplines interacted with one another and the persistence of earlier trends, including "balkanised interests and divided loyalties" that resulted in imbalances and uneven growth within interdisciplinary fields. After World War II, the increased scale and impact of the scientific enterprise in the United States provided new opportunities for researchers interested in aging. Gerontology emerged as a field of study rather than a scientific specialty. The interdisciplinary partnerships are fragile, and gerontology continues to be impeded by a lack of distinctive methods and shared understandings of the value of differing methodologies. However, by broadening its fields of vision and maintaining its interdisciplinary relationships, the field can continue to open new frontiers of knowledge on aging.

Gruman, G.J. (2003). *A History of Ideas About the Prolongation of Life.* New York: Springer.

In this influential and extensively researched monograph, Gruman, a historian, examines the history and evolution of theories and methods of life extension, coining the term *prolongevity* to indicate the significant extension of the life span by human action. This comprehensive work brings together data from a variety of fields, including mythology, religion, philosophy, and science, as well as history.

Each proponent of prolongevity has contended with apologist tendencies in most philosophical, scientific, and religious systems to accept old age and death as inevitable. These apologists argue against life extension on the basis of an inherent human inability to attain it, its perception as a violation of the natural or divine order, its undesirability due to extended old age, or the desirability of old age and death.

There is a great deal of legendary material expressing the human desire for prolonged life, including antediluvian myths, hyperborean themes, and fountain-type legends. Taoism moved prolongevity from the realm of magic into a stage of proto-science, forming life extension into an organized system of concepts and hypotheses. In contrast, life extension remained peripheral in Greek thought. Taoist practices influenced medicine and science, including gymnastic techniques, the use of pharmaceuticals, and alchemy, but was limited by primitivism and lack of objectivity. Alchemists such as Paracelsus attempted to develop elixirs of youth as well as find specific chemical remedies for particular diseases, which would eventually form the path toward modern biochemistry and chemotherapy. The personal hygiene tradition exemplified by Luigi Carnaro would give way to the ideas of social hygiene and public health in the nineteenth century. The Enlightenment thoughts on prolongevity expressed by Bacon, Franklin, Godwin, and particularly Condorcet, with his combination of optimism, objectivity, and sound methodology, would also influence the development of medicine and science.

Haber, C. (2001–2002). Anti-aging: Why now? A historical framework for understanding the contemporary enthusiasm. *Generations*, 25(4), 9–14.

Much like the fear in the early 1900s that the elderly were going to become a burden, today's fear that society cannot support an aged population has led to the resurgence of the characterization of aging as a disease against which society must fight.

Hamilton, D. (1986). *The Monkey Gland Affair*. London: Chatto & Windus.

This book provides a history of the testicle gland transplant doctors of the 1920s, focusing on Serge Voronoff, an orthodox doctor whose work on rejuvenating transplants was highly regarded in his time by both the public and the medical profession. While he did not pioneer the technique of using monkey testicle transplants in order to stop or reverse aging, he did promote and write extensively about it. The book details his life and how he and his work were eventually discredited. In particular, his direct appeals to the media, and the appropriation of his techniques by commercial quacks, helped discredit the procedures when the science failed to hold up.

Hirshbein, L.D. (1999). Masculinity, work and the fountain of youth: Irving Fisher and the Life Extension Institute, 1914–31. *Canadian Bulletin of Medical History*, 16(1), 89–124.

In 1914, the Progressive Era reformer Irving Fisher and the wealthy contractor Harold Ley founded the Life Extension Institute (LEI) to address the problems of American health. Until 1931, the LEI widely promoted its health maintenance program of annual physical examinations (mostly through life insurance companies) and health literature. Its advertised goal was to extend life without old age, and improve masculinity and good business practices through adherence to health principles. Its literature constructed a picture of healthy, vigorous, and efficient American working (middle-class) men that further separated manhood and old age. It emphasized the centrality of work and the ability to strive for ideal masculinity, and appropriated the language and urgency of the World War I effort. However, masculinity was also portrayed through the negative example of the racial/disabled other. Thus, "someone who succumbed to aging and degeneration could not be a real man" (p. 110). The opposition of physicians, the loss of life insurance clients, and the shift of physicians toward health maintenance and the treatment of disease contributed to LEI's eventual decline.

Hirshbein, L.D. (2000). The glandular solution: Sex, masculinity, and aging in the 1920s. *Journal of the History of Sexuality,* 9(3), 277–304.

The author examines the popular and medical discussions of surgical rejuvenation in the 1920s, particularly the ideal of masculinity that emerged from these discussions, and the eventual discrediting of these procedures by the popular press and the scientific community as quackery. Voronoff and Steinach attempted to augment surgically the production of the sex glands to renew youth and vitality, extrapolating from their work with rats to present masculinity as having the energy to have sex and compete with others. Old age was a series of negative experiences resulting in the loss of physical and mental health and the ability to function in one's personal and professional lives, while masculinity was connected to sexual prowess and youthful energy. At the same time, ideas of masculinity were in flux due to changes in economic structure and work conditions. Rejuvenators explicitly connected masculinity to sex and questioned the masculinity of older men, literally promising renewed masculinity. Finally, rejuvenators proposed their procedures as a way of supplying additional youthful energy, and its business implications, to the nation. Ultimately, the differences between the rejuvenators' assumptions about old age and about sex, as well as their status as Europeans, helped to discredit their procedures. Americans were uncomfortable with the public discussions of sexuality, as well as the model of sexualized old age, and were suspicious of the motivations of the European rejuvenators. The most consistent critique was that the rejuvenators used too much general publicity to promote their work. The rejuvenator model also did not fit with physicians' calls to tackle complicated diseases like cancer. By the 1930s surgical rejuvenation was no longer popular, and was condemned in the *Journal of the American Medical Association* as quackery. However, older men's relationship to sex remained an important topic in public and medical discussion. They lost the promise of rejuvenation but were "haunted by the specter of demasculinization in old age."

Katz, S. (1996). *Disciplining Old Age: The Formation of Gerontological Knowledge.* Charlottevilles and London: University Press of Virginia.

The aim of this book is to provide a critical analysis of gerontological knowledge as a discipline, with particular use of the Foucouldian theory, characterizing the search for universals about old age as a struggle, attempting to stabilize subjects (the aged) that are inherently indeterminate. This book does not address anti-aging per se, but it does explore how gerontology has maintained itself as a science and discipline of aging and how old age has become medicalized and problematized. In addition, Katz discusses the boundary work theories (relevant to gerontologists' attacks on anti-aging medicine). To achieve credibility, gerontologists portray their history in terms of medical advances, while premodern practitioners are cast as misguided, fanciful, and non-scientific. The positivist narrative reflects not the past but the present preoccupation with scientific progress. The historical transformation from premodern to modern perceptions of the aged body began with the reinterpretation of disease through a series of symptoms that portrayed the aged body as a symbol of separation from other groups. Four discursive tactics typified the dynamics of gerontology: establishing the position of gerontological researchers as experts, shaping a language of gerontology (use of scientific rhetoric, endorsement from other fields, etc.), building the disciplinary imperative, and debating the positive and negatives aspects of aging. Clinical works legitimated the aged body as a distinct subject; popular treatises continued to dramatize the idea that old age was a menace to society and national security; and multidisciplinary formats reflected on the new modern life course, connecting the medical conception of old age to such fields as psychology. Gerontologists should learn from their history and use it to deal with gerontology's lack of discipline—its role as a *nomad science* that is heterogeneous, indefinite, and potentially radical.

Lock, S. (1983). "O That I Were Young Again": Yeats and the Steinach operation. *British Medical Journal,* 287, 1964–1968.

After undergoing the reputedly rejuvenating Steinach operation (vasectomy), the poet W.B. Yeats experienced a creative and personal reawakening. This article reviews the circumstances in which this operation took place, both in Yeats' personal life and in medicine, and the link between Yeats' revived sexual desire and his relationship with the troubled Margot Ruddock. He concludes that medical treatment may improve the patient's physical condition at the expense of his spiritual life.

McGrady, P.M. (1968). *The Youth Doctors.* New York: Coward-McCann.

This detailed review, written by a journalist, of rejuvenation medicine at the time, was aimed at a popular audience. As such, it focuses on the personalities of the doctors who study/promote anti-aging medicine (often portraying them as visionaries rather than quacks) and their patients and is written in a casual, personal style. The last chapter, "The Respectables," is particularly interesting because it discusses the tension between the research gerontologists and the anti-aging practitioners, the debates over aging theories, and the politics of research funding. McGrady focuses primarily on contemporary rejuvenators, such as those working on cell therapy. His tone is optimistic rather than critical.

Sengoopta, C. (1993). Rejuvenation and the prolongation of life: Science or quackery? *Perspectives in Biology and Medicine*, 37(1), 55–66.

Although the rejuvenation doctors of the early twentieth century are now generally dismissed as quacks, and although their science was certainly flawed, much of their research was in line with accepted scientific theory of the time. The theories on aging and the therapies promoted by Metchnikoff (who popularized yogurt) and Voronoff (who conducted monkey gland transplants) were based on evolutionary biology, while Steinach's vasectomies were based on theories of blood circulation. Metchnikoff's theory of aging was immunological, based on the idea that the large intestine was an evolutionary leftover that produced toxins in the body, causing the decline of higher cells. Voronoff similarly saw the endocrine hormones as energizing and protecting the higher cells from destruction. While his use of monkey transplants is ridiculed, they were used because of their close evolutionary relationship with humans. For Steinach, the sex hormones were rejuvenating because they maintained blood circulation, which would nourish the tissues and restore their function.

Shapin, S. and Martyn, C. (2000). How to live forever: Lessons of history. *British Medical Journal*, 321, 1580–1582.

Although there has been a lot of hype recently about discovering the secret to immortality, such claims have been made since ancient times, pursued by philosophers such as Descartes and Bacon as well as by physicians. However, one should not try to live forever: it is both impossible and, as suggested by Montaigne, would not be worth the price (becoming even more afraid of death). Although philosophy has become separated from science, and although scientists' projections of what can be done to define societal goals, seeking technological solutions to suffering and death "impoverishes both our resolutions and fortitude as individuals and the collective resources that underpin them."

Trimmer, E.J. (1967). *Rejuvenation: The History of an Idea*. London: The Scientific Book Club.

This book is a review of the various methods, theories, techniques, and beliefs surrounding physical rejuvenation throughout history. It is more of a popular history than a critical discussion, although it is quite detailed and draws its data not only from historical records and media accounts, but also from myth, legend, and literature. It also contains many biographical accounts of individuals, as well as some discussion of the scientific backgrounds of the various methods.

There have been many plant remedies throughout history, including mandrake, saw palmetto, and orchids, but little is known in the scientific literature of the active ingredients that might explain their reputed effects. In contrast, the use of animal products has been much more extensive, and has been associated more with sexual (rather than general) rejuvenation. The 1920s and 1930s were the height of sexual/general rejuvenation through sex glands, although Brown-Sequard's injections of guinea pig testes, Steinach's vasoligations, and Voronoff's monkey gland transplants were eventually discredited. Water cures include the Roman baths, the myth of the Fountain of Youth, and spas in the nineteenth century. *Fringe rejuvenation methods*, or quackery, are defined as those methods that are commercial rather than altruistic or scientific in nature, and make claims of exotic origin, use medical status, and exploit recent scientific thought to sell such products as royal jelly and essential oils. Metchnikoff's use of yogurt became popular but was criticized when he associated himself with a commercial enterprise based on it, and it is now largely discounted. The book concludes with maintenance rejuvenation, which comes out of conventional science and consists of routine in-depth checkups (described in detail) and treatment of diseases or conditions (often nutritional deficiencies).

Wyndham, D. (2003). Versemaking and lovemaking—W.B. Yeats' "Strange Second Puberty": Norman Haire and the Steinach rejuvenation operation. *Journal of History of the Behavioral Sciences,* 39(1), 25–50.

After the poet Yeats underwent the popular Steinach operation (vasectomy) for rejuvenation, he experienced a burst of creativity. This paper documents the context for the operation, the life histories of the surgeon who conducted it and Yeats, and the consequences of the operation itself. Yeats believed that the operation was successful, rejuvenating his creativity, sexual ability, and sense of physical and psychological health. His rejuvenation was more likely due to the placebo effects of daily attention and psychological support he received from his personal physician.

Primary Literary Sources
on Prolongevity

....

Carol C. Donley

Images of Aging in Major Western Literature

Greek Myth of Geras (Roman name: Senectus). Source of the terms *geriatric, gerontology, senescent, senile, senator,* and *senior.*

The only elderly Greek god is Geras, a minor figure who was born of Nyx (Night) and Erebos (Darkness). His name means to grow ripe, as in geriatric "ripe old age." In the *Homeric Hymn V to Aphrodite*, he is referred to as "loathsome old age" and "harsh old age." But Geras rarely appears. Nearly all the gods and goddesses are young and beautiful or else a robust middle age (like Zeus).

Homer in *The Odyssey.*

Homer uses old age as a disguise for Odysseus when he returns home to deal with the suitors of his wife, Penelope. They do not fear the old filthy tramp, who has no "skills in tasks or in strength, but is just a burden on the land" (XX.289). The elderly suffer from weakness, poor eyesight and hearing, absentmindedness, and general aches and pains. Odysseus' father, Laertes, suffers from "raw old age." King Nestor, in his garrulous senility, keeps talking and talking until younger people have to escape from his presence. When Athena wants Odysseus or Laertes to be impressive, she makes them taller, stronger, and younger.

Beckett, S. (1959). *Krapp's Last Tape.* London: Faber and Faber.

Krapp is an old man, alone with his tape-recorded memories and commentaries made at earlier times in his life. He continually eats bananas, forgetting that he just ate one, and slips on the peels as if he were a slapstick clown. As he listens to his various earlier selves describing work or love or belief, he has trouble accepting the values and goals he once thought important. The dialogue between several of his past selves (on tape) and his present self helps him recognize that death is near, as he experiences a sense of loss and uncertainty about his identity.

Eliot, T.S. (1920). "Gerontian." *Collected Poems 1909–1962.* New York: Harcourt Brace Jovanovich.

T. S. Eliot's character Gerontian (Greek for "little old man") has lost most of his senses—touch, taste, smell, sight, and hearing—as well as his mental acuity. Like the environment, he is dried up, without the refreshment water might bring. "Here I am, an old man in a dry month,/ being read to by a boy, waiting for rain. . . . / I an old man/ A dull head among windy spaces."

Forster, E.M. (1947). *The Road from Colonus.* Cambridge: Alfred A. Knopf.

The elderly Mr. Lucas, on a trip to Greece with his daughter, Ethel, compares himself to Oedipus and Ethel to Antigone (from *Oedipus at Colonus*). He finds a cool stream flowing out of a hollow tree in which a small shrine was established. When he enters the hollow, he feels connected to the stream and to all the world. He refuses to leave this magical place, but on Ethel's orders, stronger people carry him to a mule, which trots away. Back in London, he degenerates into a whimpering old man. When his daughter discovers that they would have been killed had they stayed in that place, old Mr. Lucas can't even remember it and babbles on about hating the sound of running water.

Frost, R. [1916] (1995). An Old Man's Winter Night, In *Mountain Interval.* New York: Collectors Reprints.

The scene is an isolated farmhouse at night in New England; snow drifts against the door; icicles line the roof, and the windows are caked with frost. Outside in the dark, tree branches crack with the cold; inside, floorboards creak as an aged man shuffles from room to room. An ancient farmer living by himself and wandering around trying to remember what he is looking for finally falls asleep in his chair. He is alone and near death. The poem uses archetypal seasonal, daily, and life cycle imagery to portray old age as cold, dark, and useless.

Shakespeare, W. [1606] (1948). *King Lear.* New York: Harcourt Brace Jovanovich.

This great tragedy opens with the aged King Lear foolishly giving up his kingdom, dividing it among his three daughters according to which one can prove that she loves him the most. His willful contest provokes the two older daughters to lie about their love in order to get their rewards. When the youngest is honest, Lear reacts furiously, driving her out of the country. The demented old man finds himself unwanted and cast away by his older daughters. He calls himself "a poor, infirm, weak, and despised old man." He knows his "wits begin to turn" because his "two pernicious daughters joined . . . against a head so old and white as this." When his youngest, Cordelia, returns to him, Lear is not sure who she is at first: "Pray do not

mock me. I am a very foolish fond old man . . . I fear I am not in my perfect mind." The play explores the jealous greed of adult children who want
their father's wealth but not the responsibility of caring for him. It reveals
the impetuousness and dementia associated with old age and the heart-
breaking loss of a loved child.

Sophocles [fifth century B.C.E.] (1958). *Oedipus at Colonus*, trans. Paul
Roche. New York: New American Library.

Old and weary, Oedipus, long exiled from Thebes, stops by a sacred
grove near Colonus. The chorus, composed of old men from Athens, refer
to him as a poor old man. The chorus describes old age as a condition of
loss—loss of friends, of power, of love, of health, of dignity. Oedipus has an
additional problem: his memories are full of his own disastrous behavior—
incest and murder—so he has no consolation in looking back on his life. Citizens of Colonus say that "unregarded Old Age [is] joyless, companionless
and slow, of woes the crowning woe" (1225). When Oedipus realizes he is
going to die, he greets death eagerly.

Literature About Great Longevity

Genesis stories of the patriarchs.

According to Genesis, Methuselah lived 969 years and Noah lived 950
years. Biblical scholars debate about whether this record of longevity was
actually a confusion in calendars or translations, but whatever the case may
be, Methuselah has become synonymous with long life.

Greek myth of Tiresias.

Tiresias shows up in several myths and stories, including *Oedipus Rex*
and *The Odyssey*. He is a blind seer who has lived both as a woman and as a
man. One myth reports that he was blinded by Athena because he saw her
naked; because she could not restore his sight, she gave him the power of
prophecy, the ability to understand the birds, and a long life. Tennyson uses
this version of the myth in his poem *Tiresias*. Another version says that Zeus
and Hera argued about whether a man or a woman enjoyed sex more, and
because Tiresias had been both male and female, they asked him. His
answer enraged Hera, who blinded him; to compensate, Zeus gave him long
life and the power of a seer. His long life spanned the time from the founding of Thebes by Cadmus to the fight over it by Oedipus' sons.

He belongs with the wise old man archetype that includes Mentor;
Merlin; Yoda, the 900-year-old Jedi Master of *Star Wars*; Obi-Wan Kenobi;
Gandalf, the wizard in Tolkien's *Lord of the Rings*; and Dumbledore, the
headmaster of Hogwarts in the Harry Potter novels. Portraying rare positive images of old age, they are the sages and wizards, the wise ancients who
guide and teach the youth.

Legends of elves as long-living childlike creatures.

One tradition has elves born before the fall in the Garden of Eden
(children of Adam and Lillith) and therefore not subject to punishment by
death; on the other hand, they are not redeemable because they are not

part of the fallen and therefore are without the hope of heaven. They appear in Spenser's *Fairie Queene* and Shakespeare's *Midsummer Night's Dream*. In Tolkein's *Lord of the Rings* trilogy, the elves are sad, because they can suffer and see others suffer but they do not die. In *The Fellowship of the Ring*, Galadriel tells Frodo, "Through the ages of the world we have fought the long defeat" (462).

Bacon, F. [1626] (2002). *New Atlantis*. In: Vickers, B., ed. *Francis Bacon: The Major Works*. Oxford: Oxford University Press.

Bacon believes in the ability of science to learn nature's laws and use that information for solving problems. His utopian kingdom has discovered all kinds of useful technologies, from perpetual motion machines to ways of extending life. Longevity is best achieved by hermits who live some 3 miles underground in well-accommodated caves. They live very long lives and become sources of wisdom and information for the rest of the community.

Heinlein, R. [1945] (1999). *Methuselah's Children; Time Enough for Love (1973)*. New York: Baen Books.

These science fiction novels describe the long life of Woodrow Wilson Smith (Lazarus Long), the product of a selective breeding program to extend the human life span. In *Methuselah's Children*, Long is 300 years old. He saves his family from persecution and genocide. In *Time Enough for Love*, Long is 2000 years old and ready to die, but his family persuades him to tell stories, like Sheherazade, to stay alive. All his stories focus on love and family as centers of a good life.

Hilton, J. [1933] (1991). *Lost Horizon*. New York: Pocket Books.

This novel gives us Shangri-La, a small utopia hidden in the Tibetan mountains and inhabited by people who live very long lives, blessed with harmonious relations with nature and each other. Those from the outside world who accidentally land there discover that if they leave, they can never come back. And if they take someone who looks young from Shangri-La, the person will grow as old as he or she would be in the real world.

Huxley, A. [1939] (1993). *After Many a Summer Dies the Swan*, reprint ed. Chicago, IL: Ivan R. Dee.

The rich protagonist of this work searches for a secret for longevity. He finds a diary written by one Charles Hauberk, who claims to be 200 years old because he eats the intestines of a fish that lives in ponds on his property. The rich man buys the property and discovers an underground passage where Haubert himself still lives, nearly 300 years old. But he has devolved into an animal, so longevity has a price in loss of humanity.

Janacek, L. (1926). *The Macropolous Case* (opera).

Based on Karel Capek's 1922 book *The Macropolous Case*, this opera stars a leading lady who is 337 years old, having been given an elixir when she was 16 years old by her father, who was court physician to the sixteenth-century king of Bohemia. The elixir works for only 300 years, so if she doesn't take a new dose, she will die. She decides that life loses its value if it lasts too long and dies as the formula is destroyed.

Shaw, G.B. [1918–1920] (1947). *Back to Methuselah.* Oxford: Oxford University Press.

This collection of five linked plays progresses through time from the creation to 31,920 C.E. More discussion than drama, these plays explain Shaw's philosophy of creative evolution. In the fourth play, set in 2170, people reach life spans of 300 years. Religion, politics, and other culturally constructed crutches have disappeared. In the fifth play, set in 31,920, the scientist Pygmalion (an allusion to the classical sculptor) tries to create an improved human, but his engineered eternal human machines fight with each other and kill Pygmalion.

Stoker, B. [1897] (1997). *Dracula.* New York: Signet.

The famous vampire Count Dracula lives in remote Transylvania, where he can hide in crypts, sleep in the daylight, and go out to suck blood at night. Vampires have the curse of immortality; they cannot die unless they are killed by someone they love, by driving a stake through their hearts. They are called the Un-Dead. Immortal human vampires also have supernatural strength and sexual hypnotic power, but they are forever isolated and alone.

Wells, H.G. [1895](1995). *The Time Machine,* reissue ed. New York: Tor Books.

The Time Traveler moves into the future (802,701 C.E.), expecting to find a highly advanced civilization with great technological sophistication. Instead of a utopia, he finds a dystopia; human classes have inbred until recessive traits dominate, evolving into two races: the childlike Eloi, descended from the nonworking aristocracy, who play on the surface of the Earth; and the bestial Morlocks, descended from the working class, who live underground and cannibalize the Eloi. Time travel itself can be understood as a device to achieve longevity of a sort.

Wilde, O. [1890](1992). *The Picture of Dorian Gray,* reprint ed. New York: Modern Library.

When the handsome young Dorian has his portrait painted, he wishes that he could stay that attractive forever—in a sense, he sells his soul for the hope of eternal youth. This late Victorian version of the Faust myth shows Dorian split between body and soul. While he remains physically gorgeous, his soul-reflecting portrait shows not only his aging but his corruption and evil behavior, including murder. In the end, his guilt destroys him.

Literature About Humans Creating Artificial Life (Early Versions of Cloning)

Greek/Roman myth of Pygmalion.

Pygmalion was a talented sculptor who created a stunning marble statue of a young woman. Then, like many artists, he fell in love with his own creation. In Ovid's version of the story, Pygmalion took the statue to bed with him and was so smitten with it that the goddess Venus took pity on him and turned the statue into a real woman. Later she acquired the name Galatea. Many variations on this theme occur throughout literature, including the children's story of Pinocchio. Usually some supernatural intervention is required to bring life to the doll. Shaw's *Pygmalion* became the basis of the musical *My Fair Lady*, with the transformation accomplished by teaching proper English language to a Cockney flower girl.

Jewish Kabbalistic tradition and legend of the Golem.

According to Jewish mystics of the third to sixth centuries C.E., the fundamental units of the universe were the 22 letters of the Jewish alphabet and the numbers 1 through 10. Mystic Kabbalists used this system to move closer to God; others used it as a cookbook for creating "human" beings out of clay. According to legend, they created golems, clumps of earth given life by the four holy letters of the name of God (YHVH). The Golem of Prague was created in the 1580s by Rabbi Uehuda Loew in order to destroy those who were persecuting the Jews. He made him from clay, using the four elements (earth, air, fire, and water) and the four letters. Then he gave the golem the breath of life. Some traditions say that the golem destroyed all of Israel's enemies; others say that he went insane and destroyed his creator; still others say that he was dangerous and had to be deanimated, returned to being a lump of clay. A statue of this golem stands at the entrance to the Jewish sector of Prague.

Paracelsus and the Homunculus.

Related to the golem is the homunculus, a human-like creature created by alchemists. The famous physician-alchemist Paracelsus (1493–1541) includes a detailed recipe for how to create a homunculus in his work *De Natura Reram (The Nature of Things)* (1537). Paracelsus assumed that each sperm contained a tiny human, and that by treating it with blood, dung, and a certain magical cooking apparatus, the homunculus could be generated. However, because no female "seed" was involved, the homunculus had no conscience, no virtue or soul, which normal humans get from their mothers, according to Paracelsus. Because it has no conscience, it can easily cause harm. Most authors portray the fabrication of the homunculus as a forbidden act. In Part Two of Goethe's *Faust*, Faust's assistant, Wagner, creates a homunculus in a phial.

Shelley, M. [1818] (1992). *Frankenstein*. New York: Knopf Everyman's Library.

Drawing on the traditions of the golem and the homunculus, Mary Shelley's Frankenstein collected body parts and created a monster, because, as he explained, "I succeeded in discovering the cause of generation and life; nay more, I became myself capable of bestowing life upon lifeless matter" (p. 54). In bringing life to dead body parts, Frankenstein crosses the border of natural limits, creating life or extending it far beyond its normal span. While he represents the natural human yearning to know more, to cross frontiers, he also represents the same prideful overreaching that brought down the Tower of Babel. Like some golems and homunculi, Frankenstein's monster becomes dangerous.

Literature About Immortality
(Endless Human Life on Earth)

Epic of Gilgamesh (Ancient Sumerian myth).

In the beginning, Gilgamesh tries to find immortality through young virgins who are betrothed to other men. He is stopped by Enkidu; their fight breaks the doorway to immortality. In a second major encounter, Gilgamesh battles the forest deity and uses the power of civilization to establish order. He then seeks immortality through his ancestor, Utnapishtim, who clothes him in the immortal garments; but Gilgamesh does not realize his state and loses his immortality to a serpent. Finally, he records his story on stone and the story itself lasts forever, which is another form of immortality.

Greek myth of Tithonus.

In this myth, an immortal god falls in love with a human (not a good arrangement). Eos (Aurora) loves Tithonus, the son of the king of Troy. She gets him the gift of immortality but forgets to ask for his perpetual youth, so he ages, withers, becomes demented, and begins babbling irritating nonsense. Eos turns him into a grasshopper or cicada, and we can still hear his repetitious noises on summer nights. This myth appears in *The Illiad*. Tennyson wrote a poem entitled *Tithonus*.

Greek myths of Sibyl, Endymion, and Arachne.

Ovid tells the story of how Apollo fell in love with Sibyl, daughter of Tiresias. He gave her the gift of prophecy and said she could live as long as the grains of sand in her hand, but she did not get perpetual youth and so gradually withered away to dust, though her prophetic voice remained.

Theocritus describes how the goddess Selene (moon) fell in love with the sleeping shepherd Endymion. She granted him immortality, but in order to keep him youthful and handsome, she left him asleep for eternity. Still she managed to have 50 sleepy daughters by him.

In Ovid's story, Arachne was a Lydian girl who faced the goddess Athena in a weaving contest. Arachne's tapestry revealed various love affairs between the gods and women. Athena was enraged, but as Arachne tried to hang herself, Athena changed her into a spider before she died. Arachne dangles forever on her web.

Homer [eighth century B.C.E.] (1998). *The Odyssey*, trans. Robert Fitzgerald. New York: Noonday Press.

Odysseus describes how the goddess Calypso took him in, nourished him, and "said she would make me immortal and ageless all my days, but she did not persuade the heart within my breast" (pp. 257–258). After 7 years, she finally agreed to let Odysseus build a raft and try to get home to his wife, son, and elderly father, because he valued their love and preferred mortality in the bosom of his family more than immortality with the goddess.

Myth of the Wandering Jew.

Many legends contribute to this story. Some are based on Matthew

16:28, where Jesus says that some of the people there with him will not taste of death until the Second Coming. That may be construed as a blessing. The negative versions imply that some people are cursed and punished by having to live so long. One tradition says that the Wandering Jew is Ahauserus (Xerxes) or a person who struck Jesus on the way to Golgatha. In the Koran, Moses curses Sameri for helping to build the golden calf and condemns him to wander forever.

Both Rudyard Kipling and William Wordsworth wrote variations on this theme. In Wordsworth's *Song of the Wandering Jew* (1800), the narrator laments:

> Day and night my toils redouble,
> Never nearer to the goal;
> Night and day, I feel the trouble
> Of the Wanderer in my soul.

In Kipling's short story *The Wandering Jew*, the protagonist John Hay tries to achieve immortality by rushing east around the world and gaining a day every time he crosses the international date line. He finally finds "the assurance of a blessed immortality" by hanging from the roof of his room like a pendulum and "letting the round earth swing free beneath him." Near the end of his life, he comes to doubt that his system really works.

Myth of the Flying Dutchman.

This variation on the Wandering Jew theme concerns a cursed sailor who has to sail for eternity. Every 7 years, he can land and look for his true love for 1 day in hopes of breaking that spell. *The Flying Dutchman* was Wagner's first major opera. Samuel Coleridge's *Rime of the Ancient Mariner* (1798) also belongs in this tradition, with the albatross representing the cross the mariner must bear for killing the bird. When the mariner learns the holiness of all things, the albatross drops from his neck. He then wanders the world to tell his story as an apostle of sorts.

Borges, J.L. (1988). The Immortal in *Labyrinths: Selected and Other Writings*. New York: W.W. Norton.

Borges' short story, *The Immortal*, portrays a doctor who keeps heads on tripods, connected to systems that will let them "live" indefinitely. He calls them *immortals* and tries to interest the narrator in his project. When the narrator sees them, his reaction is to panic and leave the country.

Kundera, M. (1999). *Immortality*. New York: Perennial.

Milan Kundera's novel in seven parts alternates several stories of living fictional characters and dead historical figures. For instance, Goethe, Bettina von Arnim, and Ernest Hemingway talk together in the afterlife. The narrator, named Kundera, discusses the difference between a person and his or her public image, the conflict between reality and appearance, the importance of fame and celebrity in keeping one alive in others' memories, and the quest for immortality.

Swift, J. [1726] (1991). *Gulliver's Travels*. New York: Knopf Everyman's Library.

Jonathan Swift also warns against trying to live indefinitely, especially without staying young. His Struldbrugs, in *Gulliver's Travels*, are born with a mark on their heads that signals that they will live forever. That is not a fortunate event, as Gulliver at first mistakenly thinks, because the Struldbrugs grow old just like everyone else. "When they come to fourscore years, . . . they [have] not only all the follies and infirmities of other old men, but many more which arose from the dreadful prospect of never dying. They [are] not only opinionative, peevish, covetous, morose, vain, talkative; but uncapable of friendship, and dead to all natural affection. . . . They find themselves cut off from all possibility of pleasure; and whenever they see a funeral, they lament and repine that others are gone to a harbor of rest, to which they themselves never can hope to arrive" (p. 251). They lose their memory; they look ghastly; they are a public nuisance. Learning from their disaster, Gulliver soon loses his appetite for immortality.

Vonnegut, K. (1965). Fortitude, in *Wampeters, Foma and Granfalloons*. New York: Doubleday.

In Vonnegut's story/play *Fortitude*, Dr. Frankenstein has fallen in love with a rich old woman who reminds him of his mother, so every time one of her organs wears out, Frankenstein orders a mechanical one from Westinghouse or Union Carbide. Of course, Vonnegut's Dr. Frankenstein alludes to Mary Shelley's Frankenstein. By the time the story opens, the old lady is just a head, with some mechanical arms that are designed so she cannot shoot herself to death (Frankenstein clearly was anticipating that she might have some quality-of-life issues). However, she can shoot *him*, and she does. But the twist is that after he dies, his head gets hooked up to the same machinery, so he can share the rest of his immortal life with her (at least until there is a power failure).

Wordsworth, W. [1804] (1994). Ode: Intimations on Immortality, in *William Wordsworth: Selected Poems*. New York: Penguin Classics.

Wordsworth accepts as background for this poem that the soul is immortal, and exists before the body comes into existence and continues after the body's death. Growing up is understood as a stage of dying. This idea is best captured in the famous lines "our birth is but a sleep and a forgetting/ The Soul that rises with us, our life's Star/ . . . cometh from afar:/ Not in entire forgetfulness,/ And not in utter nakedness/ But trailing clouds of glory do we come/ From God, who is our home" (stanza 5).

Literature About Forfeiting Life After Death

Faust Legends.

The Faust legends have generated many great works of literature and music. In the late sixth century C.E., a German chapbook was translated into English as "The Historie of the damnable life, and deserved death of Doctor John Faustus." Christopher Marlowe's play is based on this chapbook. About a century later, Goethe published *Faust*, Part I. Then George Lord Byron wrote *Manfred*; Turgenev wrote *Faust: A Story in Nine Letters*; and Berlioz,

Wagner, and Gounod all wrote operas on the theme. In the twentieth century, Thomas Mann contributed *Doctor Faustus: The Life of the German Composer Adrian Leverkuhn, as told by a Friend* (1947). The musical *Damn Yankees* is another variation on the theme. By the turn of the twenty-first century, Faust had even appeared in a rock opera.

Goethe, J.W.V. [1808, 1832] (1960). *Faust.* Oxford: Oxford University Press.

In this masterpiece of German literature Faust is a scholar, sunk in depression because he has limits on his learning and feels he has not accomplished anything. Meanwhile, Mephisto has made a bargain with God (somewhat like the bargain in Job): Mephisto will try to entice Faust to sell his soul forever, while God thinks Faust's soul can be saved. Mephisto enters Faust's life in the form of a black dog. He tempts Faust with knowledge and pleasures, some of which end in other people's deaths. But Faust keeps struggling to learn and to experiment. Finally, as Faust is blind and dying, he sees the light and gives all his land to the people, and his soul is saved.

Marlowe, C. [1588] (1989). *Doctor Faustus.* New York: NAL-Dutton.

Faustus is a brilliant scholar who is never satisfied with the limits on his learning. He wants the power of knowledge that Mephistophilis promises him if he gives his soul to Lucifer. Faustus does this because he does not believe in the immortality of the soul. With the help of Mephistophilis, he tricks the Pope and raises the spirit of Alexander the Great. Near the end of his 24-year agreement, he gets Mephistophilis to bring him Helen of Troy. He does not repent, and he is carried off by devils at the end.

Literature About Reversing Aging or Rejuvenation

Myth of Autochthonous.

Greek mythology describes the sons of the soil, who grow out of the soil just as plants do. According to ancient traditions, these Autochthonous come into being during times of great change when the whole universe starts moving backward. During these reversals, people grow younger and younger, until they are babies and then finally disappear into the ground. The Dead grow out of the ground as old men and live their lives backward. No one is born during these retro-ages.

Myth of Medea and Aeson.

One of the oldest stories tells of how Medea, Jason's wife, was able to restore the youth of Aeson, Jason's father, so that he could participate in the celebrations over the recovery of the Golden Fleece. Medea used incantations, invoked help from the gods, built two altars and sacrificed a black sheep, and concocted a complicated stew in a cauldron into which she put magic herbs, seeds, flowers, stones, sand, hoarfrost, a screech owl's head, and other delicacies. She stirred this with an old, dry olive branch that suddenly became green and full of young olives. Then she cut Aeson's throat, drained all his blood, and replaced it with the juices of her cauldron. He was transformed into a healthy and vigorous man 40 years younger.

Ponce de Leon.

History records that Juan Ponce de Leon, the Spanish explorer who discovered Florida, was on a quest for a rejuvenating spring. He had been on the second voyage of Columbus and had heard from Caribbean natives about a Fountain of Youth, full of a tonic water that made people younger. He did not find it apparently.

Hawthorne, N. [1837] (1982). Dr. Heidegger's Experiment, in *Nathaniel Hawthorne: Tales and Sketches*. New York: Literary Classics of the United States.

In this cautionary story, a doctor shows several of his elderly friends that if he dips a dead flower in a magic potion, it suddenly becomes a fresh, young bud. When they drink the elixir that makes them suddenly younger, they flirt awkwardly with each other as if they were teenagers. But when the elixir wears off, they grow old again and feel much worse for the contrasting experience. In a romantic rejection of mechanistic science, Hawthorne often portrays the scientific mind as having too narrow a focus (much like Blake's single vision). In his story *The Birthmark*, the obsessive scientist sees only the stain of the tiny birthmark and not the beautiful living being of his wife. His fanatic determination to remove the birthmark has the side effect of killing her.

London, J. [November 1899]. The Rejuvenation of Major Rathbone, in *Conkey's Home Journal*, 6 (1993). *The Complete Short Stories of Jack London*. Stanford, CA: Stanford University Press.

Jack London pursues a similar fountain of youth theme in *The Rejuvenation of Major Rathbone*. After using his lymph elixir to convert his decrepit old dog into a young puppy, Dover Wallingford decides to experiment on his ancient Uncle Max. The narrator of the story exclaims that "We who had started out to resuscitate a feeble old man, found upon our hands an impetuous young giant." But Max's hair and beard remains white, and although he has astonishing youthful energy, he stays irascible and stubborn, so his rejuvenation is incomplete. Most people are shocked by seeing an old man with such childish behavior. Dover realizes that "before we can foist this rejuvenator upon the world, we must also discover an antidote for it—a sort of emasculator to reduce the friskiness attendant upon the return to youth." They decide to give the lymph elixir to a bedridden old lady, who soon rises and falls in love with Max. And then "the superannuated lovers walked bravely to the altar and then went off on their honeymoon" (p. 282). London's satire is much lighter and funnier than Hawthorne's dark warning, but both indicate that many unexpected results may come from trying to rejuvenate people.

Name Index

Subject Index